Prosthetic Joint Infection: The Challenges of Prevention, Diagnosis and Treatment and Opportunities for Future Research

Prosthetic Joint Infection: The Challenges of Prevention, Diagnosis and Treatment and Opportunities for Future Research

Editors

Natividad Benito
Óscar Murillo
Jaime Lora-Tamayo

MDPI • Basel • Beijing • Wuhan • Barcelona • Belgrade • Manchester • Tokyo • Cluj • Tianjin

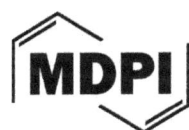

Editors

Natividad Benito
Infectious Disease Unit
Hospital de la Santa Creu i
Sant Pau
Universitat Autònoma de
Barcelona
Spain
CIBERINFEC, ISCIII

Óscar Murillo
Department of Infectious
Diseases
Hospital Universitari
Bellvitge
Universitat de Barcelona
Spain
CIBERINFEC, ISCIII

Jaime Lora-Tamayo
Department of Internal
Medicine
Hospital Universitario 12 de
Octubre
Madrid
Spain
CIBERINFEC, ISCIII

Editorial Office
MDPI
St. Alban-Anlage 66
4052 Basel, Switzerland

This is a reprint of articles from the Special Issue published online in the open access journal *Antibiotics* (ISSN 2079-6382) (available at: www.mdpi.com/journal/antibiotics/special_issues/joint_infection).

For citation purposes, cite each article independently as indicated on the article page online and as indicated below:

LastName, A.A.; LastName, B.B.; LastName, C.C. Article Title. *Journal Name* **Year**, *Volume Number*, Page Range.

ISBN 978-3-0365-7937-5 (Hbk)
ISBN 978-3-0365-7936-8 (PDF)

© 2023 by the authors. Articles in this book are Open Access and distributed under the Creative Commons Attribution (CC BY) license, which allows users to download, copy and build upon published articles, as long as the author and publisher are properly credited, which ensures maximum dissemination and a wider impact of our publications.

The book as a whole is distributed by MDPI under the terms and conditions of the Creative Commons license CC BY-NC-ND.

Contents

Preface to "Prosthetic Joint Infection: The Challenges of Prevention, Diagnosis and Treatment and Opportunities for Future Research" vii

Alba Rivera, Alba Sánchez, Sonia Luque, Isabel Mur, Lluís Puig and Xavier Crusi et al.
Intraoperative Bacterial Contamination and Activity of Different Antimicrobial Prophylaxis Regimens in Primary Knee and Hip Replacement
Reprinted from: *Antibiotics* **2020**, *10*, 18, doi:10.3390/antibiotics10010018 1

Dolors Rodríguez-Pardo, Laura Escolà-Vergé, Júlia Sellarès-Nadal, Pablo S. Corona, Benito Almirante and Carles Pigrau
Periprosthetic Joint Infection Prophylaxis in the Elderly after Hip Hemiarthroplasty in Proximal Femur Fractures: Insights and Challenges
Reprinted from: *Antibiotics* **2021**, *10*, 429, doi:10.3390/antibiotics10040429 15

Jérôme Grondin, Pierre Menu, Benoit Métayer, Vincent Crenn, Marc Dauty and Alban Fouasson-Chailloux
Intra-Articular Injections Prior to Total Knee Arthroplasty Do Not Increase the Risk of Periprosthetic Joint Infection: A Prospective Cohort Study
Reprinted from: *Antibiotics* **2021**, *10*, 330, doi:10.3390/antibiotics10030330 21

Nora Renz, Andrej Trampuz and Werner Zimmerli
Controversy about the Role of Rifampin in Biofilm Infections: Is It Justified?
Reprinted from: *Antibiotics* **2021**, *10*, 165, doi:10.3390/antibiotics10020165 31

Eric Senneville, Aurélien Dinh, Tristan Ferry, Eric Beltrand, Nicolas Blondiaux and Olivier Robineau
Tolerance of Prolonged Oral Tedizolid for Prosthetic Joint Infections: Results of a Multicentre Prospective Study
Reprinted from: *Antibiotics* **2020**, *10*, 4, doi:10.3390/antibiotics10010004 41

Eva Benavent, Laura Morata, Francesc Escrihuela-Vidal, Esteban Alberto Reynaga, Laura Soldevila and Laia Albiach et al.
Long-Term Use of Tedizolid in Osteoarticular Infections: Benefits among Oxazolidinone Drugs
Reprinted from: *Antibiotics* **2021**, *10*, 53, doi:10.3390/antibiotics10010053 53

Luis Buzón-Martín, Ines Zollner-Schwetz, Selma Tobudic, Emilia Cercenado and Jaime Lora-Tamayo
Dalbavancin for the Treatment of Prosthetic Joint Infections: A Narrative Review
Reprinted from: *Antibiotics* **2021**, *10*, 656, doi:10.3390/antibiotics10060656 63

Laura Soldevila-Boixader, Bernat Villanueva, Marta Ulldemolins, Eva Benavent, Ariadna Padulles and Alba Ribera et al.
Risk Factors of Daptomycin-Induced Eosinophilic Pneumonia in a Population with Osteoarticular Infection
Reprinted from: *Antibiotics* **2021**, *10*, 446, doi:10.3390/antibiotics10040446 75

Javier Cobo and Rosa Escudero-Sanchez
Suppressive Antibiotic Treatment in Prosthetic Joint Infections: A Perspective
Reprinted from: *Antibiotics* **2021**, *10*, 743, doi:10.3390/antibiotics10060743 83

Joan Gómez-Junyent, Jaime Lora-Tamayo, Josu Baraia-Etxaburu, Mar Sánchez-Somolinos, Jose Antonio Iribarren and Dolors Rodriguez-Pardo et al.
Implant Removal in the Management of Prosthetic Joint Infection by *Staphylococcus aureus*: Outcome and Predictors of Failure in a Large Retrospective Multicenter Study
Reprinted from: *Antibiotics* **2021**, *10*, 118, doi:10.3390/antibiotics10020118 . . . . **91**

Raquel Bandeira da Silva and Mauro José Salles
Outcomes and Risk Factors in Prosthetic Joint Infections by multidrug-resistant Gram-negative Bacteria: A Retrospective Cohort Study
Reprinted from: *Antibiotics* **2021**, *10*, 340, doi:10.3390/antibiotics10030340 . . . . **105**

Helem H. Vilchez, Rosa Escudero-Sanchez, Marta Fernandez-Sampedro, Oscar Murillo, Álvaro Auñón and Dolors Rodríguez-Pardo et al.
Prosthetic Shoulder Joint Infection by *Cutibacterium acnes*: Does Rifampin Improve Prognosis? A Retrospective, Multicenter, Observational Study
Reprinted from: *Antibiotics* **2021**, *10*, 475, doi:10.3390/antibiotics10050475 . . . . **119**

Laura Escolà-Vergé, Dolors Rodríguez-Pardo, Pablo S. Corona and Carles Pigrau
Candida Periprosthetic Joint Infection: Is It Curable?
Reprinted from: *Antibiotics* **2021**, *10*, 458, doi:10.3390/antibiotics10040458 . . . . **133**

Hugo Garlito-Díaz, Jaime Esteban, Aranzazu Mediero, Rafael Alfredo Carias-Cálix, Beatriz Toirac and Francisca Mulero et al.
A New Antifungal-Loaded Sol-Gel Can Prevent *Candida albicans* Prosthetic Joint Infection
Reprinted from: *Antibiotics* **2021**, *10*, 711, doi:10.3390/antibiotics10060711 . . . . **143**

Isabel Mur, Marcos Jordán, Alba Rivera, Virginia Pomar, José Carlos González and Joaquín López-Contreras et al.
Do Prosthetic Joint Infections Worsen the Functional Ambulatory Outcome of Patients with Joint Replacements? A Retrospective Matched Cohort Study
Reprinted from: *Antibiotics* **2020**, *9*, 872, doi:10.3390/antibiotics9120872 . . . . **159**

Preface to "Prosthetic Joint Infection: The Challenges of Prevention, Diagnosis and Treatment and Opportunities for Future Research"

Joint replacement is a common and increasingly performed surgical procedure. The most commonly replaced joints are the hip and knee, although virtually all extra-axial joints can be replaced. Prosthetic joint infections (PJIs) are devastating complications with significant patient morbidity and mortality and considerable healthcare and societal costs. Although the percentage of PJIs in patients with joint replacements could be considered low (1–3% for elective primary arthroplasties), the increasing frequency of such procedures transforms an apparently low risk into a substantial and growing burden of infection. Nevertheless, the risk of PJIs is higher in revision procedures and in specific groups of patients. Indeed, in most developed countries, PJIs are considered a major public health problem.

PJI is a paradigm of biofilm-associated infection. The presence of biofilm influences and complicates the prevention, diagnosis, and treatment of PJI. Eradication of the infection requires surgery and antimicrobial therapy. Close collaboration between all medical and surgical specialists involved is a critical component of the care of patients with PJI.

In this complex scenario, despite the considerable amount of research conducted in recent decades on the prevention, diagnosis, treatment, and outcome of PJIs, many questions remain unanswered. Indeed, most recommendations in this area are based on expert opinion due to the limitations of the available information.

This Special Issue aimed to advance knowledge and broaden our perspectives on the prevention, diagnosis, management, and outcomes of PJI.

Natividad Benito, Óscar Murillo, and Jaime Lora-Tamayo
Editors

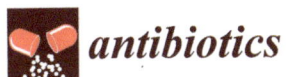

Article

Intraoperative Bacterial Contamination and Activity of Different Antimicrobial Prophylaxis Regimens in Primary Knee and Hip Replacement

Alba Rivera [1,2], Alba Sánchez [1,2], Sonia Luque [3], Isabel Mur [4,5,6], Lluís Puig [7], Xavier Crusi [8], José Carlos González [8], Luisa Sorlí [6,9,10], Aránzazu González [8], Juan Pablo Horcajada [4,9], Ferran Navarro [1,2] and Natividad Benito [4,5,6,*]

1. Department of Microbiology, Hospital de la Santa Creu i Sant Pau—Institut d'Investigació Biomèdica Sant Pau, 08025 Barcelona, Spain; mrivera@santpau.cat (A.R.); asanchezmor@santpau.cat (A.S.); FNavarror@santpau.cat (F.N.)
2. Department of Genetic and Microbiology, Universitat Autònoma de Barcelona, 08193 Barcelona, Spain
3. Department of Pharmacy, Hospital del Mar—Hospital del Mar Medical Research Institute (IMIM), 08003 Barcelona, Spain; sluque@parcdesalutmar.cat
4. Department of Medicine, Faculty of Medicine, Universitat Autònoma de Barcelona, 08193 Barcelona, Spain; imur@santpau.cat (I.M.); jhorcajada@parcdesalutmar.cat (J.P.H.)
5. Infectious Disease Unit, Department of Internal Medicine, Hospital de la Santa Creu i Sant Pau—Institut d'Investigació Biomèdica Sant Pau, 08025 Barcelona, Spain
6. Bone and Joint Infection Study Group of the Spanish Society of Infectious Diseases and Clinical Microbiology (GEIO-SEIMC), 28003 Madrid, Spain; lsorli@parcdesalutmar.cat
7. Department of Orthopedic Surgery and Traumatology, Hospital del Mar—Hospital del Mar Medical Research Institute (IMIM), 08003 Barcelona, Spain; lpuig@parcdesalutmar.cat
8. Department of Orthopedic Surgery and Traumatology, Hospital de la Santa Creu i Sant Pau—Institut d'Investigació Biomèdica Sant Pau, 08025 Barcelona, Spain; XCrusi@santpau.cat (X.C.); JGonzalezR@santpau.cat (J.C.G.); agonzalezo@santpau.cat (A.G.)
9. Department of Infectious Diseases, Hospital del Mar—Hospital del Mar Medical Research Institute (IMIM), 08003 Barcelona, Spain
10. Department of Experimental and Health Sciences, Universitat Pompeu Fabra, 08003 Barcelona, Spain
* Correspondence: nbenito@santpau.cat

Abstract: Surgical antimicrobial prophylaxis (SAP) is important for the prevention of prosthetic joint infections (PJIs) and must be effective against the microorganisms most likely to contaminate the surgical site. Our aim was to compare different SAP regimens (cefazolin, cefuroxime, or vancomycin, alone or combined with gentamicin) in patients undergoing total knee (TKA) and hip (THA) arthroplasty. In this preclinical exploratory analysis, we analyzed the results of intraoperative sample cultures, the ratio of plasma antibiotic levels to the minimum inhibitory concentrations (MICs) for bacteria isolated at the surgical wound and ATCC strains, and serum bactericidal titers (SBT) against the same microorganisms. A total of 132 surgical procedures (68 TKA, 64 THA) in 128 patients were included. Cultures were positive in 57 (43.2%) procedures (mostly for coagulase-negative staphylococci and *Cutibacterium* spp.); the rate was lower in the group of patients receiving combination SAP (adjusted OR 0.475, CI95% 0.229–0.987). The SAP regimens evaluated achieved plasma levels above the MICs in almost all of intraoperative isolates (93/94, 98.9%) and showed bactericidal activity against all of them (SBT range 1:8–1:1024), although SBTs were higher in patients receiving cefazolin and gentamicin-containing regimens. The potential clinical relevance of these findings in the prevention of PJIs remains to be determined.

Keywords: surgical antimicrobial prophylaxis; knee arthroplasty; hip arthroplasty; prosthetic joint infection; surgical site infection prevention; prosthetic joint infection prevention; intraoperative cultures; antibiotic levels; serum bactericidal titer

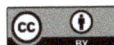

1. Introduction

Prosthetic joint infection (PJI) is a serious complication associated with substantial morbimortality and economic costs [1]. Microorganisms introduced at the time of surgery, contiguous spread from adjacent infected tissue, and hematogenous seeding from a remote site are considered the usual routes of infection, although the former is believed to be the most frequent [1]. The risk of infection developing after microbial contamination of the surgical field depends on the dose and virulence of the pathogen and the patient's resistance to infection [2]. Surgical antimicrobial prophylaxis (SAP), considered to be one of the most important preventive strategies, can help offset this by reducing the risk of surgical site infections (SSIs), including PJIs [3,4]. The goal of SAP is to eradicate bacteria inoculated into the wound at the time of surgery. From a pharmacodynamic point of view, antimicrobial levels should be maintained above the minimal inhibitory concentration (MIC) of the pathogens most likely to contaminate the surgical field for the whole duration of the operation [5–7]. Cefazolin or cefuroxime (first- and second-generation cephalosporins, respectively) and vancomycin in cases of beta-lactam allergy, are the antibiotics most commonly used and recommended in current guidelines, although there are no data supporting the superiority of one class of antimicrobials over another for SAP in total joint replacement [5,6]. Furthermore, studies have suggested that a growing proportion of SSIs (including PJIs) following arthroplasty procedures are caused by organisms resistant to first- and second-generation cephalosporins, including both Gram-positive (mainly methicillin-resistant staphylococci), and Gram-negative bacteria (such as some Enterobacterales or *Pseudomonas aeruginosa*) [8–11]. In light of this, various expanded combination SAP regimens have been proposed and analyzed in small clinical studies, with different effects but no conclusive results because of their methodological limitations [12–17]. Consequently, routine prophylactic use of dual antibiotics (such as cephalosporins and aminoglycosides or cephalosporins and vancomycin) is not currently recommended [18].

Conclusively demonstrating the superiority of one SAP regimen over another in clinical studies involves overcoming a number of problems. Ideally, randomized controlled trials would be conducted, but these would require an extraordinarily large number of participants (thousands) due to the relatively low incidence of PJI (1–2%). Furthermore, follow-up duration would be extremely long—at least two years—to take account of delayed cases of PJI. [19]. Before considering any clinical trial, therefore, the prophylactic regimens to be compared should be carefully evaluated. A preclinical exploratory analysis of potential SAP regimens using microbiological, pharmacokinetic (PK), and pharmacodynamic (PD) studies could be a very useful step. Using this approach, the aim of our study was to compare intraoperative bacterial contamination and the activity of six SAP regimens against microorganisms isolated in the surgical wounds of patients undergoing elective primary total knee (TKA) and hip (THA) arthroplasty surgery. We analyzed the following data obtained at the end of surgical procedures: (1) bacteria isolated from surgical wounds (rate and etiology); (2) free plasma antibiotic concentrations relative to the MICs of the isolated microorganisms and some reference American Type Culture Collection (ATCC) strains; and (3) serum bactericidal titers (SBTs) against the same microorganisms.

2. Patients and Methods

2.1. Setting and Patients

This prospective study was conducted at two acute care university hospitals in Barcelona, Spain (Hospital de la Santa Creu i Sant Pau and Hospital del Mar). The Institutional Review Boards of the two participating hospitals approved the study.

Patients undergoing elective primary total knee and hip replacement surgery between June 2016 and March 2020 were included. Three orthopedists recruited patients who agreed to participate in the study and provided written informed consent. Each of the four cephalosporin-containing regimens was sequentially administered to consecutively enrolled patients; penicillin-allergic patients received vancomycin or vancomycin and gentamicin. Preoperative whole-body bathing or showering with chlorhexidine soap on the day of the surgical procedure and the night before was indicated. Alcoholic 2% chlorhexidine was used as antiseptic for skin preparation before surgical incision.

A minimum follow-up of one year was planned after prosthesis implantation in order to diagnose possible postoperative PJIs; this minimum period of follow-up is still ongoing in some patients.

2.2. Surgical Antimicrobial Prophylaxis Regimens

Patients received cefazolin (2 g), cefuroxime (1.5 g), or vancomycin (15 mg/kg total body weight), alone or in combination with gentamicin (5 mg/kg total body weight) as SAP. Antibiotics were administered intravenously within 60 min prior to incision, except for vancomycin, which was given up to 120 min prior to incision.

2.3. Sample Collection

Blood samples (3–5 mL) were collected at the end of surgery in heparinized and gelose-containing tubes. After centrifugation, serum and plasma samples were stored at $-80\ °C \pm 5\ °C$ until testing for antimicrobial levels and SBT titers.

Five standard perioperative tissue samples were collected from each patient at the end of surgery and sent for culture. All samples were obtained after implantation of the prosthesis and before wound closure. In TKA surgery, two tissue samples were collected from around the femur, two from around the tibia, and one from the subcutaneous tissue. In THA surgery, two tissue samples were collected from around the acetabulum, two from around the femur, and one from the subcutaneous tissue.

2.4. Determination of Antibiotic Levels

Plasma concentrations of cefazolin and cefuroxime were determined by a validated high-performance liquid chromatography (HPLC) method with a UV-Vis spectrophotometric detector, and those of gentamicin and vancomycin by chemiluminescent microparticle immunoassay (Alinity, Abbott). For the HPLC assay, 100 µL of each plasma sample was mixed with 200 µL of methanol and vortexed for 10 s. The mixture was then centrifuged for 5 min at $15,000\times g$ in a refrigerated centrifuge and 20 µL of the supernatant was injected into the system for the assay (Alliance e2695, and 2487 HPLC Absorbance UV-Vis Detector, Waters). The method was shown to be sensitive and specific for the measurement of cefazolin and cefuroxime in plasma. The assay response was linear (coefficient of linearity >0.99) over the full range of concentrations assayed (0.5–200 mg/L for cefazolin and 0.5–100 mg/L for cefuroxime). The limit of quantification was 0.5 mg/L for both cefazolin and cefuroxime. Imprecision values were < 15% over the entire range of calibration standards, and accuracy was within the range of 85–115% for all concentrations. Total measured concentrations of cefazolin, cefuroxime and vancomycin were adjusted to free concentrations, assuming protein binding of 80%, 40% and 50%, respectively [20,21]. Protein binding of gentamicin was considered to be negligible [21,22].

Antibiotic levels were considered appropriate when their free plasma concentration was above the MIC of pathogens isolated from the wound at the time of the prosthetic joint implant surgery, or the MIC of the ATCC strains studied.

2.5. Microbiological Methods

Tissue samples were homogenized in 1 ml of sterile saline using a sterile mortar and pestle, and 100 µl volumes were inoculated onto each plate of blood agar (BioMerieux, Marcy l'Etoile, France) and chocolate agar (BioMerieux, Marcy l'Etoile, France), both incubated in aerobic conditions, and Schaedler agar (BioMerieux, Marcy l'Etoile, France) incubated in anaerobic conditions. The remaining homogenate was inoculated into thioglycollate broth. Cultures were incubated for seven days at $35 \pm 2\ °C$. Bacterial isolates were identified using MALDI-TOF (Bruker, Bremen, Germany). Antimicrobial susceptibility was determined by either gradient diffusion (Liofilchem, Roseto degli Abruzzi, Italy) or disk diffusion (Rosco Diagnostica, Taastrup, Denmark) and interpreted according to

EUCAST [23]. Bacterial isolates were tested against the antibiotics used in each prophylaxis. For staphylococci, resistance to cefazolin or cefuroxime was inferred from resistance to cefoxitin.

While microbiological diagnosis of PJI requires that at least two of a minimum of five intraoperative cultures (obtained at the surgery to treat the infection) yield the same microorganism, however the present study represented a different scenario. Prosthetic joint implantation is clean surgery, and therefore, a very low bacterial inoculum is expected in the surgical field. For this reason, we considered any growth on any of the plates as a positive culture, and a patient with a single positive culture was rated as having a positive intraoperative culture. Culture-positive results were blinded, and patients were not given antimicrobial treatment on the basis of these results. The only antibiotic administered to patients was the surgical prophylaxis.

SBT was performed with sera collected at the time of surgical closure from patients with positive intraoperative cultures and measured against the patient's respective bacterial isolates. In addition, SBT was performed with sera from patients with positive intraoperative cultures and a subset of patients with negative cultures against the reference strains *Staphylococcus epidermidis* ATCC 12228, *Staphylococcus aureus* ATCC 25923, *Escherichia coli* ATCC 25922 and *P. aeruginosa* ATCC 27853. The assays were performed by the microdilution method, according to the Clinical Laboratory Standards Institute guidelines [24], with some modifications.

Two-fold serial dilutions of patient serum were prepared in cation-adjusted Mueller Hinton broth (Thermo Scientific, USA) or Mueller Hinton supplemented with lysed horse blood (Thermo Scientific, USA). The dilution range was 1:2–1:1024. Plates were incubated at $35 \pm 2\,°C$ for 24 h or 48 h. The SBT titer was defined as the highest dilution of patient serum at which a $\geq 99.9\%$ reduction in the starting inoculum was achieved. Reciprocal SBT values were used to calculate median SBTs.

2.6. Statistical Methods

Categorical variables were summarized as percentages of the total sample for that variable, and continuous variables as means and standard deviation (SD) or median and interquartile range (IQR), depending on their homogeneity. The Wilcoxon rank-sum and Chi-squared tests (or Fisher's exact tests when appropriate) were used to evaluate group differences for continuous and categorical variables, respectively. A multivariate logistic regression model was used to identify factors independently associated with a higher risk of having positive intraoperative cultures. Any variable tested in univariate analysis with a p-value less than 0.25, together with all variables of known clinical importance, were selected as candidates for the first multivariate model. We then followed the purposeful selection of covariates method described by Hosmer and Lemeshow [25]. Final parameter estimates are shown as odds ratios (ORs) with their corresponding 95% confidence intervals (CIs). p-values of < 0.05 were considered to be significant for all statistical tests. Data were analyzed using IBM® SPSS®, version 26.0.

3. Results

3.1. Patients and Surgical Antimicrobial Prophylaxis

A total of 132 surgical procedures for joint replacement (68 TKA and 64 THA) were performed in 128 patients (four patients underwent two different procedures at different times). Seventy-two (56.3%) patients were female, and the median age was 71 years (SD 8.6) (Table 1). The SAP regimens administered were: cefazolin, in 22 (16.7%) procedures, cefuroxime in 20 (15.2%), vancomycin in 11 (8.3%), cefazolin plus gentamicin in 39 (29.5%), cefuroxime plus gentamicin in 20 (15.2%) and vancomycin plus gentamicin in 20 (15.2%).

During a median follow-up of 15 months (interquartile range, IQR, of 21), two PJIs (1.5%) were diagnosed. A 72-year-old woman with no underlying pathology, BMI 33, ASA II, and an uneventful 88-min surgery in which she received cefuroxime as prophylaxis, presented a THA infection caused by *S. aureus* (methicillin-susceptible) five weeks after prosthesis implantation. Free plasma concentration of cefuroxime at the end of the surgery was 9 mg/L. The second was a TKA infection caused by *Morganella morganii*, which occurred one month after a 100-min surgery. The patient was a 74-year-old diabetic woman, BMI 38.5 and ASA III, who received cefazolin plus gentamicin as SAP. In this case, free plasma concentration of cefazolin was 15.4 mg/L and gentamicin 15.2 mg/L. Both patients had negative intraoperative cultures during prosthesis implantation.

Table 1. Patients undergoing primary total knee and hip arthroplasty surgical procedures, with and without positive intraoperative cultures.

Variable	Intraoperative Cultures		p-Value	Multivariate Analysis	p-Value
	Positive (n = 57)	Negative (n = 75)		OR (CI 95%)	
Sex—number of males or females with positive cultures/total number of males or females, respectively (%)			0.023	2.412 (1.170–4.973)	0.017
- Male	31/57 (54.4)				
- Female	26/75 (37.7)				
Age, years—mean (SD)	71 (9.6)	72 (7.9)	0.615		
BMI—mean (SD)	29.9 (5.1)	29.1 (4.9)	0.393		
Antimicrobial prophylaxis—number of culture-positive patients with each type of prophylaxis/total of patients receiving each type of prophylaxis (%)					
- Cefazolin	9/22 (40.9)		0.293		
- Cefuroxime	13/20 (65)				
- Vancomycin	6/11 (54.5)				
- Cefazolin	9/22 (40.9)		0.698		
- Cefazolin + gentamicin	14/39 (35.9)				
- Cefuroxime	13/20 (65)		0.204		
- Cefuroxime + gentamicin	9/20 (45)				
- Vancomycin	6/11 (54.5)		0.180		
- Vancomycin + gentamicin	6/20 (30)				
- Cefazolin, cefuroxime, and vancomycin	29/79 (36.7)		0.067	0.475 (0.229–0.987)	0.046
- Cefazolin + gentamicin, cefuroxime + gentamicin and vancomycin + gentamicin	28/53 (52.8)				
Prosthesis location—number of patients with a hip or knee prosthesis and positive cultures/total number of patients with hip or knee prostheses, respectively (%)			0.406		
- Hip	30/64 (46.9)				
- Knee	27/68 (39.7)				
Surgery duration, minutes—mean (SD)	75 (18.8)	78 (20.2)	0.363		

CI, confidence interval; OR, odds ratio.

3.2. Intraoperative Cultures

At least one of the five tissue samples taken yielded positive culture results in 57 (43.2%) surgical procedures: 39.7% (27/68) were TKA and 46.9% (30/64) THA. The number of positive samples per patient ranged from one to five (median 2, IQR 1). There were no substantial differences in culture yield between subcutaneous tissue samples (20 positive culture samples from 57 procedures, 35.1%) and those from deep tissue (the four deep samples yielded positive cultures in 25, 17, 20 and 25 cases, respectively, with a mean of 21.8, 38.2%).

Table 1 shows the characteristics of patients undergoing primary THA and TKA, with and without positive intraoperative cultures. With respect to single-drug prophylaxis, patients receiving cefazolin had the lowest percentage of positive cultures, while patients with combined SAP regimens less frequently had positive intraoperative cultures than those with a single drug, although these differences were not statistically significant. In the adjusted analysis, we found that males had a two-fold higher risk of positive cultures than women, while gentamicin-containing SAP regimens were associated with a lower risk of positive cultures.

Overall, a total of 94 bacterial isolates—all of them Gram-positive bacteria—were identified. The most frequently isolated microorganisms were coagulase-negative staphylococci (CoNS), 42 (44.7%), followed by *Cutibacterium* spp., 34 (36.2%). The predominant individual species was *Cutibacterium acnes* (35.1%). Polymicrobial isolation occurred in 23 (40.4%) culture-positive surgical procedures (14 of 30 THA [46.7%] and 9 of 27 TKA [36.3%]; $p = 0.451$). *Cutibacterium* spp. or CoNS were isolated in more than half of culture-positive surgeries (Table 2). *Cutibacterium* spp. was more frequently found in THA than in TKA surgery.

Table 2. Bacterial species isolated from intraoperative samples during total hip and knee replacement surgical procedures with positive cultures.

Bacterial Species	Surgical Procedures ($n = 57$)	THA ($n = 30$)	TKA ($n = 27$)	p-Value *
Cutibacterium species—n (%)	34 (59.6)	22 (73.3)	12 (44.4)	0.026
- Cutibacterium acnes	33	21	12	
- Cutibacterium avidum	1	1	0	0.051
Coagulase-negative staphylococci—n (%)	30 (52.6)	15 (50)	15 (55.6)	0.675
- Staphylococcus epidermidis	19 (33.3)	8 (26.7)	11 (40.7)	0.399
- Staphylococcus hominis	12 (21.1)	8 (26.7)	4 (14.8)	0.441
- Staphylococcus warneri	3	1	2	
- Staphylococcus simulans	2	2	0	
- Staphylococcus capitis	1	1	0	
- Staphylococcus caprae	1	1	0	
- Staphylococcus haemolyticus	1	0	1	
- Staphylococcus pettenkoferi	1	0	1	
- Staphylococcus saccharolyticus	1	1	0	
Micrococcus luteus—n (%)	8 (14.0)	4 (13.3)	4 (14.8)	
Corynebacterium species—n (%)	4 (7.0)	3	1	
- Corynebacterium afermentans	1	0	1	
- Corynebacterium pseudodiphtheriticum	1	1	0	
- Corynebacterium accolens	1	1	0	
- Corynebacterium mucifaciens	1	1	0	
- Corynebacterium propinquum	1	1	0	
- Corynebacterium simulans	1	0	1	
Paenibacillus lautus	1	1	0	
Actinomyces neuii	1	1	0	
Dermabacter hominis	1	0	1	
Kocuria rhizophila	1	1	0	

THA, total hip arthroplasty; TKA, total knee arthroplasty. * Statistically significant differences between percentages were considered when an organism or group of organisms was isolated in more than ten surgical procedures.

3.3. Susceptibility of Bacterial Isolates and ATCC Strains, Antibiotic Plasma Levels and Serum Bactericidal Titers

Supplementary Table S1 shows in detail the following data of patients with intraoperative positive cultures: plasma levels of antibiotics used as SAP, bacteria isolated and the corresponding MICs of the antimicrobials administered, and SBT against the isolated bacteria.

Cefazolin MICs determined in 38 bacterial isolates obtained from patients receiving this antibiotic (with or without gentamicin) ranged from 0.032–64 mg/L. There were five (13.2%) cefazolin-resistant isolates, of which four were CoNS and one was *Paenibacillus lautus*. Cefuroxime MICs for 37 isolates ranged from 0.016 to 16 mg/L, one (2.6%) of which was resistant (*S. epidermidis*). MICs of vancomycin were determined in 16 isolates with a range of 0.125–2 mg/L; none of the isolates showed resistance. MICs of gentamicin for 42 strains ranged from 0.047 to 24 mg/L, with 22 (52.4%) resistant isolates (*C. acnes* and one *Staphylococcus warneri*).

Overall, 94.5% (86/91) of bacterial isolates were susceptible to the particular SAP regimen administered (or to at least one of the antibiotics in a combination regimen). With respect to single-drug cephalosporin prophylaxis, 82.3% (14/17) and 96% (24/25) of isolates were susceptible to cefazolin and cefuroxime, respectively. The rate of susceptible isolates was higher for combinations with cephalosporins plus gentamicin: 95.2% (20/21) in the case of cefazolin, and 100% (13/13) in the case of cefuroxime, although these differences were not statistically significant. Plasma levels of antimicrobials used in prophylaxis were determined in 130 (98.5%) patients (blood samples could not be obtained from two patients). Median plasma levels and ratios to MIC are shown in Table 3.

Table 3. Prophylactic plasma antimicrobial levels in culture-positive surgical procedures and ratios of these antimicrobial levels to the minimum inhibitory concentrations (MICs) for bacteria isolated in the surgical field.

Antimicrobial Used as Prophylaxis	Free Plasma Concentration (mg/L), Median (Range)	Free Plasma Concentration (mg/L)/ MIC (mg/L), Median (Range)
Cefazolin	17.3 (11.2–33.2)	44.4 (0.3–1037.5)
Cefuroxime	24.2 (11–44.2)	81.6 (1.1–1833.5)
Gentamicin	12.3 (8.5–19.4)	9.01 (0.6–323.4)
Vancomycin	7.8 (4.6–19.05)	25.6 (3.5–152.4)

Free plasma concentrations of cefazolin exceeded the MIC in 94.7% (36/38) of the isolates tested. Only two isolates (*P. lautus* and *S. warneri*) presented MICs above the plasma concentration. In the case of cefuroxime and vancomycin, free plasma concentrations were higher than the MICs in all isolates tested. Gentamicin plasma levels were higher than the MIC in all isolates except eight (seven strains of *C. acnes* and one strain of *S. warneri*), 80.9% (34/42). In all these cases, except for *S. warneri*, the plasma concentrations of antibiotic used in combination with gentamicin were above the MIC.

SBTs were performed with serum samples obtained from patients with positive intraoperative cultures against the bacteria isolated from the surgical field of each patient (Figure 1, Table 4, and Supplementary Table S1). In four patients, SBT could not be performed due to a lack of serum.

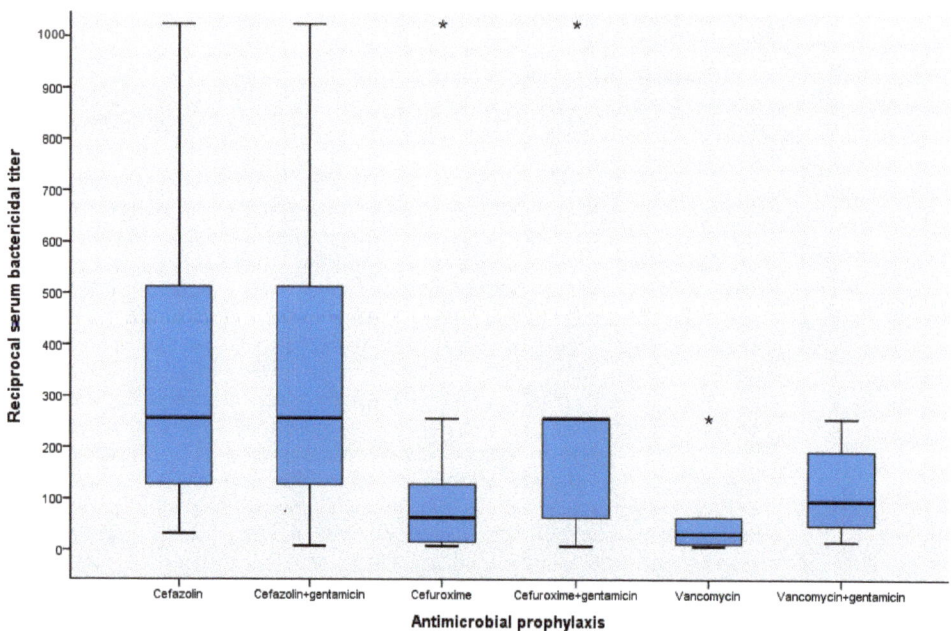

Figure 1. Reciprocal serum bactericidal titers against bacteria isolated in the surgical field for each surgical antimicrobial prophylaxis regimen. * Outliers are marked with an asterisk (*); outlier is defined as a data point that is located outside 1.5 times the interquartile range above the upper quartile and bellow the lower quartile.

Table 4. Reciprocal serum bactericidal titers against bacteria isolated in the surgical field and reference strains for each antimicrobial prophylaxis.

Antimicrobial Prophylaxis	Reciprocal Serum Bactericidal Titer—Median (Range)				
	Isolates from the Surgical Field	Staphylococcus epidermidis ATCC 12228	Staphylococcus aureus ATCC 25923	Escherichia coli ATCC 25922	Pseudomonas aeruginosa ATCC 27853
Cefazolin	256 (32–1024)	256 (32–512)	256 (64–1024)	64 (16–256)	<2 (<2)
Cefazolin+Gentamicin	256 (8–1024)	512 (32–1024)	256 (32–1024)	64 (16–256)	8 (<2–16)
Cefuroxime	64 (8–1024)	64 (16–512)	32 (8–64)	8 (2–32)	<2 (<2)
Cefuroxime+Gentamicin	256 (8–1024)	256 (64–512)	128 (8–128)	32 (16–32)	4 (<2–4)
Vancomycin	32 (8–256)	12 (8–32)	12 (8–16)	<2 (<2–2)	<2 (<2)
Vancomycin+Gentamicin	64 (16–256)	256 (256–512)	128 (32–256)	32 (16–64)	4 (4–8)

Overall, SBTs ranged from 1:8 to 1:1024. Statistically significant differences between the six SAP regimens studied ($p < 0.001$) were observed. Among patients receiving single-drug prophylaxis, SBTs were higher with cefazolin than with both cefuroxime and vancomycin ($p = 0.001$ and $p = 0.002$, respectively), while no differences were observed between cefuroxime and vancomycin ($p = 0.278$). Globally, patients receiving combined prophylaxis with gentamicin had higher SBTs than those receiving single-drug prophylaxis ($p = 0.009$), although these differences were only relevant with cefuroxime (vs. cefuroxime plus gentamicin) ($p = 0.023$) and vancomycin (vs. vancomycin plus gentamicin) ($p = 0.098$), and were not observed with cefazolin (vs. cefazolin plus gentamicin) ($p = 0.780$). Of note, serum bactericidal activity was detected (SBTs ranging from 1:16 to 1:128) in four methicillin-resistant CoNS isolates from patients who received only cefazolin or cefuroxime (despite the fact that methicillin resistance implies resistance to all beta-lactams, cephalosporins included). Moreover, an SBT of 1:16 was found against one *S. warneri* isolate, which was the only one in which plasma levels of both prophylactic antibiotics (cefazolin and gentamicin) did not exceed the MIC (Supplementary Table S1).

The bactericidal activity of each SAP regimen was also assessed by comparing SBTs performed against the reference strains S. epidermidis ATCC 12228, S. aureus ATCC 25923, E. coli ATCC 25922 and P. aeruginosa ATCC 27853 (Table 4). For this, 93 sera samples (53 from patients with positive intraoperative cultures and 40 with negative cultures) were tested. The results of SBTs against the Gram-positive bacteria S. epidermidis and S. aureus were very similar to those observed against isolates taken from the surgical field (all of them also Gram-positive bacteria). Overall, patients receiving gentamicin-containing SAP regimens had higher SBT titers than those who received single-agent prophylaxis, although this difference was not observed in the cefazolin groups. With respect to single-drug prophylaxis, the highest SBTs were found for cefazolin. Bactericidal activity against the Gram-negative bacterium, E. coli ATCC 25922, was observed with all SAP regimens, except for vancomycin alone (because of the intrinsic resistance to vancomycin of Gram-negative bacteria). SBTs against this E. coli strain followed the same pattern as for Gram-positive bacteria (highest SBT titers with cefazolin groups, and higher SBTs with gentamicin-containing cefuroxime and vancomycin regimens than with single cefuroxime and vancomycin prophylaxis); however, all SAP regimens (except vancomycin alone) showed four-fold lower median titers than against Gram-positive bacteria. Bactericidal activity against the Gram-negative bacterium P. aeruginosa ATCC 27853 was only observed in sera from patients treated with combinations with gentamicin (which correlates with the intrinsic resistance of this strain against cefazolin, cefuroxime and vancomycin), but with median SBTs four- to eight-fold lower than against E. coli ATCC 25922.

Antibiotic plasma levels and MICs of drugs used in prophylaxis against the reference strains are shown in Table 5. For P. aeruginosa ATCC 27853, none of the antibiotics except gentamicin achieved plasma levels above the MIC. For the remaining reference strains tested, all the antibiotics showed plasma levels above the MIC, except for vancomycin and E. coli ATCC 25922.

Table 5. Antibiotic plasma levels in surgical procedures with positive (n = 53) and negative (n = 40) intraoperative cultures and MICs of antimicrobial agents used in prophylaxis against ATCC reference strains.

Antimicrobial (n)	Free Plasma Concentration (mg/L), Median (Range)	MIC (mg/L)			
		Staphylococcus epidermidis ATCC 12228	Staphylococcus aureus ATCC 25923	Escherichia coli ATCC 25922	Pseudomonas aeruginosa ATCC 27853
Cefazolin (56)	17.3 (6.5–35.4)	0.5	0.5	3	>256
Cefuroxime (21)	25.7 (11–44.2)	0.75	0.5	6	>256
Gentamicin (54)	12.55 (8.5–19.4)	0.125	0.38	0.75	1.5
Vancomycin (16)	7.65 (4.6–19.05)	1.5	1	>256	>256

4. Discussion

Antimicrobial prophylaxis plays a crucial role in reducing the incidence of PJIs, although there is no consensus about antibiotic choice [26]. Some observational clinical studies have analyzed the effect of different SAP regimens on SSI/PJI rates following arthroplasty surgery, with conflicting results. Babu et al. compared five different antimicrobial prophylactic regimes in elective primary TKA and found no differences in the incidence of PJI or the pathogens involved [27]. Wyles et al. evaluated different SAPs in patients undergoing primary TKA or THA and found higher rates of PJI when non-cefazolin antibiotics were used [28]. Tornero et al. found a significant decrease in the PJI rate when teicoplanin was added to cefuroxime during primary arthroplasty, thanks to the decrease in Gram-positive bacterial infections [13]. Similar results were reported by

Barbero-Allende et al. with the addition of teicoplanin to cefazolin [17]. Another study found that the addition of gentamicin to cefazolin (or vancomycin in penicillin-allergic patients) reduced the SSI rate following THA [15]. These studies, however, have significant methodological limitations that prevent definitive conclusions from being drawn. Due to the difficulty of conducting sound clinical trials to compare the effect of different SAPs on PJI prevention, we evaluated six prophylactic regimens (cefazolin, cefuroxime and vancomycin as single agents or combined with gentamicin) in a preclinical exploratory study using microbiological and PK/PD analysis. We compared contamination of the surgical field, plasma antibiotic levels relative to the MICs of microorganisms isolated in wounds and some reference ATCC strains, and SBTs against the same bacteria.

Despite advances in preventive measures, intraoperative contamination of the surgical field in orthopedic surgery remains frequent. Contamination can originate from many sources, including the patients' microbiota, surgical personnel, surgical instruments, or the operating room environment [29–31]. Our results showed an overall intraoperative contamination rate of 43.2%, consisting of Gram-positive bacteria often found in normal cutaneous microbiota. This percentage is in the upper range limit of rates observed in prior studies [32–36], although neither the number of samples per patient, nor the collection method or specific anatomical location were standardized and indeed varied widely between studies. Furthermore, fewer samples per patient were taken and the swab was the most frequent collection method, which has lower sensitivity and specificity than tissue samples [37]. In accordance with previous studies, the most frequent organisms isolated were CoNS and *C. acnes*, both of which form part of the skin microbiota and are considered to be of low virulence, although they are a common cause of PJI, especially CoNS [9,38]. After a median follow-up of 15 months, two patients (1.5%) developed PJI. In both cases, previous intraoperative cultures were negative. According to these results, and those observed in previous studies, intraoperative contamination during primary TKA and THA surgery is common, but cannot be used to identify patients at increased risk of PJI [32–36]. On the other hand, factors such as longer duration of surgery [35] and high body mass index [32] have been associated with an increased risk of contamination. Other studies have shown that the use of iodinated drapes reduced intraoperative contamination in patients undergoing primary knee arthroplasty [39]. In our study, after adjusting for clinically relevant variables, we found that the group of patients receiving gentamicin-containing SAP combinations had a lower percentage of positive intraoperative cultures than the group that received only one drug. Nevertheless, the potential clinical relevance of these results and their influence on the risk of developing PJI remain to be determined. In fact, because the influence of intraoperative contamination on SSIs has not been conclusively proven, one publication has posited a new hypothesis about the pathogenesis of SSI [40]. The authors proposed that pathogens located in areas remote from the SSI, such as the teeth or gastrointestinal tract, could be transported in immune cells (macrophages or neutrophils) to the wound site and cause wound infection. We agree with the authors that further studies using genetic approaches can help to more clearly determine the significance of intraoperative contamination or other potential sources of infection in order to improve the SSI prevention strategies.

We analyzed the possible usefulness of SBT to evaluate the activity of antimicrobial agents used in prophylaxis. SBT assesses the antibacterial activity of a drug in the patient's serum [41,42]. These tests have been used in the past to guide antimicrobial therapy in severe infections such as endocarditis and osteomyelitis, but are practically abandoned in routine contemporary clinical practice because they are technically demanding and their usefulness has been questioned. Nevertheless, the advantage of SBT over standard antimicrobial susceptibility methods is that it integrates PK/PD factors. Indeed, some studies have breathed new life into this technique by showing its usefulness for monitoring antimicrobial therapy in patients with difficult-to-treat or multidrug-resistant infections [43–45]. Although SBT titers of 1:8 have been reported to correlate with successful outcomes of infection [41,42], the SBT titer required for surgical prophylaxis is unknown. Considering the breakpoint accepted for therapeutics, our study found that bactericidal activity was maintained throughout the surgical procedure against all isolates recovered from intraoperative samples (SBT range 1:8–1:1024), regardless of the prophylaxis used. Among the reference ATCC strains tested, staphylococci corroborated these results. For Gram-negative reference strains, bactericidal activity was observed against *E. coli* ATCC 25922 with all prophylactic regimens except vancomycin, while activity against *P. aeruginosa* ATCC 27853 was observed only with gentamicin combinations. These results correlate with the intrinsic resistance of both species to vancomycin, as well as the additional intrinsic resistance of *P. aeruginosa* to cefazolin and cefuroxime. The consistency of the results obtained using SBT supports its potential utility for assessing SAP.

Although high rates of resistance to beta-lactams have been found among pathogens causing PJI [8,10,38,46], particularly CoNS, most of the bacteria cultured from intraoperative samples in our study were susceptible to the cephalosporins administered. SAP may be able to eliminate these susceptible strains, but may also select for resistant ones that could cause PJI. Interestingly, the SBTs in patients receiving cefazolin or cefuroxime alone were particularly high against methicillin-resistant staphylococci. This could be related to our finding that antibiotic plasma levels at the end of the surgical procedure were well above the MICs for the organisms encountered in intraoperative cultures, which is considered to be the goal of SAP [5,6]. This, in conjunction with the low bacterial load, would be enough to achieve bacterial eradication. Nevertheless, bactericidal activity against Gram-positive isolates was obtained even in cases where antimicrobial plasma concentrations did not exceed or were slightly above the MIC. This was also true for methicillin-resistant staphylococci isolates, which suggests that currently recommended prophylactic regimens with cefazolin or cefuroxime continue to show activity even against these resistant Gram-positive bacteria. However, as expected, bactericidal activity was not enough against some Gram-negative isolates such as *P. aeruginosa*—intrinsically resistant to first- and second-generation cephalosporins and vancomycin—showing high MICs that greatly exceed the plasma concentration. Combination prophylaxis with gentamicin could play a role against these microorganisms or other cefazolin- or cefuroxime-resistant Gram-negative bacteria. This could be particularly relevant because some studies have reported an increased frequency of Gram-negative bacilli causing PJIs [8]. Furthermore, we found that the addition of gentamicin increased the antimicrobial activity of cefuroxime and vancomycin against bacteria isolated from surgical wounds, as well as ATCC staphylococci and *E. coli* reference strains. Cefazolin had higher activity than cefuroxime or vancomycin. Although the potential clinical implications of these findings need to be clarified, they should be borne in mind in order to design additional studies about arthroplasty surgery prophylaxis.

This study has some limitations. In the analysis of intraoperative cultures, any number of colonies was considered positive, which may have led to overestimating the positive culture rate in the surgical field. Bacterial contamination can occur at any time during analytical sample processing, and this possibility cannot be ruled out. Conversely, the lack of bacterial growth does not necessarily imply surgical site sterility because of the limitations of current techniques in detecting all bacteria present in the surgical field. We did not randomly assign patients to receive the different SAP regimens. While randomization is expected to produce comparable intervention groups and eliminate potential sources of bias in treatment assignment, this cannot be excluded in the present study. To overcome this limitation, we adjusted for clinically relevant covariates in the analysis stage; however, we cannot rule out the potential effect of unknown confounding or prognostic variables. Furthermore, although we performed an extensive microbiological and PK/PD study with different SAPs and found consistent results, its applicability in the prevention of SSIs/PJIs remains to be determined. It should also be considered that SAP is only part of the measures for prevention of SSI and that a patient's intrinsic characteristics and perioperative factors have a major influence on the development of these infections.

In conclusion, the six antimicrobial prophylactic regimens evaluated (cefazolin, cefuroxime and vancomycin, alone and combined with gentamicin) showed good activity against the microorganisms isolated from intraoperative tissue samples—including cephalosporins against methicillin-resistant CoNS—and achieved plasma levels above the MICs in almost all of them. Intraoperative bacterial contamination was less frequent in the combination group than in the group receiving single-drug prophylaxis. Although all the prophylactic regimens showed good activity against the intraoperative bacteria and staphylococcal reference strains (all of them Gram-positive bacteria), cefazolin with or without gentamicin displayed the greatest activity; cefuroxime and vancomycin as single drugs had lower activity than when combined with gentamicin. With respect to Gram-negative bacteria, SBT demonstrated, as expected, that vancomycin alone was the only SAP without activity against the *E. coli* reference strain, and that only gentamicin-containing regimens were active against the *P. aeruginosa* reference strain. The potential clinical relevance of these findings in the prevention of PJI remains to be determined. SBT was shown to be a potentially reliable tool for assessing antimicrobial surgical prophylaxis.

Supplementary Materials: The following are available online at https://www.mdpi.com/2079-6382/10/1/18/s1, Table S1: Antibiotic plasma levels of patients with intraoperative positive cultures, bacterial species from surgical samples, MICs of antimicrobials used in prophylaxis and serum bactericidal titers against the isolated bacteria.

Author Contributions: Conceptualization, A.R., F.N., J.P.H. and N.B.; methodology, A.R., A.S., S.L., F.N. and N.B.; validation, S.L., J.P.H., F.N.; formal analysis, A.R. and N.B.; investigation, A.S., S.L., I.M., L.P., X.C., J.C.G., L.S. and A.G.; data curation, L.S., I.M., L.P., X.C., J.C.G. and A.G.; writing—original draft preparation, A.R.; writing—review and editing, A.S., S.L., I.M., L.P., X.C., J.C.G., L.S., A.G., J.P.H., F.N. and N.B.; supervision, A.R. and N.B.; funding acquisition, N.B. All authors have read and agreed to the published version of the manuscript.

Funding: This research was funded by the Instituto de Salud Carlos III, Spanish Ministry of Economy and Competitiveness (grant number PI15/1026). Co-funded by European Regional Development Fund/European Social Fund "Investing in your future".

Institutional Review Board Statement: The study was conducted according to the guidelines of the Declaration of Helsinki, and approved by the Ethics Committee of the Hospital de la Santa Creu i Sant Pau and the Hospital del Mar (October 28th 2015 and March 2nd 2016, respectively).

Informed Consent Statement: Informed consent was obtained from all subjects involved in the study.

Data Availability Statement: The data presented in this study are available on request from the corresponding author.

Conflicts of Interest: The authors declare no conflict of interest.

References

1. Tande, A.J.; Patel, R. Prosthetic Joint Infection. *Clin. Microbiol. Rev.* **2014**, *27*, 302–345. [CrossRef] [PubMed]
2. Owens, C.D.; Stoessel, K. Surgical site infections: Epidemiology, microbiology and prevention. *J. Hosp. Infect.* **2008**, *70*, 3–10. [CrossRef]
3. Batty, L.M.; Lanting, B. Contemporary Strategies to Prevent Infection in Hip and Knee Arthroplasty. *Curr. Rev. Musculoskelet. Med.* **2020**, *13*, 400–408. [CrossRef] [PubMed]
4. Gallo, J.; Nieslanikova, E. Prevention of Prosthetic Joint Infection: From Traditional Approaches towards Quality Improvement and Data Mining. *J. Clin. Med.* **2020**, *9*, 2190. [CrossRef]
5. Aboltins, C.A.; Berdal, J.E.; Casas, F.; Corona, P.S.; Cuellar, D.; Ferrari, M.C.; Hendershot, E.; Huang, W.; Kuo, F.; Malkani, A.; et al. Hip and Knee Section, Prevention, Antimicrobials (Systemic): Proceedings of International Consensus on Orthopedic Infections. *J. Arthroplast.* **2019**, *34*, S279–S288. [CrossRef]
6. Bratzler, D.W.; Dellinger, E.P.; Olsen, K.M.; Perl, T.M.; Auwaerter, P.G.; Bolon, M.K.; Fish, D.N.; Napolitano, L.M.; Sawyer, R.G.; Slain, D.; et al. Clinical practice guidelines for antimicrobial prophylaxis in surgery. *Am. J. Heal. Pharm.* **2013**, *70*, 195–283. [CrossRef]
7. Talbot, T.R. Surgical Site Infections and Antimicrobial Prophylaxis. In *Mandell, Douglas, and Bennett's Principles and Practice of Infectious Diseases*; Elsevier: New York, NY, USA, 2019; pp. 3891–3904. [CrossRef]
8. Benito, N.; Franco, M.; Ribera, A.; Soriano, A.; Rodriguez-Pardo, D.; Sorli, L.; Fresco, G.; Fernandez-Sampedro, M.; del Toro, M.D.; Guio, L.; et al. Time trends in the aetiology of prosthetic joint infections: A multicentre cohort study. *Clin. Microbiol. Infect.* **2016**, *22*, 732. [CrossRef]

9. Peel, T.N.; Cheng, A.C.; Buising, K.L.; Choong, P.F.M. Microbiological aetiology, epidemiology, and clinical profile of prosthetic joint infections: Are current antibiotic prophylaxis guidelines effective? *Antimicrob. Agents Chemother.* **2012**, *56*, 2386–2391. [CrossRef]
10. Siljander, M.P.; Sobh, A.H.; Baker, K.C.; Baker, E.A.; Kaplan, L.M. Multidrug-Resistant Organisms in the Setting of Periprosthetic Joint Infection—Diagnosis, Prevention, and Treatment. *J. Arthroplast.* **2018**, *33*, 185–194. [CrossRef]
11. Berríos-Torres, S.I.; Yi, S.H.; Bratzler, D.W.; Ma, A.; Mu, Y.; Zhu, L.; Jernigan, J.A. Activity of commonly used antimicrobial prophylaxis regimens against pathogens causing coronary artery bypass graft and arthroplasty surgical site infections in the United States, 2006–2009. *Infect. Control. Hosp. Epidemiol.* **2014**, *35*, 231–239. [CrossRef]
12. Sewick, A.; Makani, A.; Wu, C.; O'Donnell, J.; Baldwin, K.D.; Lee, G.-C. Does dual antibiotic prophylaxis better prevent surgical site infections in total joint arthroplasty? *Clin. Orthop. Relat. Res.* **2012**, *470*, 2702–2707. [CrossRef] [PubMed]
13. Tornero, E.; García-Ramiro, S.; Martínez-Pastor, J.C.; Bori, G.; Bosch, J.; Morata, L.; Sala, M.; Basora, M.; Mensa, J.; Soriano, A. Prophylaxis with Teicoplanin and Cefuroxime Reduces the Rate of Prosthetic Joint Infection after Primary Arthroplasty. *Antimicrob. Agents Chemother.* **2015**, *59*, 831–837. [CrossRef] [PubMed]
14. Courtney, P.M.; Melnic, C.M.; Zimmer, Z.; Anari, J.; Lee, G.-C. Addition of Vancomycin to Cefazolin Prophylaxis Is Associated with Acute Kidney Injury After Primary Joint Arthroplasty. *Clin. Orthop. Relat. Res.* **2015**, *473*, 2197–2203. [CrossRef] [PubMed]
15. Bosco, J.A.; Tejada, P.R.R.; Catanzano, A.J.; Stachel, A.G.; Phillips, M.S. Expanded Gram-Negative Antimicrobial Prophylaxis Reduces Surgical Site Infections in Hip Arthroplasty. *J. Arthroplast.* **2016**, *31*, 616–621. [CrossRef] [PubMed]
16. Tucker, A.; Hegarty, P.; Magill, P.J.; Blaney, J.; Armstrong, L.V.; McCaffrey, J.E.; Beverland, D.E. Acute Kidney Injury After Prophylactic Cefuroxime and Gentamicin in Patients Undergoing Primary Hip and Knee Arthroplasty—A Propensity Score–Matched Study. *J. Arthroplast.* **2018**, *33*, 3009–3015. [CrossRef] [PubMed]
17. Barbero-Allende, J.M.; García-Sánchez, M.; Montero-Ruiz, E.; Vallés-Purroy, A.; Plasencia-Arriba, M.Á.; Sanz-Moreno, J. Dual prophylaxis with teicoplanin and cefazolin in the prevention of prosthetic joint infection. *Enferm. Infecc. Microbiol. Clin.* **2019**, *37*, 588–591. [CrossRef]
18. Parvizi, J.; Ghazavi, M. Committee of the Consensus Meeting M of PA. Optimal Timing and Antibiotic Prophylaxis in Periprosthetic Joint Infection (PJI): Literature Review and World Consensus (Part Three). *Shafa Orthop. J.* **2015**, *2*, e2355.
19. Yusuf, E.; Croughs, P. Vancomycin prophylaxis in prosthetic joint surgery? *Clin. Microbiol. Infect.* **2020**, *26*, 3–5. [CrossRef]
20. Rybak, M.; Lomaestro, B.; Rotschafer, J.C.; Moellering, R.; Craig, W.; Billeter, M.; Dalovisio, J.R.; Levine, D.P. Therapeutic monitoring of vancomycin in adult patients: A consensus review of the American Society of Health-System Pharmacists, the Infectious Diseases Society of America, and the Society of Infectious Diseases Pharmacists. *Am. J. Heal. Pharm.* **2009**, *66*, 82–98. [CrossRef]
21. Ulldemolins, M.; Roberts, J.A.; Rello, J.; Paterson, D.L.; Lipman, J. The effects of hypoalbuminaemia on optimizing antibacterial dosing in critically ill patients. *Clin. Pharmacokinet.* **2011**, *50*, 99–110. [CrossRef]
22. Bailey, D.N.; Briggs, J.R. Gentamicin and Tobramycin Binding to Human Serum in Vitro. *J. Anal. Toxicol.* **2004**, *28*, 187–189. [CrossRef] [PubMed]
23. The European Committee on Antimicrobial Susceptibility Testing. Breakpoint Tables for Interpretation of MICs and Zone Diameters. Version 9.0. 2019. Available online: http://www.eucast.org (accessed on 23 December 2020).
24. National Committee for Clinical and Laboratory Standards. *Methodology for the Serum Bactericidal Test.; Approved Guideline*; NCCLS document M21-A: Wayne, PA, USA, 1999.
25. Hosmer, D.W.; Lemeshow, S.; Sturdivant, R. Model-building strategies and methods for logistic regression. In *Applied Logistic Regression*; Hosmer, D.W., Lemeshow, S., Sturdivant, R., Eds.; John Wiley & Sons, Inc.: Hoboken, NJ, USA, 2013; pp. 89–152.
26. Siddiqi, A.; Forte, S.A.; Docter, S.; Bryant, D.; Sheth, N.P.; Chen, A.F. Perioperative antibiotic prophylaxis in total joint arthroplasty. *J. Bone Jt. Surg.* **2019**, *101*, 828–842. [CrossRef] [PubMed]
27. Babu, S.; Al-Obaidi, B.; Jardine, A.; Jonas, S.; Al-Hadithy, N.; Satish, V. A comparative study of 5 different antibiotic prophylaxis regimes in 4500 total knee replacements. *J. Clin. Orthop. Trauma* **2020**, *11*, 108–112. [CrossRef] [PubMed]
28. Wyles, C.C.; Hevesi, M.; Osmon, D.R.; Park, M.A.; Habermann, E.B.; Lewallen, D.G.; Berry, D.J.; Sierra, R.J. 2019 John Charnley Award: Increased risk of prosthetic joint infection following primary total knee and hip arthroplasty with the use of alternative antibiotics to cefazolin: The value of allergy testing for antibiotic prophylaxis. *Bone Jt. J.* **2019**, *101-B*, 9–15. [CrossRef] [PubMed]
29. Bitkover, C.Y.; Marcusson, E.; Ransjö, U. Spread of coagulase-negative staphylococci during cardiac operations in a modern operating room. *Ann. Thorac. Surg.* **2000**, *69*, 1110–1115. [CrossRef]
30. Parvizi, J.; Barnes, S.; Shohat, N.; Edmiston, C.E. Environment of care: Is it time to reassess microbial contamination of the operating room air as a risk factor for surgical site infection in total joint arthroplasty? *Am. J. Infect. Control.* **2017**, *45*, 1267–1272. [CrossRef]
31. Wildeman, P.; Tevell, S.; Eriksson, C.; Lagos, A.C.; Söderquist, B.; Stenmark, B. Genomic characterization and outcome of prosthetic joint infections caused by Staphylococcus aureus. *Sci. Rep.* **2020**, *10*, 1–14. [CrossRef]
32. Font-Vizcarra, L.; Tornero, E.; Bori, G.; Bosch, J.; Mensa, J.; Soriano, A. Relationship between intraoperative cultures during hip arthroplasty, obesity, and the risk of early prosthetic joint infection: A prospective study of 428 patients. *Int. J. Artif. Organs* **2011**, *34*, 870–875. [CrossRef]
33. Frank, C.B.; Adams, M.; Kroeber, M.; Wentzensen, A.; Heppert, V.; Schulte-Bockholt, D.; Guehring, T. Intraoperative subcutaneous wound closing culture sample: A predicting factor for periprosthetic infection after hip- and knee-replacement? *Arch. Orthop. Trauma Surg.* **2011**, *131*, 1389–1396. [CrossRef]

34. Haenle, M.; Podbielski, A.; Ellenrieder, M.; Mundt, A.; Krentz, H.; Mittelmeier, W.; Skripitz, R. Bacteriology swabs in primary total knee arthroplasty. *GMS Hyg. Infect. Control.* **2013**, *8*. [CrossRef]
35. Jonsson, E.Ö.; Johannesdottir, H.; Robertsson, O.; Mogensen, B. Bacterial contamination of the wound during primary total hip and knee replacement. Median 13 years of follow-up of 90 replacements. *Acta Orthop.* **2014**, *85*, 159–164. [CrossRef] [PubMed]
36. Knobben, B.A.S.; Engelsma, Y.; Neut, D.; Van Der Mei, H.C.; Busscher, H.J.; Van Horn, J.R. Intraoperative contamination influences wound discharge and periprosthetic infection. *Clin. Orthop. Relat. Res.* **2006**, *452*, 236–241. [CrossRef] [PubMed]
37. Aggarwal, V.K.; Higuera, C.; Deirmengian, G.; Parvizi, J.; Austin, M.S. Swab cultures are not as effective as tissue cultures for diagnosis of periprosthetic joint infection. *Clin. Orthop. Relat. Res.* **2013**, *471*, 3196–3203. [CrossRef] [PubMed]
38. Benito, N.; Mur, I.; Ribera, A.; Soriano, A.; Rodriguez-Pardo, D.; Sorli, L.; Cobo, J.; Fernandez-Sampedro, M.; del Toro, M.D.; Guio, L.; et al. The Different Microbial Etiology of Prosthetic Joint Infections according to Route of Acquisition and Time after Prosthesis Implantation, Including the Role of Multidrug-Resistant Organisms. *J. Clin. Med.* **2019**, *8*, 673. [CrossRef] [PubMed]
39. Scheidt, S.; Walter, S.; Randau, T.M.; Köpf, U.S.; Jordan, M.C.; Hischebeth, G.T.R. The Influence of Iodine-Impregnated Incision Drapes on the Bacterial Contamination of Scalpel Blades in Joint Arthroplasty. *J. Arthroplast.* **2020**, *35*, 2595–2600. [CrossRef]
40. Alverdy, J.C.; Hyman, N.; Gilbert, J. Re-examining causes of surgical site infections following elective surgery in the era of asepsis. *Lancet Infect. Dis.* **2020**, *20*, e38–e43. [CrossRef]
41. Stratton, C.W. The usefulness of the serum bactericidal test in orthopedic infections. *Orthopedics* **1984**, *7*, 1579–1580.
42. Harley, W.B.; Stratton, C.W. The serum bactericidal test revisited. *Infect. Dis. Newsl.* **1993**, *12*, 61–64. [CrossRef]
43. Gaibani, P.; Lombardo, D.; Bartoletti, M.; Ambretti, S.; Campoli, C.; Giannella, M.; Tedeschi, S.; Conti, M.; Mancini, R.; Landini, M.P.; et al. Comparative serum bactericidal activity of meropenem-based combination regimens against extended-spectrum beta-lactamase and KPC-producing Klebsiella pneumoniae. *Eur. J. Clin. Microbiol. Infect. Dis.* **2019**, *38*, 1925–1931. [CrossRef]
44. Spaziante, M.; Franchi, C.; Taliani, G.; d'Avolio, A.; Pietropaolo, V.; Biliotti, E.; Esvan, R.; Venditti, M. Serum bactericidal activity levels monitor to guide intravenous dalbavancin chronic suppressive therapy of inoperable staphylococcal prosthetic valve endocarditis: A case report. *Open. Forum Infect. Dis.* **2019**, *6*, 10–12. [CrossRef]
45. Zaghi, I.; Gaibani, P.; Campoli, C.; Bartoletti, M.; Giannella, M.; Ambretti, S.; Viale, P.; Lewis, R.E. Serum bactericidal titres for monitoring antimicrobial therapy: Current status and potential role in the management of multidrug-resistant Gram-negative infections. *Clin. Microbiol. Infect.* **2020**, *26*, 1338–1344. [CrossRef] [PubMed]
46. Ravi, S.; Zhu, M.; Luey, C.; Young, S.W. Antibiotic resistance in early periprosthetic joint infection. *ANZ J. Surg.* **2016**, *86*, 1014–1018. [CrossRef] [PubMed]

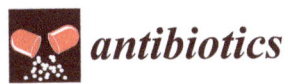

Perspective

Periprosthetic Joint Infection Prophylaxis in the Elderly after Hip Hemiarthroplasty in Proximal Femur Fractures: Insights and Challenges

Dolors Rodríguez-Pardo [1,2,3,4,*], Laura Escolà-Vergé [1,2,3], Júlia Sellarès-Nadal [1,3,4], Pablo S. Corona [2,3,4,5], Benito Almirante [1,2,4] and Carles Pigrau [1,2,3]

1. Infectious Diseases Department, Vall d'Hebron Hospital Universitari, Vall d'Hebron Barcelona Hospital Campus, Passeig Vall d'Hebron 119-129, 08035 Barcelona, Spain; lauraescola@gmail.com (L.E.-V.); juliasellares@gmail.com (J.S.-N.); balmiran@vhebron.net (B.A.); cpigrau@vhebron.net (C.P.)
2. Spanish Network for Research in Infectious Diseases (REIPI RD16/0016/0003), Instituto de Salud Carlos III, 28029 Madrid, Spain; pcorona@vhebron.net
3. Study Group on Osteoarticular Infections of the Spanish Society of Clinical Microbiology and Infectious Diseases (GEIO-SEIMC), 28003 Madrid, Spain
4. Medicina Interna, Universitat Autònoma de Barcelona, 08193 Bellaterra, Spain
5. Septic and Reconstructive Surgery Unit (UCSO), Orthopaedic Surgery Department, Vall d'Hebron Hospital Universitari, Vall d'Hebron Barcelona Hospital Campus, Passeig Vall d'Hebron 119-129, 08035 Barcelona, Spain
* Correspondence: dolorodriguez@vhebron.net; Tel.: +34-93-2746090; Fax: +34-93-4894091

Abstract: We review antibiotic and other prophylactic measures to prevent periprosthetic joint infection (PJI) after hip hemiarthroplasty (HHA) surgery in proximal femoral fractures (PFFs). In the absence of specific guidelines, those applied to these individuals are general prophylaxis guidelines. Cefazolin is the most widely used agent and is replaced by clindamycin or a glycopeptide in beta-lactam allergies. A personalized antibiotic scheme may be considered when colonization by a multidrug-resistant microorganism (MDRO) is suspected. Particularly in methicillin-resistant *Staphylococcus aureus* (MRSA) colonization or a high prevalence of MRSA-caused PJIs a glycopeptide with cefazolin is recommended. Strategies such as cutaneous decolonization of MDROs, mainly MRSA, or preoperative asymptomatic bacteriuria treatment have also been addressed with debatable results. Some areas of research are early detection protocols in MDRO colonizations by polymerase-chain-reaction (PCR), the use of alternative antimicrobial prophylaxis, and antibiotic-impregnated bone cement in HHA. Given that published evidence addressing PJI prophylactic strategies in PFFs requiring HHA is scarce, PJIs can be reduced by combining different prevention strategies after identifying individuals who will benefit from personalized prophylaxis.

Keywords: hip hemiarthroplasty; proximal femur fracture; antibiotic prophylaxis; periprosthetic joint infection; decolonization

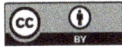

1. Introduction

Antimicrobial prophylaxis (AP) is crucial in preventing surgical site infections (SSIs) after orthopedic surgery, with a reduction by up to 81% in the relative risk of infection and 8% in the absolute risk [1]. In proximal femoral fractures (PFFs) with internal fixation, two metanalyses showed that AP reduced the incidence of SSIs compared to either non-prophylaxis or placebo [2,3]. The standard care AP in orthopedic surgery has traditionally been first-generation cephalosporins. This is due to their adequate spectrum for the general population, safety profile, and low price [1]. However, this approach may not always be adequate, particularly for institutionalized patients who have skin flora alterations and multidrug-resistant organisms (MDROs) colonization [4]. For this reason, some physicians may consider it more appropriate to provide them with individualized prophylaxis.

Other strategies such as cutaneous and nasal *Staphylococcus aureus* decolonization have proven to be effective in reducing early SSIs in orthopedic surgery [5–7]. However, their implementation may not be easy, their effectiveness is sometimes controversial, particularly with a low incidence of *S. aureus* SSIs, and it has not been specifically addressed in PFF in the elderly.

We aim to undertake a critical appraisal on current periprosthetic joint infection (PJI) prophylaxis strategies in PFFs requiring HHA surgery and exploring future research areas.

2. Current Antibiotic Prophylaxis in Proximal Femur Fractures Requiring Hip Hemiarthroplasty

Single-dose or continuation for less than 24 h AP is recommended for hip fracture repair in procedures involving prosthetic replacement or internal fixation [1,8]. Surgical AP should be administered within 120 min before incision. However, it is recommended that when using short half-life beta-lactams (e.g., first-generation cephalosporin drugs), they be administered within 60 min [1,8]. Single-dose or regimens of <24 h duration antibiotics that ensure drug concentrations during surgery will be appropriate [1].

The antimicrobial agent most commonly used in orthopedic procedure prophylaxis [1,8] is cefazolin. Even though cefuroxime has been used in PFF surgery in the elderly [9], second and third-generation cephalosporins are not routinely recommended here due to adverse events (i.e., *Clostridioides difficile*-associated diarrhea) and potential to cause antibiotic resistance [1].

In the case of beta-lactam type 1 (immunoglobulin E (IgE)-mediated) allergy, methicillin-resistant *S. aureus* (MRSA) colonization or a high prevalence of nosocomial MRSA SSI, clindamycin, or a glycopeptide (vancomycin or teicoplanin) may be used [1,8,10]. Although cross-allergic reactions between penicillin and cephalosporins are uncommon, cephalosporins should not be used for surgical prophylaxis in patients with documented or presumed IgE-mediated penicillin allergy [1]. Vancomycin is less effective than cefazolin for preventing SSIs caused by methicillin-susceptible *S. aureus* (MSSA). However, it is recommended with cefazolin in non-allergic patients [11]. Likewise, the addition of teicoplanin to cefazolin in arthroplasty surgery reduced PJIs thanks to a decrease in Gram-positive bacterial infections [12].

When there is an increased risk of Gram-negative bacilli (GNB) SSIs (i.e., colonized or recently infected patients), published guidelines recommend glycopeptides added to (1) cefazolin or cefuroxime in the absence of beta-lactam allergies and (2) aztreonam, gentamicin, or single-dose fluoroquinolone if there are allergies [1,8]. Although studies are not specific on PFFs requiring HHA, these recommendations are followed in the absence of more specific ones.

3. Current Challenges to Optimize Antibiotic Prophylaxis in Proximal Femur Fractures Requiring Hip Hemiarthroplasty

Patients with PFFs undergoing HHA are usually elderly, frail, comorbid, recently hospitalized, or even institutionalized. Consequently, standard AP may not be as effective as expected and should be individualized according to local epidemiology and antimicrobial susceptibility patterns [8]. Hence, the usefulness of strategies such as MDROs decolonization or individualized AP should be considered.

Regarding skin decolonization, there is considerable experience in *S. aureus* [5–7] which is the first cause of acute PJIs after total joint and HHA. Thus, a cohort study including 19 hospitals in Spain [13] showed a total of 7.9% (95% CI: 6.8–9.1%) MRSA-caused PJIs. Decolonization with intranasal mupirocin prevents SSIs in orthopedic surgery in patients with documented *S. aureus* [1,5,6]. However, identifying and specifically treating colonized individuals is a costly and challenging process. It requires a complex structure that allows screening, obtaining the results, and performing five days of nasal decolonization treatment with mupirocin before surgery. These steps are complicated to coordinate and done on time since PFFs require emergency surgeries. In this context, universal decolonization is the suggested alternative despite the risk of developing resistance to mupirocin which has been considered low [14]. Other noteworthy approaches are universal preoperative nasal and skin decolonization with chlorhexidine bathing in addition to the alcohol-based nasal antiseptic application [15] or chlorhexidine washcloths and oral rinse and intranasal application of povidone-iodine solution the night before and the morning of scheduled surgery [7]. Both strategies reduced PJI rates, associated morbidity, and costs thus avoiding resistance to mupirocin. However, although preoperative chlorhexidine bathing is widely performed in real-world practice, nasal decolonization is not, which probably allows for improvement in this strategy's outcomes.

In the Spanish study [13] mentioned above, a statistically significant rising linear trend was observed for those PJIs caused by aerobic GNB (25% in 2003–2004, 33.3% in 2011–2012; $p = 0.024$) globally and also by MDR-GNB (from 5.3% in 2003–2004 to 8.2% in 2011–2012; $p = 0.032$). We have also published our experience regarding PJIs in patients undergoing HHA secondary to PFFs [16]. Among a total cohort of 381 patients included between 2011 and 2013, PJIs were diagnosed in 21 (5.51%), with a significantly higher incidence of SSIs among chronic institutionalized vs. non-institutionalized (9.52% vs. 3.99%; $p = 0.04$). Remarkably, GNB were the principal pathogens involved (67% of all PJIs). These observations suggest that asymptomatic bacteriuria (ASB) and fecal and urinary incontinence, both common among the elderly, support skin colonization either before the surgery or in the immediate postoperative period. Different authors have addressed the relationship between ASB treatment and PJIs in hip or knee surgeries with controversial outcomes. Sousa et al. [17] found that ASB was an independent risk factor for PJIs, with no correlation found between previously isolated bacteria in the urine and PJIs, while Honkanen et al. [18] did not find any relation between preoperative bacteriuria and PJIs in primary hip or knee replacement surgeries. Besides, Cordero et al. [19] did not identify any PJIs of urinary origin in patients with ASB. All these studies included both patients undergoing total hip arthroplasties and HHA. However, when the analyzed cohort is reduced to geriatric patients undergoing PFF surgery, the results are more contentious, and some authors conclude that prevalent bacteriuria treatment decreases the risk of SSI [9,20]. We evaluated the clinical impact of preoperative ASB treatment with a single dose of 3 g of oral fosfomycin between 24 and 6 h before surgery vs. no treatment on the reduction of early-PJI after HHA in an open-label, multicenter randomized clinical trial (BARIFER CT, Eudra CT 2016-001108-47). A total of 594 patients were enrolled (mean age 84.3 years), of whom 152 (25%) had ASB (77 treated with fosfomycin and 75 not treated), and 442 (75%) controls did not have ASB. It was found that neither preoperative ASB nor its treatment are independent risk factors of early-PJI in HHA surgery. Therefore, we consider that routine screening and preoperative ASB treatment should not be recommended.

Some literature has been published regarding skin decolonization in patients with MDR-GNB (extended-spectrum beta-lactamase (ESBL) or carbapenemase-producing Enterobacterales). Huttner et al. [21] carried out a study in adults with an ESBL-producing Enterobacterales (ESBL-E) positive rectal swab. Fifty-eight patients were allocated 1:1 to either placebo or colistin sulfate (50 mg four times per day) or neomycin sulfate (250 mg four times per day) for up to ten days plus nitrofurantoin (100 mg three times a day) for up to five days in the presence of ESBL-E bacteriuria. It was observed that this regimen temporarily suppressed ESBL-E carriage but had no long-term effect after seven days. Given its limited efficacy and the time needed to implement the protocol, these strategies are not applicable in emergency surgeries such as HHAs for PFF. On that basis, some authors and guidelines support extending AP in high-risk of being colonized by MDR-GNB individuals [1,8].

A recently published experience by Cuchi et al. [22] evaluates the role of previous skin and urine colonization in the development of deep SSIs after PFF surgery. It failed to find a relationship between skin colonization, urine culture, and deep SSI.

As observed, it appeared that patients would not benefit from modifying current AP in HHA and ASB. Regarding cutaneous MDR-GNB colonization, there is no strong evidence but a small cohort of patients' and experts' opinions advising extending AP in patients at risk of MDR-GNB skin colonization. However, we would advise caution and act accordingly only when MDRO colonization is confirmed.

4. Future Scenarios to Optimize Prosthetic Joint Infection Prophylaxis in Proximal Femur Fractures Requiring Hip Hemiarthroplasty

Strategies for MDRO screening and decolonization need to be optimized. Recently, new molecular tools have been developed to rapidly identify MDROs in different clinical samples such as skin and rectal screening swabs by real-time polymerase-chain-reaction (PCR) and sequencing techniques. These can detect targeted genes within a few hours which is relevant in urgent surgeries such as HHA in PFFs. These highly sensitive and specific methods would rapidly determine not only MRSA/MSSA colonization [23] but also ESBL-E [24] and carbapenemase-producing Enterobacterales [25] carriers. Standardization of such techniques would allow individualized prophylaxis covering MDROs only in patients with proven colonization. As experience accumulates, it will be assessed whether this individualized prophylaxis reduces GNB infection risk and whether it is a cost-effective strategy.

Another field of study is the use of alternative antibiotic regimens. In our experience, trimethoprim/sulfamethoxazole in monotherapy (800/160 mg of cotrimoxazole during anesthesia induction followed by another dose after 12 h) is effective. It prevents MRSA infections among chronic institutionalized patients undergoing HHA [16]. Besides, it is easy to handle and shows good tolerability.

There is a lack of information about the need to address candiduria or candidal intertrigo when they are detected before HHA surgery. These are quite common in elderly individuals who need diapering because of incontinence. In our experience, 34 (79.1%) out of 43 patients analyzed with *Candida* PJIs had at least one risk factor for *Candida* infection (six had concomitant intertrigo, and four showed candiduria before surgery) [26]. These data suggest that treating candidal intertrigo before HHA surgery could prevent PJIs easily. In contrast, it is not obvious whether candiduria should be addressed once we have observed that treating bacteriuria has no impact on reducing early-PJIs after HHA surgery.

Finally, the role of antibiotic-impregnated cement in primary HHA surgery is controversial. Antibiotic-impregnated bone cement is used as a spacer or during reimplantation surgery to treat infected total hip arthroplasties. A recent meta-analysis concluded it reduces infection rates by approximately 50% [27]. It has also been reported that high-dose dual antibiotic-impregnated (vancomycin and gentamicin) bone cement decreases PJIs rates in hip fractures [28]. Their use has recently become widespread in Spanish hospitals. This was reviewed during our multicenter randomized trial which assessed the impact of a PJI prevention strategy in patients with a PFF requiring HHA surgery (BARIFER CT data, Eudra CT 2016-001108-47). It was observed that 65.46% of HHA implant cases were cemented with antibiotics (64% with single and 36% with dual antibiotics). Given that some of the participating sites used them without changes in their specific AP, we hypothesize that this could justify a reduction in early-PJI rates compared to those previously reported between 2011 and 2013 (up to 9.52% among institutionalized patients) [16] and also in hospitals in our area [29]. Therefore, we encourage the use of antimicrobial-impregnated bone cement, and we also consider it interesting to be standardized in high-risk patients.

One of the major limitations of the opinion we share here is that the highest strength of evidence cannot always support recommendations due to the scarcity of published studies. Although certain antibiotics and prophylactic strategies may be discouraged or supported, final approaches should be tailored to local epidemiology and the antimicrobial stewardship programs at each center. We suggest a targeted preventive strategy, given that a broad-spectrum antibiotic regimen (i.e., meropenem plus linezolid or daptomycin), although covering possible MDROs, may result in new resistances (i.e., carbapenemases expression in Enterobacterales) and invalidate its future use.

5. Conclusions

Cefazolin might not be adequate for elderly and fragile patients with recent hospitalizations or institutionalization. In this scenario, our recommendations are (1) to expand AP to address MRSA or MDR-GNB in colonized or recently infected patients with such microorganism, (2) to perform universal preoperative nasal and skin decolonization accordingly the night before and the morning of surgery limiting the use of mupirocin for MRSA colonized patients and (3) to use dual antibiotic-impregnated (vancomycin and gentamicin) bone cement in primary HHA surgery. Thus, PJIs can be reduced by combining all these strategies after identifying those patients who may benefit from using personalized SSIs prophylaxis.

Author Contributions: D.R.-P. contributed to its conception, funding acquisition, methodology, data curation, writing of the original draft, and writing of the review and editing with the assistance of a medical writer. C.P., P.S.C., L.E.-V., J.S.-N., and B.A. contributed to the review and editing of the manuscript. All authors have read and agreed to the published version of the manuscript.

Funding: This work was supported by the ISCIII-Subdirección General de Evaluación y Fomento de la Investigación, through the project PI15/02161 and by the Plan Nacional de I+D+i 2013-016 and ISCIIII, Subdirección General de Redes y Centros de Investigación Cooperativa, Ministerio de Economia, Industria y Competitividad, Spanish Network for Research in Infectious Diseases (REIPI RD16/0016/0003)-co-financed by European Development Regional Fund "A way to achieve Europe", Operative program Intelligent Growth 2014–2020.

Data Availability Statement: Data presented in this study regarding BARIFER CT, Eudra CT 2016-001108-47 are available upon request from the corresponding author. BARIFER randomized clinical trial manuscript has been recently accepted for publication in the European Journal of Clinical Microbiology & Infectious Diseases.

Acknowledgments: We thank Maria Romero (Trialance, S.C.C.L.) for the medical writing support.

Conflicts of Interest: The authors declare no conflict of interest.

References

1. Bratzler, D.W.; Dellinger, E.P.; Olsen, K.M.; Perl, T.M.; Auwaerter, P.G.; Bolon, M.K.; Fish, D.N.; Napolitano, L.M.; Sawyer, R.G.; Slain, D.; et al. Clinical practice guidelines for antimicrobial prophylaxis in surgery. *Am. J. Health Pharm.* **2013**, *70*, 195–283. [CrossRef]
2. Gillespie, W.J.; Walenkamp, G. Antibiotic prophylaxis for surgery for proximal femoral and other closed long bone fractures. In *Cochrane Database of Systematic Reviews*; John Wiley & Sons, Ltd: Hoboken, NJ, USA, 2001; p. CD000244. [CrossRef]
3. Southwell-Keely, J.P.; Russo, R.R.; March, L.; Cumming, R.; Cameron, I.; Brnabic, A.J.M. Antibiotic Prophylaxis in Hip Fracture Surgery: A Metaanalysis. *Clin. Orthop. Relat. Res.* **2004**, 179–184. [CrossRef] [PubMed]
4. Peel, T.N.; Cheng, A.C.; Buising, K.L.; Choong, P.F.M. Microbiological aetiology, epidemiology, and clinical profile of prosthetic joint infections: Are current antibiotic prophylaxis guidelines effective? *Antimicrob. Agents Chemother.* **2012**, *56*, 2386–2391. [CrossRef]
5. Bode, L.G.M.; Kluytmans, J.A.J.W.; Wertheim, H.F.L.; Bogaers, D.; Vandenbroucke-Grauls, C.M.J.E.; Roosendaal, R.; Troelstra, A.; Box, A.T.A.; Voss, A.; van der Tweel, I.; et al. Preventing Surgical-Site Infections in Nasal Carriers of Staphylococcus aureus. *N. Engl. J. Med.* **2010**, *362*, 9–17. [CrossRef]
6. Barbero Allende, J.M.; Romanyk Cabrera, J.; Montero Ruiz, E.; Vallés Purroy, A.; Melgar Molero, V.; Agudo López, R.; Gete García, L.; López Álvarez, J. Resultados de una intervención de descolonización de Staphylococcus aureus en pacientes portadores a los que se indica una prótesis articular. *Enferm. Infecc. Microbiol. Clin.* **2015**, *33*, 95–100. [CrossRef] [PubMed]
7. Bebko, S.P.; Green, D.M.; Awad, S.S. Effect of a preoperative decontamination protocol on surgical site infections in patients undergoing elective orthopedic surgery with hardware implantation. *JAMA Surg.* **2015**, *150*, 390–395. [CrossRef] [PubMed]
8. Del Toro López, M.D.; Arias Díaz, J.; Balibrea, J.M.; Benito, N.; Canut Blasco, A.; Esteve, E.; Horcajada, J.P.; Ruiz Mesa, J.D.; Manuel Vázquez, A.; Muñoz Casares, C.; et al. Executive summary of the Consensus Document of the Spanish Society of Infectious Diseases and Clinical Microbiology (SEIMC) and of the Spanish Association of Surgeons (AEC) in antibiotic prophylaxis in surgery. *Cir. Esp.* **2021**, *99*, 11–26. [CrossRef]
9. Li, Y.; Wang, J.; Wang, W. Peri-Operative Antibiotic Treatment of Bacteriuria Reduces Early Deep Surgical Site Infections in Geriatric Patients with Proximal Femur Fracture: Is It Related? Springer: Berlin/Heidelberg, Germany, 2018; Volume 42, pp. 719–720. [CrossRef]
10. Bryson, D.J.; Gulihar, A.; Aujla, R.S.; Taylor, G.J.S. The hip fracture best practice tariff: Early surgery and the implications for MRSA screening and antibiotic prophylaxis. *Eur. J. Orthop. Surg. Traumatol.* **2015**, *25*, 123–127. [CrossRef] [PubMed]

11. Bull, A.L.; Worth, L.J.; Richards, M.J. Impact of vancomycin surgical antibiotic prophylaxis on the development of methicillin-sensitive staphylococcus aureus surgical site infections: Report from Australian surveillance data (VICNISS). *Ann. Surg.* **2012**, *256*, 1089–1092. [CrossRef]
12. Barbero-Allende, J.M.; García-Sánchez, M.; Montero-Ruiz, E.; Vallés-Purroy, A.; Plasencia-Arriba, M.Á.; Sanz-Moreno, J. Dual prophylaxis with teicoplanin and cefazolin in the prevention of prosthetic joint infection. *Enferm. Infecc. Microbiol. Clin.* **2019**, *37*, 588–591. [CrossRef]
13. Benito, N.; Franco, M.; Ribera, A.; Soriano, A.; Rodriguez-Pardo, D.; Sorlí, L.; Fresco, G.; Fernández-Sampedro, M.; Dolores del Toro, M.; Guío, L.; et al. Time trends in the aetiology of prosthetic joint infections: A multicentre cohort study. *Clin. Microbiol. Infect.* **2016**, *22*, 732.e1–732.e8. [CrossRef]
14. Hetem, D.J.; Bootsma, M.C.J.; Bonten, M.J.M.; Weinstein, R.A. Prevention of Surgical Site Infections: Decontamination with Mupirocin Based on Preoperative Screening for Staphylococcus aureus Carriers or Universal Decontamination? *Clin. Infect. Dis.* **2016**, *62*, 631–636. [CrossRef]
15. Franklin, S. A safer, less costly SSI prevention protocol—Universal versus targeted preoperative decolonization. *Am. J. Infect. Control* **2020**, *48*, 1501–1503. [CrossRef]
16. Gallardo-Calero, I.; Larrainzar-Coghen, T.; Rodriguez-Pardo, D.; Pigrau, C.; Sánchez-Raya, J.; Amat, C.; Lung, M.; Carrera, L.; Corona, P.S. Increased infection risk after hip hemiarthroplasty in institutionalized patients with proximal femur fracture. *Injury* **2016**, *47*. [CrossRef] [PubMed]
17. Sousa, R.; Muñoz-Mahamud, E.; Quayle, J.; Da Costa, L.D.; Casals, C.; Scott, P.; Leite, P.; Vilanova, P.; Garcia, S.; Ramos, M.H.; et al. Is asymptomatic bacteriuria a risk factor for prosthetic joint infection? *Clin. Infect. Dis.* **2014**, *59*, 41–47. [CrossRef]
18. Honkanen, M.; Jämsen, E.; Karppelin, M.; Huttunen, R.; Huhtala, H.; Eskelinen, A.; Syrjänen, J. The impact of preoperative bacteriuria on the risk of periprosthetic joint infection after primary knee or hip replacement: A retrospective study with a 1-year follow up. *Clin. Microbiol. Infect.* **2018**, *24*, 376–380. [CrossRef]
19. Cordero-Ampuero, J.; González-Fernández, E.; Martínez-Vélez, D.; Esteban, J. Are antibiotics necessary in hip arthroplasty with asymptomatic bacteriuria? Seeding risk with/without treatment. *Clin. Orthop. Relat. Res.* **2013**, *471*, 3822–3829. [CrossRef]
20. Langenhan, R.; Bushuven, S.; Reimers, N.; Probst, A. Peri-operative antibiotic treatment of bacteriuria reduces early deep surgical site infections in geriatric patients with proximal femur fracture. *Int. Orthop.* **2018**, *42*, 741–746. [CrossRef]
21. Huttner, B.; Haustein, T.; Uçkay, I.; Renzi, G.; Stewardson, A.; Schaerrer, D.; Agostinho, A.; Andremont, A.; Schrenzel, J.; Pittet, D.; et al. Decolonization of intestinal carriage of extended-spectrum B-lactamase-producing Enterobacteriaceae with oral colistin and neomycin: A randomized, double-blind, placebo-controlled trial. *J. Antimicrob. Chemother.* **2013**, *68*, 2375–2382. [CrossRef] [PubMed]
22. Cuchí, E.; García, L.G.; Jiménez, E.; Haro, D.; Castillón, P.; Puertas, L.; Matamala, A.; Anglès, F.; Pérez, J. Relationship between skin and urine colonization and surgical site infection in the proximal femur fracture: A prospective study. *Int. Orthop.* **2020**, *44*, 1031–1035. [CrossRef] [PubMed]
23. Valour, F.; Blanc-Pattin, V.; Freydière, A.M.; Bouaziz, A.; Chanard, E.; Lustig, S.; Ferry, T.; Laurent, F.; Perpoint, T.; Boibieux, A.; et al. Rapid detection of Staphylococcus aureus and methicillin resistance in bone and joint infection samples: Evaluation of the GeneXpert MRSA/SA SSTI assay. *Diagn. Microbiol. Infect. Dis.* **2014**, *78*, 313–315. [CrossRef]
24. Blanc, D.S.; Poncet, F.; Grandbastien, B.; Greub, G.; Senn, L.; Nordmann, P. Evaluation of the performance of rapid tests for screening carriers of acquired ESBL-producing Enterobacterales and their impact on turnaround time. *J. Hosp. Infect.* **2021**, *108*, 19–24. [CrossRef]
25. Baeza, L.L.; Pfennigwerth, N.; Hamprecht, A. Rapid and easy detection of carbapenemases in enterobacterales in the routine laboratory using the new GenePOC Carba/Revogene Carba C Assay. *J. Clin. Microbiol.* **2019**, *57*. [CrossRef]
26. Escolà-Vergé, L.; Rodríguez-Pardo, D.; Lora-Tamayo, J.; Morata, L.; Murillo, O.; Vilchez, H.; Sorli, L.; Carrión, L.G.; Barbero, J.M.; Palomino-Nicás, J.; et al. Candida periprosthetic joint infection: A rare and difficult-to-treat infection. *J. Infect.* **2018**, *77*, 151–157. [CrossRef] [PubMed]
27. Parvizi, J.; Saleh, K.J.; Ragland, P.S.; Pour, A.E.; Mont, M.A. Efficacy of antibiotic-impregnated cement in total hip replacement: A meta-analysis. *Acta Orthop.* **2008**, *79*, 335–341. [CrossRef]
28. Sprowson, A.P.; Jensen, C.; Chambers, S.; Parsons, N.R.; Aradhyula, N.M.; Carluke, I.; Inman, D.; Reed, M.R. The use of high-dose dual-impregnated antibiotic-laden cement with hemiarthroplasty for the treatment of a fracture of the hip the fractured hip infection trial. *Bone Jt. J.* **2016**, *98-B*, 1534–1541. [CrossRef] [PubMed]
29. Vigilància de la Infecció Nosocomial als Hospitals de Catalunya (VINCat), Informe 2017. Available online: https://catsalut.gencat.cat/web/.content/minisite/vincat/documents/informes/informe-2017.pdf (accessed on 10 April 2021).

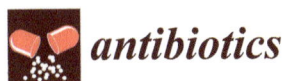

Article

Intra-Articular Injections Prior to Total Knee Arthroplasty Do Not Increase the Risk of Periprosthetic Joint Infection: A Prospective Cohort Study

Jérôme Grondin [1,2], Pierre Menu [1,2,3,4], Benoit Métayer [5], Vincent Crenn [6,7], Marc Dauty [1,2,3,4] and Alban Fouasson-Chailloux [1,2,3,4,*,†]

1. CHU Nantes, Service de Médecine Physique et de Réadaptation Locomotrice, University Hospital of Nantes, 44093 Nantes, France; jerome.grondin@chu-nantes.fr (J.G.); pierre.menu@chu-nantes.fr (P.M.); marc.dauty@chu-nantes.fr (M.D.)
2. CHU Nantes, Service de Médecine du Sport, University Hospital of Nantes, 44093 Nantes, France
3. INSERM UMR U1229/RMeS, Regenerative Medicine and Skeleton, Nantes University, 44000 Nantes, France
4. IRMS, Institut Régional de Médecine du Sport, Hôpital Saint Jacques, 44093 Nantes, France
5. CHU Nantes, Service de Rhumatologie, University Hospital of Nantes, 44093 Nantes, France; benoit.metayer@chu-nantes.fr
6. CHU de Nantes, Clinique Chirurgicale Orthopédique et Traumatologique, Hôtel-Dieu, 44093 Nantes, France; vincent.crenn@chu-nantes.fr
7. Physos, Inserm UMR 1238, Nantes University, 44000 Nantes, France
* Correspondence: alban.fouassonchailloux@chu-nantes.fr; Tel.: +33-240-846-211
† Current address: MPR Locomotrice et Respiratoire, CHU de Nantes, Hôpital St Jacques, 85 rue Saint Jacques, 44093 Nantes, France.

Citation: Grondin, J.; Menu, P.; Métayer, B.; Crenn, V.; Dauty, M.; Fouasson-Chailloux, A. Intra-Articular Injections Prior to Total Knee Arthroplasty Do Not Increase the Risk of Periprosthetic Joint Infection: A Prospective Cohort Study. *Antibiotics* **2021**, *10*, 330. https://doi.org/10.3390/antibiotics10030330

Academic Editor: Jaime Esteban

Received: 3 March 2021
Accepted: 19 March 2021
Published: 21 March 2021

Publisher's Note: MDPI stays neutral with regard to jurisdictional claims in published maps and institutional affiliations.

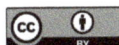

Copyright: © 2021 by the authors. Licensee MDPI, Basel, Switzerland. This article is an open access article distributed under the terms and conditions of the Creative Commons Attribution (CC BY) license (https://creativecommons.org/licenses/by/4.0/).

Abstract: Periprosthetic joint infections (PJI) occur in 0.5 to 2.8% of total knee arthroplasties (TKA) and expose them to an increase of morbidity and mortality. TKA are mainly performed after failure of non-surgical management of knee osteoarthritis, which frequently includes intra-articular injections of corticosteroids or hyaluronic acid. Concerning the potential impact of intra-articular injections on TKA infection, literature provides a low level of evidence because of the retrospective design of the studies and their contradictory results. In this prospective cohort study, we included patients after a total knee arthroplasty, at the time of their admission in a rehabilitation center, and we excluded patients with any prior knee surgery. 304 patients were included. Mean follow-up was 24.9 months, and incidence proportion of PJI was 2.6%. After multivariate logistic regression, male was the only significant risk factor of PJI (OR = 19.6; p = 0.006). The incidence of PJI did not differ between patients who received prior intra-articular injections and others, especially regarding injections in the last 6 months before surgery. The use of intra-articular injection remains a valid therapeutic option in the management of knee osteoarthritis, and a TKA could still be discussed.

Keywords: knee; total knee arthroplasty; infection; intra-articular injection

1. Introduction

Periprosthetic Joint Infection (PJI) constitutes one of the most feared complications after total knee arthroplasties (TKA) [1]. PJI increases mortality, with a 71.7% overall survival five years after PJI diagnosis [2] and exposes them to the complications of challenging surgical and medical treatments [3–5]. It also reduces physical function and impairs quality of life [6,7]. Its incidence ranges from 0.5 to 2.8% according to the studies [8–10]. TKA is a frequent surgical procedure, increasing in number every year [11]. There is a great concern about prevention of PJI, and different recommendations have been published [12,13]. Yet, despite these recommendations, the rate of PJI apparently does not decrease over time [2].

TKA improves primary outcomes of knee osteoarthritis (KOA) such as pain and function [14], and is mainly performed after failure of medical treatment. Intra-articular injection remains an usual treatment of non-surgical KOA in the absence of absolute contraindications such as infectious arthritis and drug hypersensitivity [15], but guidelines are contradictory regarding its efficiency and safety [16,17]. During the procedure of intra-articular injections, a contamination of the joint may happen and potentially induce a PJI if an arthroplasty is secondarily performed [1]. In 2017, the Centers for Disease Control and Prevention (CDC) broached the topic, but the issue was considered unresolved, and no recommendation was made [13]. In clinical practice, intra-articular infiltrations of corticosteroids (CS) or hyaluronic acid (HA) are frequently performed [18], and around 30% of the patients who underwent TKA had previously had an intra-articular steroid injection [19]. In this context, many studies have been performed, but have provided a low level of evidence because of their retrospective design and contradictory results [10,19–25] (Supplementary Materials Table S1). Among them, three studies based on large databases have highlighted an increased risk of PJI if prior intra-articular injections had been performed in the few months preceding the surgery [10,19,20], but they were exposed to common limitations with large database studies. A few meta-analyses were performed on PJI after TKA or Total Hip Arthroplasty (THA) [18,26–28], also with contradictory results, and emphasizing the low level of evidence of available studies and the need for prospective trials.

Thus, we aimed to prospectively assess the impact of prior intra-articular injections on the occurrence of periprosthetic joint infection after TKA.

2. Results

Between January 2016 and May 2019, 304 patients were included, and 279 (91.8%) eventually followed, while 25 patients (8.2%) were lost to follow-up (Figure 1). Mean follow-up was 24.9 months ± 3.8.

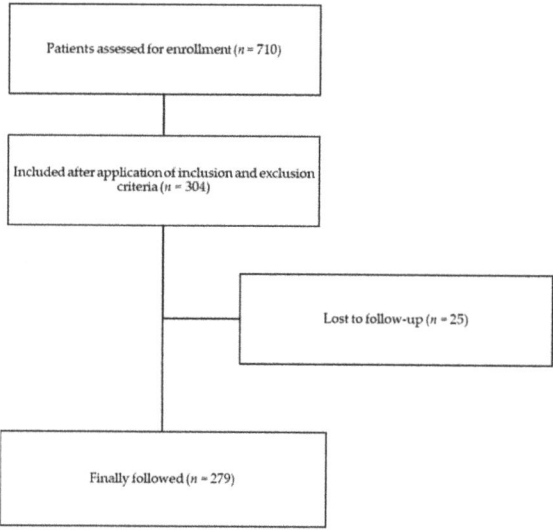

Figure 1. Flow-chart.

Most of the patients were females (72.4%; $n = 220$), and mean age was 71.8 years ± 8.9. Mean body mass index (BMI) was 30.9 kg/m^2 ± 5.3 and 85.5% ($n = 260$) of the patients were overweight (BMI > 25) or obese (BMI > 30) at the time of the surgery (35.8% overweight ($n = 109$), 49.7% obese ($n = 151$)) (Table 1). Mean American Society of Anesthesiologists (ASA) score was 2.3 ± 0.6. Two patients were deceased 5 and 7 months after the arthroplasty (1 heart failure due to myocardial ischemia, and 1 cerebral stroke). 68.1% ($n = 207$) of the patients received infiltration before surgery, 48.8% (*n* = 101) of them with hyaluronic acid alone, 15.5% (*n* = 32) with corticosteroids, and 24.6% (*n* = 51) received both.

Table 1. Demographic characteristics.

Characteristics	Patients (*n* = 304)
Mean age, years ± SD [min–max]	71.8 ± 8.9 [31–91]
Sex: -Female, *n* (%) -Male, *n* (%)	 220 (72.4) 84 (27.6)
Mean weight, kg ± SD [min–max]	82.0 ± 16.3 [46–149]
Mean height, cm ± SD [min–max]	162.9 ± 9.3 [136–190]
Mean BMI, kg/m^2 ± SD [min–max]	30.9 ± 5.3 [19.4–47.6]
Diabetes mellitus: -Type 1, *n* (%) -Type 2, *n* (%) -None, *n* (%)	 7 (2.3) 43 (14.1) 254 (83.6)
Smoking: -Active, *n* (%) -Cessation, *n* (%) -None, *n* (%)	 14 (4.6) 49 (16.1) 241 (79.3)
Alcoholism: -Active, *n* (%) -Cessation, *n* (%) -None, *n* (%)	 23 (7.5) 5 (1.7) 276 (90.8)
Mean ASA Score, mean ± SD [min–max]	2.3 ± 0.6 [1–4]
Prior IA injection, *n* (%): -CS -HA -CS+HA -Unknown	207 (68.1) 32 (15.5) 101 (48.8) 51 (24.6) 23 (11.1)
No prior IA injection, *n* (%)	97 (31.9)

SD: Standard-deviation; BMI: Body mass index; ASA: American society of anesthesiologists; IA: Intra-articular; CS: Corticosteroids; HA: Hyaluronic acid.

Table 2 summarizes the cases of PJI, mainly males (6 out of 8). Most of the infections (7/8) occurred in the first 6 weeks following arthroplasty and were caused by Staphylococcus aureus (6/8) or Staphylococcus capitis (1/8). The remaining case concerns a patient who initially received a surgery consisting of irrigation and debridement in a context of infectious endocarditis due to a persistent PJI, and a one-stage exchange was secondly performed. One patient died from myocardial ischemia 5 months after diagnosis of PJI. Other surgical and medical strategies performed were all considered successful, and no additional surgery was necessary.

Table 2. Cases of periprosthetic joint infections.

Patients	Age Years	Sex F/M	BMI	Diabetes	Smoking	Alcoholism	ASA	DTS	Infiltrations Medication	n	Delay Surgery-PJI	Surgery	Bacteria	Antibiotic Therapy Type	Duration
1	73	M	32.3	No	No	Yes	1	14 m	CS	1	11 d	Debridement, implant retention, replacement of exchangeable components	Methi-S Staph. aureus	Levofloxacin + Rifampicin	12 w
2	64	F	33.3	Type 2	No	No	3	-	-	0	4 w	One-Stage Arthroplasty Exchange	Methi-S Staph. aureus	Levofloxacin + Rifampicin	12 w
3	88	M	20.4	No	Former smoker	No	2	1 m	HA	9	5 w	One-Stage Arthroplasty Exchange	Methi-S Staph. aureus	Levofloxacin + Rifampicin	12 w
4	78	F	37.5	No	No	No	3	-	-	0	5 w	Debridement, implant retention, replacement of exchangeable components	Methi-S Staph. aureus	Levofloxacin + Clindamycin	12 w
5	85	M	28.7	No	No	No	3	4 m	CS	3	4 w	Debridement, implant retention, replacement of exchangeable components	Methi-S Staph. aureus	Levofloxacin + Rifampicin	12 w
6	53	M	26.9	No	No	No	2	12 m	HA	unknown	12 d	Debridement, implant retention, replacement of exchangeable components	Staph. capitis	Levofloxacin + Rifampicin	8 w
7	77	M	24.4	No	Former smoker	No	3	10 m	CS + HA	7	5 m	Initially irrigation and debridement, then 4 months later 1-Stage Arthroplasty Exchange	Strep. oralis	Moxifloxacin + Amoxicillin after lavage; Moxifloxacin + Clindamycin after 1-stage exchange	12 w
8	74	M	29.4	No	Current smoker	No	3	4 m	CS + HA	7	14 d	Debridement, implant retention, replacement of exchangeable components	Methi-R Staph. aureus	Cotrimoxazole + fusidic acid, then Clindamycin + fusidic acid (renal insufficiency)	12 w

F: Female; M: Male; BMI: Body mass index; ASA: American society of anesthesiologists; DTS: Delay to surgery; m: Months; d: Days; w: Weeks; CS: Corticosteroids; HA: Hyaluronic acid; PJI: Periprosthetic Joint Infections; Methi-S: Methicillin sensitive; Methi-R: Methicillin resistant, Staph.: Staphylococcus; Strep.: Streptococcus.

The overall incidence of infection was 2.6% (8/304). Comparisons of incidence of PJI were completed with Fisher's exact test depending on the "injection" status. Incidence was 2.1% (2/97) in patients without prior injection, and 2.9% (6/207) if any prior intra-articular injection had been performed, OR = 1.42 (CI 95% = 0.28–7.16; p = 0.67). It increased to 7.1% (3/42) if injection had been performed within 6 months before surgery, OR = 3.95, but without statistical significance (CI 95% 0.91–17.21; p = 0.08).

In univariate regression, the "sex" variable was the only one to be significantly associated with PJI, with an increased risk of infection in males. A trend was found concerning "injection < 6 months" with an OR of 3.46 (p = 0.09) (Table 3). Based on these findings, we have investigated potential differences between males and females that could explain the increased risk of PJI in males (Table 4). Therefore, we have highlighted significant differences between the two groups: Smoking, diabetes, alcoholism, and ASA score were significantly higher in males than in females.

Table 3. Univariate logistic regression according to patients' characteristics.

Independent Variables	Odds-Ratio	CI 95%	p
Age	1.03	0.94–1.12	0.48
Sex	0.05	0.006–0.41	0.005
BMI	0.93	0.8–1.08	0.35
Smoking	2.36	0.54–10.1	0.24
Diabetes mellitus	0.72	0.08–5.98	0.76
Alcoholism	1.77	0.2–15.1	0.59
ASA	2.12	0.6–7.43	0.23
Injection < 6 months	3.46	0.79–15	0.09

CI: Confidence interval; BMI: Body mass index; ASA: American society of anesthesiologists.

Table 4. Comparison between males and females.

Characteristics	Males n = 84	Females n = 220	p
Mean age, years ± SD	70.5 ± 8.8	72.3 ± 8.9	0.12 [a]
Mean BMI, kg/m^2 ± SD	30.6 ± 5.2	30.9 ± 5.4	0.71 [a]
Smoking (Active or cessation), n	35	28	0.001 [b]
Diabetes mellitus, n	21	29	0.01 [b]
Active alcoholism, n	19	4	0.0001 [b]
ASA ≥ 3, n	37	60	0.01 [b]
Injection < 6 months, n	12	30	0.88 [b]

[a] t-test; [b] χ^2-test. SD: Standard-deviation; BMI: Body mass index; ASA: American society of anesthesiologists.

Multivariate logistic regressions were performed considering differences between males and females. In the total population, only sex was significantly associated with occurrence of infection (OR = 19.6; CI95%: 2.4–164; p = 0.006). Knowing existing differences between males and females in our population, we performed multivariate logistic regressions analyzing these 2 groups separately: No factor was significantly associated with PJI occurrence.

3. Discussion

In this study, the risk of PJI did not significantly increase between patients who had previously received knee infiltration and patients who had not [OR = 1.42 (CI 95% = 0.28–7.16; p = 0.67)]. Many studies have been performed concerning the safety of intra-articular infiltrations in the pre-operative period, with a retrospective design and conflicting results [10,19–25]. Four of these studies did not bring out significant associations. However, 3 studies based on large retrospective databases suggested an increased risk of PJI in patients who had received an infiltration in the 3 months preceding surgery [10,19] or even in the preceding 7 months [20]. These findings explain why we compared the occurrence of infection between patients who had received an infiltration in the 6 months preceding surgery to the others. There was no significant difference, but a trend toward an increased risk in patients who had received an infiltration in the 6 months preceding surgery (OR = 3.95; CI 95% 0.91–17.21; p = 0.08). As discussed below, this trend requires further investigation with larger cohorts in prospective studies. Thus, special attention should be paid to the benefit/risk assessment of a knee infiltration if a surgery is to be scheduled in the next months.

In previous retrospective studies based on large prospective databases, confounding factors such as male sex, BMI, tobacco smoking, prior surgery, and inflammatory arthritis may have been involved in the significant association reported between PJI and prior intra-articular injections [10,19,20]. As recommended in previous systematic reviews [28], we clearly excluded patients with major risk factors of infection: Any prior surgery or septic arthritis of the knee, history of rheumatoid arthritis or hemophilia, and immunosuppressive or immunomodulatory drugs. We also adjusted the results on potential confounding factors previously reported: Male sex, age < 60 years, BMI > 25 kg/m^2, diabetes, previous or current tobacco smoking, ASA $\geq$ 3 [29–32]. In our cohort, male sex was the unique risk factor associated with infection. Smoking, diabetes, alcoholism, and ASA score were significantly higher for males than females. In multivariate logistic regression, excluding male sex, no factor was significantly associated with PJI. Further analysis focusing on male population did not bring out significant results, especially regarding prior intra-articular injection in the 6 months preceding surgery.

Thus, despite conflicting evidence regarding the potential association between PJI and pre-operative joint injection, some pathophysiological hypotheses were suggested: An infectious risk due to the prolonged immunosuppressive effect of glucocorticoids injected [10,24,33], or direct inoculation from the infiltration procedure due to insufficient sterile precautions [10,24]. To investigate these hypotheses, we planned a 24 month-follow-up. Indeed, the first 2 years are the greatest risk period and represent 60 to 70% of PJI [11,34], and studies with shorter follow-ups have reported lower incidence of infection [8]. Furthermore, early (<3 months) and delayed infections (between 3 and 24 months after surgery) are often exogenous, early infections caused by more virulent organisms than delayed ones; whereas late-onset infections (>24 months) are frequently due to hematogenous infection [1,11], except in cases of very indolent infections due to very low-virulent bacteria [11]. These pathophysiological hypotheses are unlikely to explain late-onset hematogenous infections, which is why we did not follow patients for more than 2 years. In our cohort, every infection occurred within 6 months after surgery, most of them within 6 weeks, consistent with the hypotheses of exogenous pathogenesis.

We selected a telephone follow-up, for it produces higher response rates than postal survey or mail/internet surveys [35–37]. However, the telephone mode brings more positive responses to subjective items than other modes [37], but this bias does not apply in our case, since the interview was closed-ended to detect the occurrence of PJI. A memorization bias may be suggested in principle, but patients would unlikely forget a Periprosthetic Joint Infection with its devastating consequences, revision surgeries, and extended antibiotic therapy.

This study has limitations. Indeed, our cohort was formed with patients admitted in a Physical and Rehabilitation Medicine Hospital, which are usually different from those discharged home directly after surgery: They are usually older, with a higher BMI, and are more frequently females [38]. In our cohort as well, patients were mostly females (72.4%) with a mean BMI of 30.9. Periprosthetic joint infections are usually estimated between 1 and 2% after TKA [30], but may range over 2% [9,10]. In this study, the incidence proportion was 2.6%, which seems consistent with literature knowing that we included more fragile patients. The main limitation was the size of the cohort (around 300 patients), which may have reduced its ability to detect a statistically significant association between intra-articular infiltrations and PJI. However, at the beginning of the study, we calculated that 276 patients were required to detect a doubling of the incidence of infection. Therefore, we included 304 patients and eventually followed 279 of them, but our initial projection may be challenged. The number of patients needed to improve the power and allowing recommendations depends on the incidence of PJI in the population, on the difference in incidence proportion that we aimed to detect, and on the pre-specified power (usually 80%). Further prospective studies should be performed in larger cohorts to clearly establish the safety of intra-articular injections before total knee arthroplasty, in order to improve sensitivity and power. Yet, a single institution is unlikely to sustain such a study. A multicentric study proves to be necessary [28], but exposes us to specific bias of multicentric designs, such as unrecognized heterogeneity across centers [39].

Another limitation is the diagnosis and classification of PJI which are challenging and not consensual [40]. In this study, we used the definition of the International Consensus Meeting on Periprosthetic Joint Infection, and every case fulfilled at least one of the two major criteria of PJI [41,42]. Different classifications exist, mainly based on timing of clinical presentation leading to different surgical strategies [40,43], and therefore decreasing comparability between studies.

Finally, the telephone follow-up might have failed to detect some PJI signs, especially in case of indolent infections due to low-virulent bacteria, which usually provide few clinical manifestations. Indeed, clinical, radiological, and biological parameters may have been more sensitive.

4. Materials and Methods

4.1. Participants

Patients were included in the few days following the arthroplasty (2 to 7 days), at the time of their admission in the rehabilitation center. Surgery was performed in the University Hospital of Nantes or in other clinics of Nantes' region, France. Inclusion criteria were: Age > 18 years old, patients hospitalized for rehabilitation after TKA. Exclusion criteria were: Any prior ipsilateral knee surgery, any prior infectious arthritis of the knee, history of rheumatoid arthritis or hemophilia, and immunosuppressive or immunomodulatory drugs.

At the time of the inclusion, we systematically collected the following data: Age, sex, weight, height, BMI, diabetes, tobacco smoking, alcoholism, ASA Score, other significant medical and surgical antecedents, date and place of surgery, prior intra-articular infiltration of the knee: Number, date, and type of medication injected.

4.2. Outcome

The primary outcome was the incidence of PJI. Every case of infection was reviewed and defined as a PJI if it fulfilled the definition provided by the International Consensus Meeting on Periprosthetic Joint Infection (at least one of the two major criteria: Two positive growths of the same organism using standard culture methods, or sinus tract with evidence of communication to the joint or visualization of the prosthesis) [41,42]. First, we compared incidences of infection between patients who had received prior intra-articular injections and others, and then we focused on patients who had had an intra-articular injection in the 6 months preceding surgery.

4.3. Follow-Up

Follow-up was performed at 24 months after surgery. A phone call was performed, and occurrences of an infection or an additional surgery were checked based on following questions: "Do you feel any persistent knee pain, erythema and oedema?", "Have you noticed any wound drainage?", "Has a diagnosis of prosthetic infection or any infection of your knee been established? "Have you got any additional surgery?". If any of these occurred, medical, surgical, and bacteriological reports were gathered. If a patient was not able to answer these questions, his general practitioner was called.

4.4. Statistical Analyses

Statistical analyses were performed using software SPSS 23.0 IBM Corp, Armonk, NY, USA. Comparisons of incidence proportions of PJI were performed with a Fisher's exact test. Logistic regressions were performed with PJI as dichotomous dependent variable, and independent variables were sex, age, BMI, ASA, diabetes, smoking, alcoholism, prior infiltration (Yes/No), infiltration < 6 months (Yes/No). First, we analyzed the association between dependent and independent variables in univariate regression, and then we performed a multivariate logistic regression with forward selection (Wald). We compared demographic characteristics between males and females using t-test. $p < 0.05$ was considered significant. To evaluate the number of subjects required, we defined a power of 80%, an alpha risk of 5%, a theoretical incidence of PJI of 2.8% [10], and aimed to detect a doubling of the incidence. We calculated that 276 patients were required.

4.5. Ethics

This research was conducted in our institution from January 2016 to June 2019. Due to the non-interventional nature of the study, no ethics committee was necessary at the time of the beginning of the study. Yet, necessary processes were performed with the "Direction de la Recherche Clinique" (DRC) of the University Hospital of Nantes, France, and the "Commission Nationale de l'Informatique et des Libertés" (CNIL); the study was registered under the number RC16_0039. The database was anonymized, and all the patients provided their verbal consent and got an information document.

5. Conclusions

This study showed no evidence of the causality of prior intra-articular injections in Periprosthetic Joint Infection occurrence, even in the 6 months preceding surgery. In clinical practice, wise use of intra-articular injection remains a valid therapeutic option in the management of knee osteoarthritis, and a total knee replacement could still be discussed.

Supplementary Materials: The following are available online at https://www.mdpi.com/2079-6382/10/3/330/s1, Table S1: Literature review of the impact of intraarticular injection before surgery on the occurrence of infection.

Author Contributions: Conceptualization, A.F.-C., M.D.; methodology, J.G., A.F.-C. and M.D.; Formal analysis, J.G., A.F.-C. and M.D.; data curation, J.G., A.F.-C., P.M., B.M., V.C. and M.D.; investigation, J.G., A.F.-C., P.M., B.M., V.C. and M.D.; writing—original draft preparation, J.G., A.F.-C. and M.D.; writing—review and editing, J.G., A.F.-C., P.M., B.M., V.C. and M.D. All authors have read and agreed to the published version of the manuscript.

Funding: This research received no external funding.

Institutional Review Board Statement: The study was conducted according to the guidelines of the Declaration of Helsinki, and due to the non-interventional nature of the study, no ethics committee was necessary at the time of the beginning of the study. The study was declared to the "Direction de la Recherche Clinique" (DRC) of the University Hospital of Nantes, France, and was registered under the number RC16_0039. Necessary processes were performed with the "Commission Nationale de l'Informatique et des Libertés" (CNIL).

Informed Consent Statement: All the patients gave their oral consent and got an information document. All data were anonymized.

Data Availability Statement: The datasets generated and/or analyzed during the current study are available from the corresponding author on reasonable request.

Acknowledgments: We would like to thank Annie Chailloux for proofreading the manuscript.

Conflicts of Interest: The authors declare no conflict of interest.

References

1. Parvizi, J.; Shohat, N.; Gehrke, T. Prevention of Periprosthetic Joint Infection: New Guidelines. *Bone Jt. J.* **2017**, *99-B*, 3–10. [CrossRef]
2. Kurtz, S.M.; Lau, E.C.; Son, M.-S.; Chang, E.T.; Zimmerli, W.; Parvizi, J. Are We Winning or Losing the Battle With Periprosthetic Joint Infection: Trends in Periprosthetic Joint Infection and Mortality Risk for the Medicare Population. *J. Arthroplast.* **2018**, *33*, 3238–3245. [CrossRef] [PubMed]
3. Hartzler, M.A.; Li, K.; Geary, M.B.; Odum, S.M.; Springer, B.D. Complications in the Treatment of Prosthetic Joint Infection. *Bone Jt. J* **2020**, *102-B*, 145–150. [CrossRef] [PubMed]
4. Perez, S.; Dauchy, F.-A.; Salvo, F.; Quéroué, M.; Durox, H.; Delobel, P.; Chambault, R.; Ade, M.; Cazanave, C.; Desclaux, A.; et al. Severe Adverse Events during Medical and Surgical Treatment of Hip and Knee Prosthetic Joint Infections. *Med. Mal. Infect.* **2020**. [CrossRef] [PubMed]
5. Lemaignen, A.; Bernard, L.; Marmor, S.; Ferry, T.; Grammatico-Guillon, L.; Astagneau, P. Epidemiology of Complex Bone and Joint Infections in France Using a National Registry: The CRIOAc Network. *J. Infect.* **2021**, *82*, 199–206. [CrossRef] [PubMed]
6. Cahill, J.; Shadbolt, B.; Scarvell, J.; Smith, P. Quality of Life after Infection in Total Joint Replacement. *J. Orthop. Surg.* **2008**, *16*, 58–65. [CrossRef] [PubMed]
7. Mur, I.; Jordán, M.; Rivera, A.; Pomar, V.; González, J.C.; López-Contreras, J.; Crusi, X.; Navarro, F.; Gurguí, M.; Benito, N. Do Prosthetic Joint Infections Worsen the Functional Ambulatory Outcome of Patients with Joint Replacements? A Retrospective Matched Cohort Study. *Antibiotics* **2020**, *9*, 872. [CrossRef]
8. Healthcare-Associated Infections: Surgical Site Infections—Annual Epidemiological Report for 2017. Available online: https://www.ecdc.europa.eu/en/publications-data/healthcare-associated-infections-surgical-site-infections-annual-1 (accessed on 29 January 2021).
9. Kurtz, S.M.; Lau, E.; Watson, H.; Schmier, J.K.; Parvizi, J. Economic Burden of Periprosthetic Joint Infection in the United States. *J. Arthroplast.* **2012**, *27*, 61–65.e1. [CrossRef]
10. Richardson, S.S.; Schairer, W.W.; Sculco, T.P.; Sculco, P.K. Comparison of Infection Risk with Corticosteroid or Hyaluronic Acid Injection Prior to Total Knee Arthroplasty. *J. Bone Jt. Surg. Am.* **2019**, *101*, 112–118. [CrossRef]
11. Tande, A.J.; Patel, R. Prosthetic Joint Infection. *Clin. Microbiol. Rev.* **2014**, *27*, 302. [CrossRef] [PubMed]
12. WHO. Global Guidelines on the Prevention of Surgical Site Infection. Available online: http://www.who.int/gpsc/ssi-prevention-guidelines/en/ (accessed on 31 January 2021).
13. Berríos-Torres, S.I.; Umscheid, C.A.; Bratzler, D.W.; Leas, B.; Stone, E.C.; Kelz, R.R.; Reinke, C.E.; Morgan, S.; Solomkin, J.S.; Mazuski, J.E.; et al. Centers for Disease Control and Prevention Guideline for the Prevention of Surgical Site Infection, 2017. *JAMA Surg.* **2017**, *152*, 784. [CrossRef]
14. Charlesworth, J.; Fitzpatrick, J.; Perera, N.K.P.; Orchard, J. Osteoarthritis-a Systematic Review of Long-Term Safety Implications for Osteoarthritis of the Knee. *BMC Musculoskelet. Disord.* **2019**, *20*. [CrossRef]
15. Caldwell, J.R. Intra-Articular Corticosteroids. Guide to Selection and Indications for Use. *Drugs* **1996**, *52*, 507–514. [CrossRef]
16. Bannuru, R.R.; Osani, M.C.; Vaysbrot, E.E.; Arden, N.K.; Bennell, K.; Bierma-Zeinstra, S.M.A.; Kraus, V.B.; Lohmander, L.S.; Abbott, J.H.; Bhandari, M.; et al. OARSI Guidelines for the Non-Surgical Management of Knee, Hip, and Polyarticular Osteoarthritis. *Osteoarthr. Cartil.* **2019**, *27*, 1578–1589. [CrossRef]
17. Kolasinski, S.L.; Neogi, T.; Hochberg, M.C.; Oatis, C.; Guyatt, G.; Block, J.; Callahan, L.; Copenhaver, C.; Dodge, C.; Felson, D.; et al. 2019 American College of Rheumatology/Arthritis Foundation Guideline for the Management of Osteoarthritis of the Hand, Hip, and Knee. *Arthritis Care Res.* **2020**, *72*, 149–162. [CrossRef] [PubMed]
18. Marsland, D.; Mumith, A.; Barlow, I.W. Systematic Review: The Safety of Intra-Articular Corticosteroid Injection Prior to Total Knee Arthroplasty. *Knee* **2014**, *21*, 6–11. [CrossRef] [PubMed]
19. Cancienne, J.M.; Werner, B.C.; Luetkemeyer, L.M.; Browne, J.A. Does Timing of Previous Intra-Articular Steroid Injection Affect the Post-Operative Rate of Infection in Total Knee Arthroplasty? *J. Arthroplast.* **2015**, *30*, 1879–1882. [CrossRef]
20. Bedard, N.A.; Pugely, A.J.; Elkins, J.M.; Duchman, K.R.; Westermann, R.W.; Liu, S.S.; Gao, Y.; Callaghan, J.J. The John N. Insall Award: Do Intraarticular Injections Increase the Risk of Infection After TKA? *Clin. Orthop. Relat. Res.* **2017**, *475*, 45–52. [CrossRef] [PubMed]
21. Joshy, S.; Thomas, B.; Gogi, N.; Modi, A.; Singh, B.K. Effect of Intra-Articular Steroids on Deep Infections Following Total Knee Arthroplasty. *Int. Orthop.* **2006**, *30*, 91–93. [CrossRef] [PubMed]
22. Desai, A.; Ramankutty, S.; Board, T.; Raut, V. Does Intraarticular Steroid Infiltration Increase the Rate of Infection in Subsequent Total Knee Replacements? *Knee* **2009**, *16*, 262–264. [CrossRef] [PubMed]
23. Horne, G.; Devane, P.; Davidson, A.; Adams, K.; Purdie, G. The Influence of Steroid Injections on the Incidence of Infection Following Total Knee Arthroplasty. *N. Z. Med. J.* **2008**, *121*, U2896. [PubMed]
24. Papavasiliou, A.V.; Isaac, D.L.; Marimuthu, R.; Skyrme, A.; Armitage, A. Infection in Knee Replacements after Previous Injection of Intra-Articular Steroid. *J. Bone Jt. Surg. Br.* **2006**, *88*, 321–323. [CrossRef]
25. Amin, N.H.; Omiyi, D.; Kuczynski, B.; Cushner, F.D.; Scuderi, G.R. The Risk of a Deep Infection Associated With Intraarticular Injections Before a Total Knee Arthroplasty. *J. Arthroplast.* **2016**, *31*, 240–244. [CrossRef] [PubMed]
26. Wang, Q.; Jiang, X.; Tian, W. Does Previous Intra-Articular Steroid Injection Increase the Risk of Joint Infection Following Total Hip Arthroplasty or Total Knee Arthroplasty? A Meta-Analysis. *Med. Sci. Monit.* **2014**, *20*, 1878–1883. [CrossRef]

27. Xing, D.; Yang, Y.; Ma, X.; Ma, J.; Ma, B.; Chen, Y. Dose Intraarticular Steroid Injection Increase the Rate of Infection in Subsequent Arthroplasty: Grading the Evidence through a Meta-Analysis. *J. Orthop. Surg. Res.* **2014**, *9*. [CrossRef]
28. Pereira, L.C.; Kerr, J.; Jolles, B.M. Intra-Articular Steroid Injection for Osteoarthritis of the Hip Prior to Total Hip Arthroplasty: Is It Safe? A Systematic Review. *Bone Jt. J.* **2016**, *98-B*, 1027–1035. [CrossRef] [PubMed]
29. Lenguerrand, E.; Whitehouse, M.R.; Beswick, A.D.; Kunutsor, S.K.; Foguet, P.; Porter, M.; Blom, A.W. Risk Factors Associated with Revision for Prosthetic Joint Infection Following Knee Replacement: An Observational Cohort Study from England and Wales. *Lancet Infect. Dis.* **2019**, *19*, 589–600. [CrossRef]
30. Kapadia, B.H.; Berg, R.A.; Daley, J.A.; Fritz, J.; Bhave, A.; Mont, M.A. Periprosthetic Joint Infection. *Lancet* **2016**, *387*, 386–394. [CrossRef]
31. Sadr Azodi, O.; Bellocco, R.; Eriksson, K.; Adami, J. The Impact of Tobacco Use and Body Mass Index on the Length of Stay in Hospital and the Risk of Post-Operative Complications among Patients Undergoing Total Hip Replacement. *J. Bone Jt. Surg. Br.* **2006**, *88*, 1316–1320. [CrossRef]
32. Cizmic, Z.; Feng, J.E.; Huang, R.; Iorio, R.; Komnos, G.; Kunutsor, S.K.; Metwaly, R.G.; Saleh, U.H.; Sheth, N.; Sloan, M. Hip and Knee Section, Prevention, Host Related: Proceedings of International Consensus on Orthopedic Infections. *J. Arthroplast.* **2019**, *34*, S255–S270. [CrossRef]
33. Kaspar, S.; de V de Beer, J. Infection in Hip Arthroplasty after Previous Injection of Steroid. *J. Bone Jt. Surg. Br.* **2005**, *87*, 454–457. [CrossRef] [PubMed]
34. Kurtz, S.M.; Ong, K.L.; Lau, E.; Bozic, K.J.; Berry, D.; Parvizi, J. Prosthetic Joint Infection Risk after TKA in the Medicare Population. *Clin. Orthop. Relat. Res.* **2010**, *468*, 52–56. [CrossRef] [PubMed]
35. Hox, J.J.; De Leeuw, E.D. A Comparison of Nonresponse in Mail, Telephone, and Face-to-Face Surveys. *Qual. Quant.* **1994**, *28*, 329–344. [CrossRef]
36. Sinclair, M.; O'Toole, J.; Malawaraarachchi, M.; Leder, K. Comparison of Response Rates and Cost-Effectiveness for a Community-Based Survey: Postal, Internet and Telephone Modes with Generic or Personalised Recruitment Approaches. *BMC Med. Res. Methodol.* **2012**, *12*, 132. [CrossRef]
37. Feveile, H.; Olsen, O.; Hogh, A. A Randomized Trial of Mailed Questionnaires versus Telephone Interviews: Response Patterns in a Survey. *BMC Med. Res. Methodol.* **2007**, *7*, 27. [CrossRef] [PubMed]
38. Gwam, C.U.; Mohamed, N.S.; Dávila Castrodad, I.M.; George, N.E.; Remily, E.A.; Wilkie, W.A.; Barg, V.; Gbadamosi, W.A.; Delanois, R.E. Factors Associated with Non-Home Discharge after Total Knee Arthroplasty: Potential for Cost Savings? *Knee* **2020**, *27*, 1176–1181. [CrossRef]
39. Localio, A.R.; Berlin, J.A.; Ten Have, T.R.; Kimmel, S.E. Adjustments for Center in Multicenter Studies: An Overview. *Ann. Intern. Med.* **2001**, *135*, 112–123. [CrossRef] [PubMed]
40. Pellegrini, A.; Legnani, C.; Meani, E. A New Perspective on Current Prosthetic Joint Infection Classifications: Introducing Topography as a Key Factor Affecting Treatment Strategy. *Arch. Orthop. Trauma Surg.* **2019**, *139*, 317–322. [CrossRef] [PubMed]
41. Parvizi, J.; Gehrke, T.; Chen, A.F. Proceedings of the International Consensus on Periprosthetic Joint Infection. *Bone Jt. J.* **2013**, *95-B*, 1450–1452. [CrossRef] [PubMed]
42. Shohat, N.; Bauer, T.; Buttaro, M.; Budhiparama, N.; Cashman, J.; Della Valle, C.J.; Drago, L.; Gehrke, T.; Marcelino Gomes, L.S.; Goswami, K.; et al. Hip and Knee Section, What Is the Definition of a Periprosthetic Joint Infection (PJI) of the Knee and the Hip? Can the Same Criteria Be Used for Both Joints?: Proceedings of International Consensus on Orthopedic Infections. *J. Arthroplast.* **2019**, *34*, S325–S327. [CrossRef]
43. Zimmerli, W.; Trampuz, A.; Ochsner, P.E. Prosthetic-Joint Infections. *N. Engl. J. Med.* **2004**, *351*, 1645–1654. [CrossRef] [PubMed]

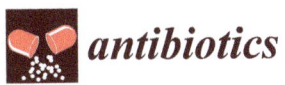

Perspective

Controversy about the Role of Rifampin in Biofilm Infections: Is It Justified?

Nora Renz [1,2], Andrej Trampuz [1,*] and Werner Zimmerli [3]

1. Center for Musculoskeletal Surgery, Charité-Universitätsmedizin, Corporate Member of Freie Universität Berlin, Humboldt-Universität zu Berlin, and Berlin Institute of Health, 10117 Berlin, Germany; nora.renz@charite.de
2. Department of Infectious Diseases, Bern University Hospital, University of Bern, 3010 Bern, Switzerland
3. Interdisciplinary Unit of Orthopaedic Infections, Kantonsspital Baselland, 4410 Liestal, Switzerland; werner.zimmerli@unibas.ch
* Correspondence: andrej.trampuz@charite.de

Abstract: Rifampin is a potent antibiotic against staphylococcal implant-associated infections. In the absence of implants, current data suggest against the use of rifampin combinations. In the past decades, abundant preclinical and clinical evidence has accumulated supporting its role in biofilm-related infections. In the present article, experimental data from animal models of foreign-body infections and clinical trials are reviewed. The risk for emergence of rifampin resistance and multiple drug interactions are emphasized. A recent randomized controlled trial (RCT) showing no beneficial effect of rifampin in patients with acute staphylococcal periprosthetic joint infection treated with prosthesis retention is critically reviewed and data interpreted. Given the existing strong evidence demonstrating the benefit of rifampin, the conduction of an adequately powered RCT with appropriate definitions and interventions would probably not comply with ethical standards.

Keywords: rifampin; biofilm; prosthetic joint infection

1. Introduction

Rifampin is one of the first-line drugs against tuberculosis. In addition, it has been used against non-mycobacterial microorganisms, mainly staphylococci, for at least 50 years [1]. However, its place in severe staphylococcal infections not involving an implanted device remained unclear for decades because no systematic comparative studies had been performed. In the meantime, few studies have been published on this topic. In five randomized controlled trials and two retrospective cohort studies in patients with *Staphylococcus aureus* bacteremia, no difference of mortality could be shown [2]. A recent multicenter, randomized, double-blind placebo-controlled trial confirmed these data in 758 patients [3]. In the study of Rieg et al. [4], only the subgroup of patients with implants had less late complications related to *S. aureus* bacteremia when treated with combination therapy (4.5% vs. 10.6%, $p = 0.03$). Most of them were treated with a rifampin combination regimen, suggesting a benefit of antibiofilm activity compared to treatment without rifampin. In contrast, the addition of rifampin to standard therapy showed no advantage in patients with native valve infective endocarditis caused by *S. aureus* [5]. Thus, the latest data advocate against the uncritical use of rifampin combination therapy in patients with severe staphylococcal infections in absence of implants.

In contrast, the benefit of rifampin in patients with staphylococcal implant-associated infection is well documented based on abundant in-vitro, animal, and clinical data, as summarized in a recent review [6]. Until recently, only one randomized controlled trial (RCT) existed, in which the added value of rifampin was shown in patients with orthopedic implant-associated staphylococcal infections [7]. In 2020, a second RCT in patients with periprosthetic joint infection (PJI) was published, using different combination therapy regimens, which did not show a better outcome with addition of rifampin to standard treatment [8]. These unexpected data may unsettle clinicians with limited experience in the field of implant-associated infections. Therefore, possible reasons for the failure of demonstrating the benefit of adding rifampin in this trial will be discussed herein in the light of available evidence, including animal data and clinical trials.

2. Short History of Rifampin Use in Patients with Implant-Associated Staphylococcal Infection

In 1982, the use of rifampin in the treatment of non-tuberculous infections has been initially presented in a large symposium, followed by the publication in a supplemental edition of the Reviews of Infectious Diseases, edited by Merle A. Sande [9]. The special interest in rifampin was based on its unique mode of action, i.e., its inactivation of the bacterial DNA-dependent RNA polymerase. Its main drawback is the single-step mutation of the rifampin-binding enzyme occurring with a frequency of 10^{-6} to 10^{-7} [10]. This high risk of emergence of resistance explains its occasional failure in infections characterized by a high bacterial load, such as in infective endocarditis or persistent *S. aureus* bacteremia [5,11,12]. Studies of rifampin in non-mycobacterial infection were retarded by the fear that its widespread use could result in resistance to rifampin in *Mycobacterium tuberculosis*.

One of the first observations of the successful use of rifampin combination therapy in implant-associated infections is the report of two patients with *S. epidermidis* infection, one with prosthetic valve endocarditis and the other with ventriculoperitoneal shunt-associated infection [13]. In a case series, Karchmer et al. [14] reported a good outcome with a vancomycin-rifampin, but not betalactam–rifampin combination (87% vs. 43%, $p = 0.025$) for treatment of prosthetic valve endocarditis caused by methicillin-resistant *S. epidermidis*. These data suggest that the combination partner of rifampin matters.

Based on our observation that rifampin could not only prevent, but also cure experimental staphylococcal implant-associated infections [15], we performed additional animal experiments with rifampin combination therapy [16], followed by observational studies and one randomized controlled trial in patients with orthopedic implant-associated infections [7,17–19]. Later, rifampin combination therapy has shown to improve the outcome in patients with other types of implant-associated infections such as staphylococcal prosthetic valve endocarditis [14,20], deep sternal wound infections [21] and vascular graft associated infections [22,23]. However, data from randomized controlled trials are still not available in patients with non-orthopedic implant-associated infections.

3. Evidence for the Efficacy of Rifampin in Animal Studies

The first observation of the biofilm activity of rifampin has been made >35 years ago in the guinea pig tissue cage model [15]. With four doses of rifampin, implant-associated *S. aureus* infection could be cured in 100% of the tissue cages, if therapy was started up to 12 h after inoculation. If the delay was prolonged to 24 h, the cure rate decreased to 57%. These results unequivocally demonstrate that rifampin is able to eliminate surface-adhering biofilm staphylococci. However, it also shows that the efficacy of a short-term therapy is limited to a young biofilm. A clear definition of the limit between young and mature (tolerant) biofilm is still lacking. It depends on the microorganism, the antibiotic, and the duration of therapy [24]. Table 1 summarizes several experimental studies with the subcutaneous tissue cage animal model in guinea pigs. In each experimental series, rifampin combinations were significantly more active than other antibiotics [16,25–30]. This animal model does not simulate orthopedic device-related infection. However, it allows following an ongoing infection with the most relevant endpoint, namely complete elimination of the biofilm. Other groups investigated the role of rifampin in animal models of implant-associated osteomyelitis, and corroborated the antibiofilm effect of rifampin, as summarized in a recent review [6].

Table 1. Cure rate in the guinea pig tissue cage infection model (copyright© American Society for Microbiology, Antimicrob Agents Chemother 63(2), e01746-18, 2019 [6]).

Microorganism	Antibiotic Regime	Cure Rate	p [a]	Reference
S. epidermidis B3972 (clinical strain)	Ciprofloxacin Ciprofloxacin + Rifampin	0% 100%	<0.01	Widmer et al. 1990 [16]
S. aureus ATCC 29,213 (MSSA)	Vancomycin Vancomycin + Rifampin Ciprofloxacin Ciprofloxacin + Rifampin	0% 75% 17% 92%	<0.01 <0.001	Zimmerli et al. 1994 [25]
S. aureus ATCC 29,213 (MSSA)	Levofloxacin Levofloxacin + Rifampin Levofloxacin + ABI-0043 [b]	0% 88% 92%	<0.001	Trampuz et al. 2007 [26]
S. aureus ATCC 43,300 (MRSA)	Linezolid Linezolid + Rifampin Levofloxacin + Rifampin	0% 60% 91%	<0.001	Baldoni et al. 2009 [27]
S. aureus ATCC 43,300 (MRSA)	Daptomycin Daptomycin + Rifampin	0% 67%	<0.001	John et al. 2009 [28]
S. aureus ATCC 43,300 (MRSA)	Dalbavancin Dalbavancin + Rifampin	0% 36%	<0.001	Baldoni et al. 2013 [29]
S. aureus ATCC 43,300 (MRSA)	Fosfomycin Fosfomycin + Rifampin	0% 83%	<0.001	Mihailescu et al. 2014 [30]

[a] Fisher's exact test for categorical variables, statistical significance is defined as $p < 0.05$. [b] ABI-0043 is a derivative of Rifalazil, which is a rifamycin derivative.

4. Role of Rifampin in Clinical Studies Involving Orthopedic Implant-Associated Infections

Based on the animal data showing an impressive antibiofilm activity of rifampin against staphylococci, we started to treat patients with orthopedic device-related infection (ODRI) with rifampin combination in clinical routine. In a first case series, 10 patients with staphylococcal ODRI undergoing debridement and implant retention (DAIR), the success rate was 80% [17]. In this and many subsequent studies, no direct comparison is possible, because either none or all patients were treated with rifampin combinations. In patients treated with DAIR without rifampin combination therapy, the success rates were as low as 31% to 35% [31,32]. However, in these studies, the Infectious Diseases Society of America (IDSA) guidelines regarding the indication for DAIR have not been considered [33].

In the study of Holmberg et al. [34], patients with staphylococcal knee PJI had a better failure-free survival, when treated with a rifampin combination than without rifampin (81% vs. 41%, $p = 0.01$). Similarly, in a study from the Mayo Clinic, patients treated with DAIR according to the IDSA-guidelines including a rifampin-regimen had a better outcome than patients in a historical control group treated without rifampin (93% vs. 63%) [35]. However, in this study, most of the patients received long-term suppressive antimicrobial therapy.

In several studies, all patients undergoing DAIR for staphylococcal PJI were treated with a rifampin-regimen. The failure-free survival ranged between 80% and 100% in patients treated according to the IDSA-guidelines, in whom the rifampin combination could be given for a prolonged time (generally >2 months) [36–43]. In a study, in which 29 patients with acute PJI were treated with ciprofloxacin plus rifampin, the success rate was 83% [39]. Interestingly, in the mentioned Norwegian randomized trial, in which rifampin-combination therapy did not show superiority, another regimen has been used, namely cloxacillin or vancomycin with or without rifampin [8]. Possible reasons for the low success rates and the lack of improvement by the addition of rifampin are presented below. Indeed, diligent choice of antimicrobial agents may be crucial. In the observational study of Puhto et al. [44] in patients with PJI treated with DAIR, treatment success was significantly higher in patients with ciprofloxacin/rifampin as compared to those with another combination partner or a regimen without rifampin.

Despite the overwhelming evidence for the antibiofilm activity of rifampin, there are a few studies, in which no beneficial effect of rifampin was shown. Bouaziz et al. [45] showed that non-compliance with IDSA guidelines was a risk factor for treatment failure in patients with hip or knee PJI. However, rifampin as single factor was not advantageous because of the strong association between surgical therapy and outcome. Thus, rifampin combination therapy should only be used in patients qualifying for DAIR [33,46]. In an observational study of patients with acute PJI treated with DAIR and linezolid with or without rifampin, patients receiving rifampin did not have an improved outcome. The confounder in this study may be the high prevalence of polymicrobial infection in both groups (41% and 35%, respectively) indicating that many patients may have had wound healing disturbance or even a sinus tract during therapy [47].

Rifampin long-term therapy is complicated by its frequent gastrointestinal side effects, and its strong induction of isoenzymes of cytochrome P450 [6,10]. This is a major clinical challenge, as the effect of rifampin can only be considered in patients in whom it can be given for a sufficient duration. Enzyme induction by rifampin leading to drug-drug interactions requires specific attention prior to and at the end of treatment. However, the interaction of rifampin and other antibiotics in vitro is difficult to interpret, because synergism/antagonism in vitro does not correlate with the effect in vivo [48]. Based on experimental data, the antibiofilm effect seems to be a class effect of all rifamycin derivatives [26,49,50]. First clinical data suggest that rifabutin is a valuable alternative to rifampin with less adverse events and less drug-drug interactions [51].

5. Critical Appraisal of a Randomized Controlled Trial (RCT) Showing no Effect of Rifampin

The above mentioned RCT compared the outcome of patients with acute staphylococcal PJI treated with prosthesis retention and either monotherapy without rifampin or rifampin combination [8]. In this multicenter study conducted from 2006 to 2012 in eight centers, 48 patients with acute PJI were included in the final analysis. PJI was caused by methicillin-susceptible staphylococci in 38 episodes (among them 36 were *S. aureus*) and 10 by methicillin-resistant staphylococci (of which all were *S. epidermidis*). Twenty-five patients were randomized to receive monotherapy, i.e., cloxacillin (two weeks intravenous, followed by four weeks oral) or vancomycin (six weeks intravenous) and 23 patients received rifampin in addition to the anti-staphylococcal treatment regimen mentioned above.

All patients underwent "soft tissue" revision with retention of the prosthesis. Re-revision with isolation of any pathogen was considered confirmed failure, while clinical signs of infection without revision surgery or isolation of pathogen were categorized as probable failure. Using the Kaplan–Meier method, the infection-free survival rate was similar in the monotherapy group (72%) and rifampin combination group (74%) at two years follow-up (median, 27 months). Success rate in PJI caused by methicillin-susceptible staphylococci was 78% with rifampin combination and 65% with monotherapy. In PJI caused by methicillin-resistant staphylococci, monotherapy was successful in all five patients (100%), whereas rifampin-vancomycin-combination had a success of 60% (three of five). No statistically significant difference was observed in any comparison. The authors conclude that adding rifampin to standard antibiotic treatment in acute staphylococcal PJIs does not improve the outcome.

In view of the above presented role of rifampin as biofilm-active antibiotic, the results of this RCT unsettled clinicians with limited experience in the field. Therefore, some critical points in this study should be highlighted for correct interpretation of the results.

First, the originally registered study protocol at ClinicalTrials.gov (NCT00423982) differs from the published manuscript, suggesting that relevant modifications were performed during the study. In contrast to the initial protocol, in addition to patients with early postoperative PJI those with acute hematogenous PJI were included. In late hematogenous PJI, the duration of infection is less well defined, because it may manifest only delayed after seeding. This may explain that the success rate of PJI treated with DAIR has shown to be significantly lower in late acute staphylococcal infection as compared to early postoperative infections [52]. Unfortunately, the distribution of the two clinical entities in the analyzed cohort is not provided, making the interpretation of the results of the heterogeneous study population difficult.

Second, the surgical treatment is described in the Methods in detail. Whereas in the trial registration protocol, only a "soft tissue" revision is mentioned, in the manuscript additionally exchange of modular parts, irrigation with 9 L of saline and placement of two gentamicin-containing sponges (10 × 10 cm^2) is stated, exceeding the procedure of a soft tissue revision. The adherence to this strict surgical protocol throughout the six-year study in eight study centers is questionable, as inclusion in the study took place most likely only after identification of the causing pathogen. Exchange of mobile parts being a proxy for a thorough debridement was shown to be among most relevant factors for successful outcome in several previous studies in case of retained infected prosthesis [36,53–55]. Noteworthy, no dropouts due to deviating surgical treatment were reported.

Third, the antimicrobial combination partner for rifampin is crucial, as mentioned by the authors in the Discussion. In this study, unusual combinations with oral cloxacillin (low oral bioavailability (37%), poor bone penetration, low maximal dose orally compared to intravenous route [56]) and prolonged intravenous vancomycin (toxic, poorly penetrating into the bone, barely bactericidal, non-therapeutic levels upon initiation of treatment) in case of methicillin-resistance were administered. Substances recommended as antimicrobial combination partner for rifampin are those with a high oral bioavailability and a good bone penetration, such as quinolones, trimethoprim-sulfamethoxazole, doxycycline or clindamycin, none of which was used in the present study. In addition, an unusual rifampin dosage (300 mg three times daily) was used, which is neither approved nor recommended for any indication.

Fourth, the absence of infectious diseases specialists in the author list suggests lack of an interdisciplinary team approach to the management of PJI, which is another important factor determining the treatment success of PJI [57,58]. After discharge, adequate intake or administration of antibiotics, patient compliance and modification in case of intolerance should be ensured. Rifampin is often discontinued due to intolerance or toxicity, as shown by the high number of dropouts (n = 7) due to rifampin discontinuation in this study. The accompaniment by an infectious diseases specialist during the treatment period could probably counteract the high dropout rate and potential selection bias.

Fifth, probably the most relevant drawback of the study is the low number of included patients. The final analysis with 48 patients in eight centers during six years indicates a reluctant recruitment. Since staphylococci are the most frequent pathogens of acute PJI [59,60], the average of one patient per center per year implies that the participating centers are not explicitly centers specialized in septic surgery and that the included patients represent a subgroup of patients bearing the risk of selection bias.

Sixth, due to the low number of included subjects, the study is underpowered, and thus does not allow any conclusion on the effect of rifampin on the outcome of acute staphylococcal PJI. The sample size calculation required at least 62 patients in each group to statistically prove an increase in cure rate of 20% (assuming a high cure rate of 70% in the monotherapy group). The authors aimed to include at least 100 subjects in each group. Only focusing on methicillin-susceptible staphylococci, the success rate with monotherapy was 65% (13 out of 20 patients), whereas the rifampin combination led to treatment success in 78% (14 out of 18 patients). Based on theoretical considerations, by increasing the number sample size sixfold (120 patients in the monotherapy group, 108 patients in the combination group) and assuming the same proportion of success in each group, the results would reach statistical significance. Unfortunately, the study was prematurely stopped without mentioning the reason for discontinuation. Only by increasing the sample size the beneficial effect of rifampin could have probably been shown, if there is one, as suggested by multiple above-mentioned studies.

Finally, there are a few imprecisions regarding the outcome evaluation, the reader should consider while interpreting the study results. It remains unclear to what extend the "probable" failures were true septic failures. Furthermore, it is not indicated, whether non-microbiological criteria (synovial fluid leukocyte count and periprosthetic tissue histopathology) for infection were fulfilled in these cases. In addition, the meticulous analysis of failures to discriminate relapse or infection caused by a new pathogen (superinfection) is missing, however, of utmost importance. The fact that the study was conducted several years ago would have allowed for assessment of long-term follow-up. However, only two-year follow-up was reported. Taking all these aspects into consideration, the discussed study does not allow any deduction on the effect of rifampin on the outcome of acute staphylococcal PJI treated with DAIR.

6. Conclusions

Taken together, the controversy about the role of rifampin in biofilm infections is not justified. There is abundant data from in-vitro and animal experiments, as well as clinical studies confirming its antibiofilm effect in patients with staphylococcal orthopedic implant-associated infections undergoing DAIR. Thus, one study with multiple weaknesses should not unsettle clinicians. An RCT with appropriate sample size, optimal choice of antimicrobials, standardized surgical interventions and accurate definition of treatment failure would be desirable. However, given the existing strong evidence demonstrating the benefit of rifampin, the conduction of such a clinical study would not comply with ethical standards and would probably not be approved by ethics committees.

Author Contributions: N.R., A.T. and N.R. discussed the outline. N.R. and W.Z. performed the literature review and wrote the manuscript. A.T. discussed and critically revised the manuscript. All authors have read and agreed to the published version of the manuscript.

Funding: This research received no external funding.

Data Availability Statement: Data is contained within the article.

Conflicts of Interest: The authors declare no conflict of interest interpretation of data, in the writing of the manuscript, or in the decision to publish the results.

References

1. Mandell, G.L.; Vest, T.K. Killing of intraleukocytie *Staphylococcus aureus* by rifampin: In-vitro and in-vivo studies. *J. Infect. Dis.* **1972**, *125*, 486–490. [CrossRef]
2. Ma, H.; Cheng, J.; Peng, L.; Gao, Y.; Zhang, G.; Luo, Z. Adjunctive rifampin for the treatment of *Staphylococcus aureus* bacteremia with deep infections: A meta-analysis. *PLoS ONE* **2020**, *15*, e0230383. [CrossRef]
3. Thwaites, G.E.; Scarborough, M.; Szubert, A.; Nsutebu, E.; Tilley, R.; Greig, J.; Wyllie, S.A.; Wilson, P.; Auckland, C.; Cairns, J.; et al. Adjunctive rifampicin for *Staphylococcus aureus* bacteraemia (ARREST): A multicentre, randomised, double-blind, placebo-controlled trial. *Lancet* **2018**, *391*, 668–678. [CrossRef]
4. Rieg, S.; Joost, I.; Weiß, V.; Peyerl-Hoffmann, G.; Schneider, C.; Hellmich, M.; Seifert, H.; Kern, W.V.; Kaasch, A. Combination antimicrobial therapy in patients with *Staphylococcus aureus* bacteraemia—A post hoc analysis in 964 prospectively evaluated patients. *Clin. Microbiol. Infect.* **2017**, *23*, 406.e1–406.e8. [CrossRef]
5. Riedel, D.J.; Weekes, E.; Forrest, G.N. Addition of rifampin to standard therapy for treatment of native valve infective endocarditis caused by *Staphylococcus aureus*. *Antimicrob. Agents Chemother.* **2008**, *52*, 2463–2467. [CrossRef]
6. Zimmerli, W.; Sendi, P. Role of Rifampin against Staphylococcal Biofilm Infections In Vitro, in Animal Models, and in Orthopedic-Device-Related Infections. *Antimicrob. Agents Chemother.* **2019**, *63*. [CrossRef]
7. Zimmerli, W.; Widmer, A.F.; Blatter, M.; Frei, R.; Ochsner, P.E.; For the Foreign-Body Infection (FBI) Study Group. Role of rifampin for treatment of orthopedic implant-related staphylococcal infections: A randomized controlled trial. *JAMA* **1998**, *279*, 1537–1541. [CrossRef]
8. Karlsen, Ø.E.; Borgen, P.; Bragnes, B.; Figved, W.; Grøgaard, B.; Rydinge, J.; Sandberg, L.; Snorrason, F.; Wangen, H.; Witsøe, E.; et al. Rifampin combination therapy in staphylococcal prosthetic joint infections: A randomized controlled trial. *J. Orthop. Surg. Res.* **2020**, *15*. [CrossRef] [PubMed]
9. Sande, M.A. The use of rifampin in the treatment of nontuberculous infections: An overview. *Rev. Infect. Dis.* **1983**, *5* (Suppl. S3), S399–S401. [CrossRef] [PubMed]
10. Rothstein, D.M. Rifamycins, Alone and in Combination. *Cold Spring Harb. Perspect. Med.* **2016**, *6*, a027011. [CrossRef] [PubMed]

11. Liu, W.L.; Hung, Y.L.; Lin, S.H.; Lee, P.I.; Hsueh, P.R. Fatal bacteraemia and infective endocarditis due to meticillin-resistant *Staphylococcus aureus* (MRSA) with rapid emergence of rifampicin resistance during vancomycin/rifampicin combination treatment. *Int. J. Antimicrob. Agents* **2010**, *35*, 615–616. [CrossRef]
12. Lai, C.C.; Tan, C.K.; Lin, S.H.; Liao, C.H.; Huang, Y.T.; Hsueh, P.R. Emergence of rifampicin resistance during rifampicin-containing treatment in elderly patients with persistent methicillin-resistant *Staphylococcus aureus* bacteremia. *J. Am. Geriatr. Soc.* **2010**, *58*, 1001–1003. [CrossRef]
13. Archer, G.L.; Tenenbaum, M.J.; Haywood, H.B., III. Rifampin therapy for *Staphylococcus epidermidis*. Use in infections from indwelling artificial devices. *JAMA* **1978**, *240*, 751–753. [CrossRef]
14. Karchmer, A.W.; Archer, G.L.; Dismukes, W.E. Rifampin treatment of prosthetic valve endocarditis due to *Staphylococcus epidermidis*. *Rev. Infect. Dis.* **1983**, *5* (Suppl. S3), S543–S548. [CrossRef]
15. Tshefu, K.; Zimmerli, W.; Waldvogel, F.A. Short-term administration of rifampin in the prevention or eradication of infection due to foreign bodies. *Rev. Infect. Dis.* **1983**, *5* (Suppl. S3), S474–S480. [CrossRef] [PubMed]
16. Widmer, A.F.; Frei, R.; Rajacic, Z.; Zimmerli, W. Correlation between in vivo and in vitro efficacy of antimicrobial agents against foreign body infections. *J. Infect. Dis.* **1990**, *162*, 96–102. [CrossRef]
17. Widmer, A.F.; Gaechter, A.; Ochsner, P.E.; Zimmerli, W. Antimicrobial treatment of orthopedic implant-related infections with rifampin combinations. *Clin. Infect. Dis.* **1992**, *14*, 1251–1253. [CrossRef] [PubMed]
18. Giulieri, S.G.; Graber, P.; Ochsner, P.E.; Zimmerli, W. Management of infection associated with total hip arthroplasty according to a treatment algorithm. *Infection* **2004**, *32*, 222–228. [CrossRef] [PubMed]
19. Laffer, R.R.; Graber, P.; Ochsner, P.E.; Zimmerli, W. Outcome of prosthetic knee-associated infection: Evaluation of 40 consecutive episodes at a single centre. *Clin. Microbiol. Infect.* **2006**, *12*, 433–439. [CrossRef] [PubMed]
20. Baddour, L.M.; Wilson, W.R.; Bayer, A.S.; Fowler, V.G., Jr.; Tleyjeh, I.M.; Rybak, M.J.; Barsic, B.; Lockhart, P.B.; Gewitz, M.H.; Levison, M.E.; et al. Infective Endocarditis in Adults: Diagnosis, Antimicrobial Therapy, and Management of Complications: A Scientific Statement for Healthcare Professionals From the American Heart Association. *Circulation* **2015**, *132*, 1435–1486. [CrossRef]
21. Khanlari, B.; Elzi, L.; Estermann, L.; Weisser, M.; Brett, W.; Grapow, M.; Battegay, M.; Widmer, A.F.; Flückiger, U. A rifampicin-containing antibiotic treatment improves outcome of staphylococcal deep sternal wound infections. *J. Antimicrob. Chemother.* **2010**, *65*, 1799–1806. [CrossRef] [PubMed]
22. Erb, S.; Sidler, J.A.; Elzi, L.; Gurke, L.; Battegay, M.; Widmer, A.F.; Weisser, M. Surgical and antimicrobial treatment of prosthetic vascular graft infections at different surgical sites: A retrospective study of treatment outcomes. *PLoS ONE* **2014**, *9*, e112947. [CrossRef]
23. Legout, L.; Delia, P.; Sarraz-Bournet, B.; Rouyer, C.; Massongo, M.; Valette, M.; Leroy, O.; Haulon, S.; Senneville, E. Factors predictive of treatment failure in staphylococcal prosthetic vascular graft infections: A prospective observational cohort study: Impact of rifampin. *BMC Infect. Dis.* **2014**, *14*, 228. [CrossRef]
24. Stewart, P.S. Antimicrobial Tolerance in Biofilms. *Microbiol. Spectr.* **2015**, *3*. [CrossRef] [PubMed]
25. Zimmerli, W.; Frei, R.; Widmer, A.F.; Rajacic, Z. Microbiological tests to predict treatment outcome in experimental device-related infections due to *Staphylococcus aureus*. *J. Antimicrob. Chemother.* **1994**, *33*, 959–967. [CrossRef] [PubMed]
26. Trampuz, A.; Murphy, C.K.; Rothstein, D.M.; Widmer, A.F.; Landmann, R.; Zimmerli, W. Efficacy of a novel rifamycin derivative, ABI-0043, against *Staphylococcus aureus* in an experimental model of foreign-body infection. *Antimicrob. Agents Chemother.* **2007**, *51*, 2540–2545. [CrossRef] [PubMed]
27. Baldoni, D.; Haschke, M.; Rajacic, Z.; Zimmerli, W.; Trampuz, A. Linezolid alone or combined with rifampin against methicillin-resistant *Staphylococcus aureus* in experimental foreign-body infection. *Antimicrob. Agents Chemother.* **2009**, *53*, 1142–1148. [CrossRef] [PubMed]
28. John, A.K.; Baldoni, D.; Haschke, M.; Rentsch, K.; Schaerli, P.; Zimmerli, W.; Trampuz, A. Efficacy of daptomycin in implant-associated infection due to methicillin-resistant *Staphylococcus aureus*: Importance of combination with rifampin. *Antimicrob. Agents Chemother.* **2009**, *53*, 2719–2724. [CrossRef]
29. Baldoni, D.; Tafin, U.F.; Aeppli, S.; Angevaare, E.; Oliva, A.; Haschke, M.; Zimmerli, W.; Trampuz, A. Activity of dalbavancin, alone and in combination with rifampicin, against meticillin-resistant *Staphylococcus aureus* in a foreign-body infection model. *Int. J. Antimicrob. Agents* **2013**, *42*, 220–225. [CrossRef]
30. Mihailescu, R.; Tafin, U.F.; Corvec, S.; Oliva, A.; Betrisey, B.; Borens, O.; Trampuz, A. High activity of Fosfomycin and Rifampin against methicillin-resistant *Staphylococcus aureus* biofilm in vitro and in an experimental foreign-body infection model. *Antimicrob. Agents Chemother.* **2014**, *58*, 2547–2553. [CrossRef] [PubMed]
31. Brandt, C.M.; Sistrunk, W.W.; Duffy, M.C.; Hanssen, A.D.; Steckelberg, J.M.; Ilstrup, D.M.; Osmon, D.R. *Staphylococcus aureus* prosthetic joint infection treated with debridement and prosthesis retention. *Clin. Infect. Dis.* **1997**, *24*, 914–919. [CrossRef]
32. Deirmengian, C.; Greenbaum, J.; Lotke, P.A.; Booth, R.E., Jr.; Lonner, J.H. Limited success with open debridement and retention of components in the treatment of acute *Staphylococcus aureus* infections after total knee arthroplasty. *J. Arthroplast.* **2003**, *18*, 22–26. [CrossRef]
33. Osmon, D.R.; Berbari, E.F.; Berendt, A.R.; Lew, D.; Zimmerli, W.; Steckelberg, J.M.; Rao, N.; Hanssen, A.; Wilson, W.R. Diagnosis and management of prosthetic joint infection: Clinical practice guidelines by the Infectious Diseases Society of America. *Clin. Infect. Dis.* **2013**, *56*, e1–e25. [CrossRef]

34. Holmberg, A.; Thórhallsdóttir, V.G.; Robertsson, O.; W-Dahl, A.; Stefánsdóttir, A. 75% success rate after open debridement, exchange of tibial insert, and antibiotics in knee prosthetic joint infections. *Acta Orthop.* **2015**, *86*, 457–462. [CrossRef] [PubMed]
35. El Helou, O.C.; Berbari, E.F.; Lahr, B.D.; Eckel-Passow, J.E.; Razonable, R.R.; Sia, I.G.; Virk, A.; Walker, R.C.; Steckelberg, J.M.; Wilson, W.R.; et al. Efficacy and safety of rifampin containing regimen for staphylococcal prosthetic joint infections treated with debridement and retention. *Eur. J. Clin. Microbiol. Infect. Dis.* **2010**, *29*, 961–967. [CrossRef]
36. Lora-Tamayo, J.; Murillo, O.; Iribarren, J.A.; Soriano, A.; Sanchez-Somolinos, M.; Baraia-Etxaburu, J.M.; Rico, A.; Palomino, J.; Rodriguez-Pardo, D.; Horcajada, J.P.; et al. A large multicenter study of methicillin-susceptible and methicillin-resistant *Staphylococcus aureus* prosthetic joint infections managed with implant retention. *Clin. Infect. Dis.* **2013**, *56*, 182–194. [CrossRef]
37. Lora-Tamayo, J.; Euba, G.; Cobo, J.; Horcajada, J.P.; Soriano, A.; Sandoval, E.; Pigrau, C.; Benito, N.; Falgueras, L.; Palomino, J.; et al. Short- versus long-duration levofloxacin plus rifampicin for acute staphylococcal prosthetic joint infection managed with implant retention: A randomised clinical trial. *Int. J. Antimicrob. Agents* **2016**, *48*, 310–316. [CrossRef]
38. Sendi, P.; Lötscher, P.O.; Kessler, B.; Graber, P.; Zimmerli, W.; Clauss, M. Debridement and implant retention in the management of hip periprosthetic joint infection: Outcomes following guided and rapid treatment at a single centre. *Bone Jt. J.* **2017**, *99-B*, 330–336. [CrossRef]
39. Berdal, J.E.; Skråmm, I.; Mowinckel, P.; Gulbrandsen, P.; Bjørnholt, J.V. Use of rifampicin and ciprofloxacin combination therapy after surgical debridement in the treatment of early manifestation prosthetic joint infections. *Clin. Microbiol. Infect.* **2005**, *11*, 843–845. [CrossRef] [PubMed]
40. Puhto, A.P.; Puhto, T.; Syrjala, H. Short-course antibiotics for prosthetic joint infections treated with prosthesis retention. *Clin. Microbiol. Infect.* **2012**, *18*, 1143–1148. [CrossRef] [PubMed]
41. Tschudin-Sutter, S.; Frei, R.; Dangel, M.; Jakob, M.; Balmelli, C.; Schaefer, D.J.; Weisser, M.; Elzi, L.; Battegay, M.; Widmer, A.F. Validation of a treatment algorithm for orthopaedic implant-related infections with device-retention—Results from a prospective observational cohort study. *Clin. Microbiol. Infect.* **2016**, *22*, 457.e1–457.e9. [CrossRef]
42. Senneville, E.; Joulie, D.; Legout, L.; Valette, M.; Dezeque, H.; Beltrand, E.; Rosele, B.; d'Escrivan, T.; Loiez, C.; Caillaux, M.; et al. Outcome and Predictors of Treatment Failure in Total Hip/Knee Prosthetic Joint Infections Due to *Staphylococcus aureus*. *Clin. Infect. Dis.* **2011**, *53*, 334–340. [CrossRef]
43. Lesens, O.; Ferry, T.; Forestier, E.; Botelho-Nevers, E.; Pavese, P.; Piet, E.; Pereira, B.; Montbarbon, E.; Boyer, B.; Lustig, S.; et al. Should we expand the indications for the DAIR (debridement, antibiotic therapy, and implant retention) procedure for *Staphylococcus aureus* prosthetic joint infections? A multicenter retrospective study. *Eur. J. Clin. Microbiol. Infect. Dis.* **2018**, *37*, 1949–1956. [CrossRef]
44. Puhto, A.P.; Puhto, T.; Niinimäki, T.; Ohtonen, P.; Leppilahti, J.; Syrjälä, H. Predictors of treatment outcome in prosthetic joint infections treated with prosthesis retention. *Int. Orthop.* **2015**, *39*, 1785–1791. [CrossRef] [PubMed]
45. Bouaziz, A.; Uçkay, I.; Lustig, S.; Boibieux, A.; Lew, D.; Hoffmeyer, P.; Neyret, P.; Chidiac, C.; Ferry, T. Non-compliance with IDSA guidelines for patients presenting with methicillin-susceptible *Staphylococcus aureus* prosthetic joint infection is a risk factor for treatment failure. *Med. Mal. Infect.* **2018**, *48*, 207–211. [CrossRef] [PubMed]
46. Zimmerli, W.; Trampuz, A.; Ochsner, P.E. Prosthetic-joint infections. *N. Engl. J. Med.* **2004**, *351*, 1645–1654. [CrossRef] [PubMed]
47. Morata, L.; Senneville, E.; Bernard, L.; Nguyen, S.; Buzelé, R.; Druon, J.; Tornero, E.; Mensa, J.; Soriano, A. A Retrospective Review of the Clinical Experience of Linezolid with or Without Rifampicin in Prosthetic Joint Infections Treated with Debridement and Implant Retention. *Infect. Dis. Ther.* **2014**, *3*, 235–243. [CrossRef]
48. Perlroth, J.; Kuo, M.; Tan, J.; Bayer, A.S.; Miller, L.G. Adjunctive use of rifampin for the treatment of *Staphylococcus aureus* infections: A systematic review of the literature. *Arch. Intern. Med.* **2008**, *168*, 805–819. [CrossRef]
49. Albano, M.; Karau, M.J.; Greenwood-Quaintance, K.E.; Osmon, D.R.; Oravec, C.P.; Berry, D.J.; Abdel, M.P.; Patel, R. In Vitro Activity of Rifampin, Rifabutin, Rifapentine, and Rifaximin against Planktonic and Biofilm States of Staphylococci Isolated from Periprosthetic Joint Infection. *Antimicrob. Agents Chemother.* **2019**, *63*. [CrossRef]
50. Fisher, C.R.; Schmidt-Malan, S.M.; Ma, Z.; Yuan, Y.; He, S.; Patel, R. In vitro activity of TNP-2092 against periprosthetic joint infection-associated staphylococci. *Diagn. Microbiol. Infect. Dis.* **2020**, *97*, 115040. [CrossRef]
51. Doub, J.B.; Heil, E.L.; Ntem-Mensah, A.; Neeley, R.; Ching, P.R. Rifabutin Use in *Staphylococcus* Biofilm Infections: A Case Series. *Antibiotics* **2020**, *9*, 326. [CrossRef] [PubMed]
52. Wouthuyzen-Bakker, M.; Sebillotte, M.; Huotari, K.; Sánchez, R.E.; Benavent, E.; Parvizi, J.; Fernandez-Sampedro, M.; Barbero-Allende, J.M.; Garcia-Cañete, J.; Trebse, R.; et al. Lower Success Rate of Débridement and Implant Retention in Late Acute versus Early Acute Periprosthetic Joint Infection Caused by *Staphylococcus* spp. Results from a Matched Cohort Study. *Clin. Orthop. Relat. Res.* **2020**, *478*, 1348–1355. [CrossRef] [PubMed]
53. Choi, H.R.; von Knoch, F.; Zurakowski, D.; Nelson, S.B.; Malchau, H. Can implant retention be recommended for treatment of infected TKA? *Clin. Orthop. Relat. Res.* **2011**, *469*, 961–969. [CrossRef] [PubMed]
54. Zhang, T.; Yan, C.H.; Chan, P.K.; Ng, F.Y.; Chiu, K.Y. Polyethylene Insert Exchange Is Crucial in Debridement for Acute Periprosthetic Infections following Total Knee Arthroplasty. *J. Knee Surg.* **2017**, *30*, 36–41. [CrossRef] [PubMed]
55. Hirsiger, S.; Betz, M.; Stafylakis, D.; Götschi, T.; Lew, D.; Uçkay, I. The Benefice of Mobile Parts' Exchange in the Management of Infected Total Joint Arthroplasties with Prosthesis Retention (DAIR Procedure). *J. Clin. Med.* **2019**, *8*, 226. [CrossRef] [PubMed]
56. Nauta, E.H.; Mattie, H. Dicloxacillin and cloxacillin: Pharmacokinetics in healthy and hemodialysis subjects. *Clin. Pharmacol. Ther.* **1976**, *20*, 98–108. [CrossRef] [PubMed]

57. Karczewski, D.; Winkler, T.; Renz, N.; Trampuz, A.; Lieb, E.; Perka, C.; Muller, M. A standardized interdisciplinary algorithm for the treatment of prosthetic joint infections. *Bone Jt. J.* **2019**, *101-B*, 132–139. [CrossRef]
58. Vasoo, S.; Chan, M.; Sendi, P.; Berbari, E. The Value of Ortho-ID Teams in Treating Bone and Joint Infections. *J. Bone Jt. Infect.* **2019**, *4*, 295–299. [CrossRef]
59. Zeller, V.; Kerroumi, Y.; Meyssonnier, V.; Heym, B.; Metten, M.A.; Desplaces, N.; Marmor, S. Analysis of postoperative and hematogenous prosthetic joint-infection microbiological patterns in a large cohort. *J. Infect.* **2018**, *76*, 328–334. [CrossRef]
60. Wouthuyzen-Bakker, M.; Sebillotte, M.; Lomas, J.; Taylor, A.; Palomares, E.B.; Murillo, O.; Parvizi, J.; Shohat, N.; Reinoso, J.C.; Sánchez, R.E.; et al. Clinical outcome and risk factors for failure in late acute prosthetic joint infections treated with debridement and implant retention. *J. Infect.* **2019**, *78*, 40–47. [CrossRef]

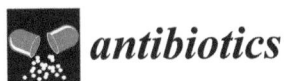

Article

Tolerance of Prolonged Oral Tedizolid for Prosthetic Joint Infections: Results of a Multicentre Prospective Study

Eric Senneville [1,2,3,*], Aurélien Dinh [4,5], Tristan Ferry [6,7], Eric Beltrand [3,8], Nicolas Blondiaux [3,9] and Olivier Robineau [1,2,3]

1. Infectious Diseases Department, Gustave Dron Hospital, 59000 Lille, France; orobineau@ch-tourcoing.fr
2. Faculty of Medicine Henri Warembourg, Lille University, 59000 Lille, France
3. French National Referent Centre for Complex Bone and Joint Infections, CRIOAC Lille-Tourcoing, 59000 Lille, France; ebeltrand@ch-tourcoing.fr (E.B.); nblondiaux@ch-tourcoing.fr (N.B.)
4. Infectious Diseases Department, Ambroise Paré Hospital, 92100 Boulogne-Billancourt, France; aurelien.dinh@aphp.fr
5. French National Referent Centre for Complex Bone and Joint Infections, CRIOAC Paris-Ambroise, 75000 Paré, France
6. Infectious Diseases Department, Croix-Rousse Hospital, 69004 Lyon, France; tristan.ferry@univ-lyon1.fr
7. French National Referent Centre for Complex Bone and Joint Infections, CRIOAC Lyon, 69000 Lyon, France
8. Orthopaedic Surgery Department, G. Dron Hospital Tourcoing, 59200 Tourcoing, France
9. Microbiology Laboratory, G. Dron Hospital Tourcoing, 59200 Tourcoing, France
* Correspondence: esenneville@ch-tourcoing.fr; Tel.: +33-0-32694848; Fax: +33-0-32694496

Abstract: Objectives: Data on clinical and biological tolerance of tedizolid (TZD) prolonged therapy are lacking. Methods: We conducted a prospective multicentre study including patients with prosthetic joint infections (PJIs) who were treated for at least 6 weeks but not more than 12 weeks. Results: Thirty-three adult patients of mean age 73.3 ± 10.5 years, with PJI including hip ($n = 19$), knee ($n = 13$) and shoulder ($n = 1$) were included. All patients were operated, with retention of the infected implants and one/two stage-replacements in 11 (33.3%) and 17/5 (51.5%/15.2%), respectively. Staphylococci and enterococci were the most prevalent bacteria identified. The mean duration of TZD therapy was 8.0 ± 3.27 weeks (6–12). TZD was associated with another antibiotic in 18 patients (54.5%), including rifampicin in 16 cases (48.5). Six patients (18.2%) had to stop TZD therapy prematurely because of intolerance which was potentially attributable to TZD ($n = 2$), early failure of PJI treatment ($n = 2$) or severe anaemia due to bleeding ($n = 2$). Regarding compliance with TZD therapy, no cases of two or more omissions of medication intake were recorded during the whole TZD treatment duration. Conclusions: These results suggest good compliance and a favourable safety profile of TZD, providing evidence of the potential benefit of the use of this agent for the antibiotic treatment of PJIs.

Keywords: tedizolid; prosthetic joint infections; prolonged oral treatment; tolerance; compliance

Citation: Senneville, E.; Dinh, A.; Ferry, T.; Beltrand, E.; Blondiaux, N.; Robineau, O. Tolerance of Prolonged Oral Tedizolid for Prosthetic Joint Infections: Results of a Multicentre Prospective Study. *Antibiotics* **2021**, *10*, 4. https://dx.doi.org/10.3390/antibiotics10010004

Received: 6 December 2020
Accepted: 21 December 2020
Published: 23 December 2020

Publisher's Note: MDPI stays neutral with regard to jurisdictional claims in published maps and institutional affiliations.

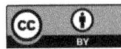

Copyright: © 2020 by the authors. Licensee MDPI, Basel, Switzerland. This article is an open access article distributed under the terms and conditions of the Creative Commons Attribution (CC BY) license (https://creativecommons.org/licenses/by/4.0/).

1. Introduction

Prosthetic joint infection (PJI) is a serious and complex complication following arthroplasty at an incidence rate after hip or knee replacement of 1 to 2% [1]. The aims of the management of patients with PJIs are to restore satisfactory joint function and to eliminate infection. Surgical options include debridement antibiotics and implant retention (DAIR), one- or two-stage replacement, arthroplastic resection and, sometimes, amputation. Given the increasing burden of these infections, especially among the elderly population, developing new therapies such as cell therapy to prevent the progression of osteo-arthritis, and thus, the need for total joint arthroplasty, is an important field of research [2–5]. The antibiotic treatment of patients with PJIs is limited by the tolerance of its prolonged administration and the resistance level of some pathogens [6,7]. Gram-positive cocci, especially coagulase-negative staphylococci (CoNS), are predominant bacteria which are responsible for infections in and around orthopaedic devices [8]. In this context, the use of the oxazolidinone agent linezolid (LZD) has been validated, but potential bone-marrow, neurologic, and metabolic toxicity limit treatment duration to no more than two to three weeks [9–11]. Additionally, the wide use of LZD has resulted in the emergence of CoNS carrying *cfr* genes which are responsible for high levels of LZD resistance [12]. The combination of rifampicin with LZD leads to a reduction in LZD blood concentration, which is associated with a lower rate of adverse hematologic effects but also with lower clinical remission rates [13,14]. Tedizolid (TZD) phosphate is a second generation oxazolidinone which is indicated for the treatment of acute bacterial skin and skin structure infections in adults [15–18]. In the Establish 1 and 2 studies, gastrointestinal disorders and bone marrow toxicity were less frequent in TZD than in LZD patients [19,20]. However, the duration of TZD treatment did not exceed six days. TZD has a high oral bioavailability and can be administered once-daily; furthermore, drug–drug interactions with mono-amine oxidase inhibitors (MAOI), serotonin-reuptake inhibitors (SRI) or rifampicin are unlikely, although the latter has recently been questioned [21,22]. Recent in vitro and animal studies suggested that the addition of rifampicin to TZD was likely to achieve a synergistic effect against methicillin-resistant *Staphylococcus aureus* (MRSA) and *S. epidermidis*, and prevent the emergence of rifampicin-resistant mutants [23,24]. While TZD appears to be an attractive candidate for the treatment of PJIs due to gram-positive cocci, and has shown satisfactory efficacy and tolerability in clinical trials, data about its tolerability and compliance in long-term treatments are lacking. The aim of the present multicentre prospective cohort study was to assess the long-term safety profile and compliance of oral TZD in monotherapy or in combination therapy for the treatment of PJIs.

2. Results

Thirty-three adult patients (sex ratio female/male 17/16) of mean age 73.3 ± 10.5 years were included from August 2018 to November 2019. A total of 17 patients (51.5%) were enrolled at the Tourcoing Centre, 13 (39.4%) at the Ambroise Paré Centre and 3 (9.1%) at the Lyon Centre. Patient characteristics are presented in Table 1. Despite chronic infection, three patients were treated with a debridement antibiotic and implant retention (DAIR) because of their age and general status which contraindicated the replacement of the implant. TZD use was used to avoid LZD potential toxicities or drug–drug interactions in 16 patients (48.5%), or because of previous, LZD-related adverse events in three patients (9.1%). Among these three patients, one had experienced thrombocytopenia, one anaemia and one gastro-intestinal intolerance. No included patients were receiving MAOI or SRI concomitantly with TZD therapy. Staphylococci were the most prevalent bacterium identified in our patients, accounting for 58% of the total number, and including 21 (42%) methicillin-resistant strains (Table 2). Infection was polymicrobial in 18 cases (54.5%) among which five were associated with gram-negative rods, all of which were susceptible to fluoroquinolones. Geometric mean MIC values for linezolid, as determined by E-test methods, were 1.24 ± 0.83 mg/L, 1.5 ± 0.7 mg/L and 1.64 ± 0.48 mg/L for *Staphylococcus* spp., *Streptococcus* spp. and *Enterococcus* spp., respectively. MIC measurements or TZD blood levels were not routinely performed for tedizolid in this study.

Following postoperative empirical antibiotic therapy (PEAT) of median duration of 7 days (range 4 to 14 days), the mean duration of TZD therapy was 8.0 ± 3.27 weeks (ranging from 6–12 weeks). Among the 27 out of 33 patients (81.8%) who completed the planned therapy, the mean duration of TZD was 8.77 weeks ± 2.79 (range 6–12 weeks). The mean total duration of the antibiotic treatment including PEAT and targeted therapy was 9.15 ± 3.43 weeks (7–12). TZD was associated with another antibiotic in 18 patients (54.5%), e.g., rifampicin in 16 cases (48.5%).

Table 1. Demographic data of 33 patients with periprosthetic joint infections.

Patient Characteristics	Values and Number of Patients (%)
Age, years in mean ± SD	73.3 ± 10.5
Sex ratio (female/male)	17/16
Body mass index, kg/m^2 mean ± SD (>30)	29.7 ± 6.2 (51.5)
Comorbidities *	19 (57.6)
- Diabetes mellitus	10 (30.3)
- Cancer	5 (15.2)
- Liver cirrhosis	1 (3.0)
- Chronic obstructive pulmonary disease	4 (12.1)
- Rheumatoid polyarthritis	1 (3.0)
- Chronic renal failure	2 (6.0)
American Society of Anaesthesiologists score ≥2 [range]	27 (81.2) [1–3]
Previous surgical revision of the prosthesis ≥1 [range]	12 (36.4) [1–10]
Total joint arthroplasty	
- Total hip prosthesis	19 (57.6)
- Total knee prosthesis	13 (39.4)
- Total shoulder prosthesis	1 (3.0)
Age of the prosthesis, months mean ± SD [range]	24.5 ± 39.0 [1–180]
Type of infection	
- Early postinterventional	6 (18.2)
- Chronic	25 (75.8)
- Acute haematogenous	2 (6.1)
Surgical intervention	
- Drainage and retention of the implant	11 (33.3)
- One-stage replacement	17 (51.5)
- Two-stage replacement	5 (15.2)
Fever (temperature > 38.0 °C)	4 (12.1)
Fistula	12 (36.4)
C-reactive protein at baseline, mg/L mean ± SD [range; IQR]	42.16 ± 34.9 [5.8–111; 52]
White blood cells at baseline, G/L mean ± SD [range; IQR]	8.34 ± 2.5 [4.3–15.6; 3.2]

SD: standard deviation. *: 4 patients had ≥2 comorbidities.

In total, 20 patients (60.6%) experienced at least one adverse event during TZD therapy. A list of adverse events (AE) potentially attributable to tedizolid is shown in Table 3; the most frequent AE were anaemia (n = 4) and pruritus (n = 4). Six patients (18.2%) had to stop TZD therapy prematurely because of (i) intolerance which was potentially attributable to TZD (n = 2), (ii) early failure of PJI treatment (n = 2) or (iii) severe anaemia (n = 2). TZD-attributable discontinuation episodes consisted of inflammatory arthritis of the wrist and knee in one patient who also received doxycycline and did not improve after stopping doxycycline but partially recovered after discontinuation of TZD, and vomiting in another patient who received TZD alone (Appendix A Table A1). According to the definitions used to describe the bone marrow toxicity profile of TZD, 8 patients (24.2%) experienced haematological adverse events including anaemia in 4 cases, 2 of which presented acute haemorrhage, leukopenia in 2 cases and thrombocytopenia in 2 cases (Table A1). With the exception of the two patients with acute haemorrhage, none of these adverse events resulted in withdrawing TZD therapy. Although a gastric haemorrhage in one patient and a hematoma at the surgical site in another patient resulted in acute severe anaemia which was most probably unrelated to TZD therapy, the treatment was discontinued. Haematological adverse events were mild and resolved spontaneously during TZD therapy except in the two patients with severe anaemia who received a blood transfusion. Non haematological adverse events were recorded in 13 (39.4%) patients for whom no premature discontinuation of TZD therapy was required, and were mostly pruritus ($n = 4$), headache ($n = 2$) and insomnia ($n = 2$) (Table A1). There was no safety signal for TZD-associated optic or peripheral neurologic toxicity or metabolic disorder. Overall, the proportion of patients who experienced TZD-attributable adverse event did not differ significantly in patients treated with a combination of antibiotics or with TZD alone [13/18 (72.2%) versus 8/15 (52.3%), respectively; $p = 0.45$], nor did it vary according to the use of rifampicin in combination with TZD or the total duration of TZD therapy (Table 4).

Table 2. Microbiology of 33 patients with periprosthetic joint infections.

Bacteria	N° of Strains (%)
Gram positive cocci	43 (86.0)
- *Staphylococcus aureus* (MRSA = 7)	13 (26)
- *Staphylococcus epidermidis* (MRSE = 14)	15 (30)
- *Staphylococcus caprae* (MR = 2)	1 (2)
- *Streptococcus agalactiae*	2 (4)
- *Corynebacterium striatum*	4 (8)
- *Enterococcus faecalis*	7 (14)
- *Enterococcus gallinarum*	1 (2)
Gram negative bacilli	5 (10)
- *Escherichia coli*	2 (4)
- *Klebsiella pneumoniae*	1 (2)
- *Pseudomonas aeruginosa*	1 (2)
- *Pasteurella multocida*	1 (2)
Anaerobes	2 (4)
- *Cutibacterium acnes*	2 (4)
Total number of bacterial strains	50 (100)

Legend: MRSA: Methicillin-resistant *Staphylococcus aureus*; MRSE: Methicillin-resistant *Staphylococcus epidermidis*; MR: Methicillin-resistant.

Table 3. Episodes of adverse effects reported in 33 patients during tedizolid therapy.

Adverse Event (N° of Discontinuation of Tedizolid Therapy)	N° of Episodes of Adverse Effects *
anemia (2)	4
asthenia	1
leukopenia	2
thrombocytopenia	2
headache	2
pruritus	4
abdominal pain	1
nausea/vomiting (1)	2
vertigo	1
xerosis	1
dysgeusia	1
epistaxis	1
arthralgia (1)	2
thrush	1
insomnia	2
intermittent blurred vision	1
Total	28

* Five patients had more than one episode of adverse effects.

Table 4. Adverse events according to the duration and the antibiotic regimen in 33 patients treated with tedizolid.

Patients' Characteristics	N° of Patients (%), Total = 33	p
≥1 adverse event	20 (60.6)	
Any combination therapy		0.8
- Yes (n = 18)	11 (61.1)	
- No (n = 15)	9 (60)	
Rifampicin combination therapy		0.9
- Yes (n = 16)	9 (56.3)	
- No (n = 17)	11 (64.7)	
Duration of treatment ≤6 weeks		0.8
- Yes (n = 13)	7 (53.8)	
- No (n = 20)	13 (65)	

The follow-up of the haematological parameters showed a significant increase of haemoglobin blood levels between baseline and week 6 followed by stabilisation, as well as a significant decrease in platelets, leukocytes and neutrophils counts between baseline and week 6 followed by stabilisation until the end of the treatment (Figure 1A–D).

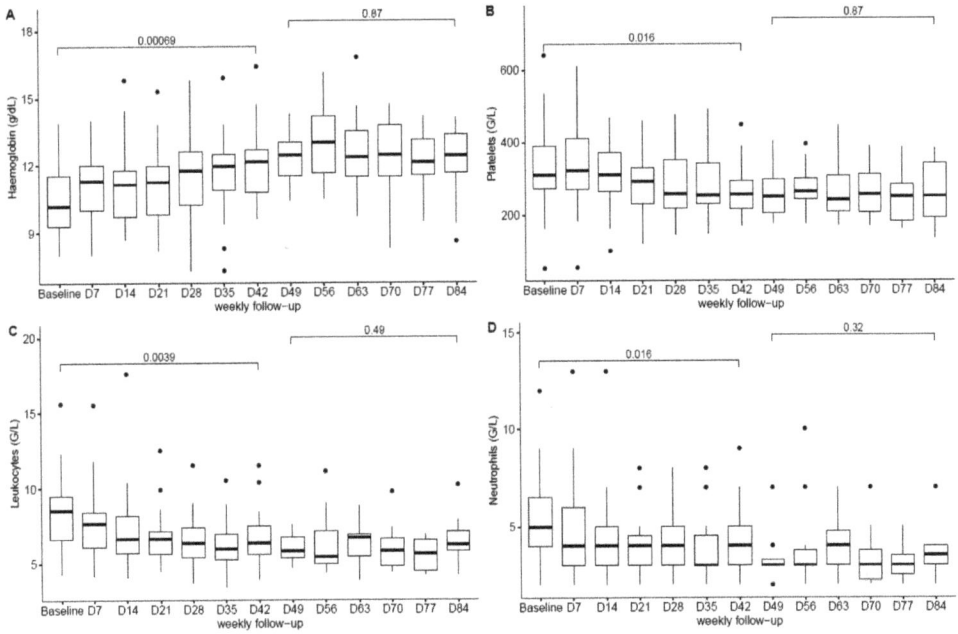

Figure 1. Boxplot of the haematological parameters ((**A**): Haemoglobin, (**B**): Platelets, (**C**): Leukocytes, (**D**): Neutrophils) during Tedizolid therapy. Each box represents median, interquartile range, largest, smallest and outside (point) values.

Regarding compliance to TZD therapy, no cases of two or more omissions of medication intake during TZD treatment were recorded, in accordance with the number of pills present in the returned boxes. Six failures (18.2%), including two early cases, were recorded at one-year following the end of TZD therapy.

3. Discussion

We report the first prospective cohort study to date providing data on the safety and compliance of prolonged use (i.e., ≥6 weeks) of oral TZD phosphate at a 200-mg, once-daily dose for the treatment of PJIs. As our safety results suggest, oral TZD therapy administered for 6 to 12 weeks according to the current recommendations [25] can be considered for the treatment of PJIs. The overall proportion of patients who experienced an adverse event (60.6%) may appear high, but this may be explained by the design of the study which allowed us to report an exhaustive list of adverse events. Despite the nonoptimal profile regarding the general status of our patients, the tolerance of prolonged oral TZD therapy allowed us to complete the therapy in more than 80% of the cases. Indeed, 19 patients (57.6%) had comorbidities and 27 (81.2%) had an ASA score ≥ 2, which is significantly different from the populations of patients evaluated in other, pivotal clinical trials [19,20]. Our results are close to those reported by Kim et al. on a series of 25 patients with nontuberculous mycobacterial infections treated with a median duration of TZD therapy of 91 days [26]. Eleven of their patients (44%) experienced an adverse event including gastrointestinal intolerance in five patients (20%) and thrombocytopenia in one (4%); no case of anaemia was recorded, while peripheral neuropathy was reported in five patients (20%). The attribution of an adverse event to TZD was, however, difficult, as almost all patients were receiving multidrug therapy. The mean age of our patients was 73.3 years, which is quite high with regard to the risk of developing bone marrow toxicity to LZD, as reported by several authors [9,10]. The correction of LZD-induced bone marrow toxicity after switching to TZD observed in one of our patients has already been reported elsewhere [27,28]. Overall, we only recorded a few significant haematological abnormalities which did not result in discontinuation of TZD therapy, except in patients with acute haemorrhage. There were no differences in safety, especially with regard to haematological laboratory changes, between patients receiving TZD in combination with rifampicin versus patients receiving TZD alone (full data are available upon request), as reported with LZD-rifampicin combination [9,10]. We hypothesise that the increase of haemoglobin values during TZD treatment represents a restoration process after blood spoliation secondary to the surgical intervention, while the decrease of platelets and WBC during TZD treatment might be related to the resolution of the infectious process. The incidence of digestive disorders reported in our patients is close to the results of a meta-analysis by Lan et al., noting, however, that the duration of TZD therapy in the studies included was six days, as recommended for the treatment of acute bacterial skin and skin structure infections [29].

The main limitations of the present pilot study are the small size of the studied population and the assessment of the patients' adherence to TDZ treatment, which was based on the return of the pillboxes and on patient self-reporting. The strengths of the present study are its prospective design and the selection criteria which allowed investigators to include patients in a real-life setting. We strongly believe that the inclusion of patients, regardless of age and risk factors for bone marrow toxicity, enhanced the external validity of our conclusions regarding the tolerance of prolonged oral TZD therapy in patients treated with PJIs.

4. Materials and Methods

The purpose of the present study was to obtain reliable data on the tolerance, compliance and efficacy of prolonged (i.e., ≥6 weeks) use of TZD alone or in combination therapy for the treatment of PJIs. We present herein data about adherence and tolerance. As post-treatment follow-ups are currently underway, we present data only for the one-year follow-up. We conducted a prospective multicentre cohort study in three French national centres for the management of complex bone and joint infections (also called CRIOAc): Lille-Tourcoing, Paris-Ambroise Paré and Lyon [30].

4.1. Definitions

Adult patients with PJIs defined according to the MSIS 2018 [31] criteria and for whom TZD treatment was indicated according to the investigator's decision were prospectively included. All patients gave their written informed consent after an explanation of the protocol by the investigating physician. PJIs were characterised according to: acute haematogenous (infection with three-week duration or less of symptoms after an uneventful postoperative period), early postinterventional (infection that manifested within one month after implantation) and chronic (infection with symptoms that persisted for >3 weeks, i.e., beyond the early postinterventional period) according to Zimmerli's definition [32].

Patients demographic data (age, gender, body mass index), comorbidities, microbiology, prior use of LZD and reason for TZD use (e.g., failure and/or toxicity of previous treatment, need to avoid linezolid toxicity or drug–drug interactions), treatment duration, concomitant antibiotics, potential adverse events attributable to TZD were recorded. Laboratory data were recorded at baseline, weekly and at the end of treatment, including haemoglobin, white blood count (WBC), platelet count, alanine aminotransferase (ALT), aspartate aminotransferase (AST) and Protein-C reactive (PCR).

Clinically significant laboratory changes were defined as: (1) anaemia, decrease in haemoglobin $\geq$2 g/L from baseline after TZD initiation and classified as severe if haemoglobin was <8 g/dL, (2) leukopenia, white blood count (WBC) of <4 G/L after TZD initiation and classified as mild (low limit normal to 3 G/L), moderate ($\geq$2-<3 G/L) and severe (<2 G/L), (3), neutropenia, absolute neutrophil count of <1.5 G/L after TZD initiation, (4) thrombocytopenia, platelet count of <150 G/L after TZD initiation and classified as mild (75–150 G/L), moderate (50-<75 G/L) or severe (<50 G/L); for patients with a baseline platelet count of <150 G/L, thrombocytopenia was defined as a reduction of 25% from the baseline, and (5) elevated AST or ALT 3 times above the upper limit of normal.

Microbiological documentation was based on joint aspiration and/or intraoperative culture samples. During surgical procedures, at least three tissue samples were taken in different areas suspected of infection, using a separate sterile instrument for each sample. The antibiotic susceptibility profile of all pathogens was assessed either by the Vitek 2 cards (BioMérieux, Marcy l'Etoile, France) or by agar diffusion technique using the procedure and interpretation criteria proposed by the Comité de l'Antibiogramme de la Société Française de Microbiologie (CA-SFM EUCAST 2018) (http://www.sfm-microbiologie.org). Methicillin resistance was confirmed by the detection of the *mecA* gene if required.

Adverse events (AEs) were identified from patients' medical records and laboratory data. Associations of adverse events with TZD and related antibiotics were assessed as suggested by the patient's physician and confirmed by the principal investigator according to the chronology of events, as were the need to reduce the daily dosage of the potentially problematic antibiotic, data from any attempt to reintroduce such a mode of treatment, and the type of recorded toxicity (e.g., anaemia, thrombocytopenia and peripheral neuropathy for TZD, tendonitis, and myalgia for levofloxacin and drug–drug interaction for rifampicin). To be attributable to a given antibiotic, a reduction in the daily dosage and/or discontinuation due to intolerance had to be recorded as well as temporal association with event resolution after discontinuation or dose reduction of the agent in question.

4.2. Antibiotic Treatment

TZD was administered orally at a once daily dose of 200 mg (i.e., one tablet) as a single antibiotic therapy or in combination therapy with another agent with proven activity against the involved pathogen(s) according to the physician's choice. The duration of antibiotic therapy ranged from 6 to 12 weeks. Exclusion criteria were pregnant women or women of childbearing age who were not using contraception, breastfeeding intolerance to TZD, allergy to oxazolidinone, the detection of bacteria which were nonsusceptible to TZD, patients with uncertainty regarding the possibility of achieving a one-year follow-up after the end of treatment or the absence of written consent. Patients were examined during consultations every 3 weeks during treatment and at 6 months and one year after the EOT.

During treatment, special attention was paid to potential neurological and optical side effects, as well as to possible drug–drug interactions.

4.3. Statistics

Data are presented as numbers (percentages) for qualitative variables and as medians (interquartile range: IQR) or means (SD) for quantitative variables. We compared biological variable that might have been affected by the use of oxazolidinone between baseline and day 42 and between day 49 and day 84 using the Student t-test, with $p = 0.05$ being set as the threshold of significance.

4.4. Ethics

Research was conducted in accordance with the Declaration of Helsinki and national and institutional standards. The study was recorded on clinicaltrial.gov under the number NCT03378427, in the EudraCT database under the number 2017-001238-24 and was approved by the French Sud Mediterranean IV *Committee* of *Protection* of the *People* in Biomedical Research on 21 November 2017 under the number 17 10 09. This interventional survey was declared to the National Agency for Medicines and Safety of Health Products under the number 17060A-43. Tedizolid was supplied by *Merck Sharp & Dohme*, Inc.

5. Conclusions

The results of the present study suggest good compliance and a favourable safety profile of TZD, providing evidence of the potential benefit of the use of this agent for the antibiotic treatment of PJIs.

Author Contributions: E.S., E.B. and O.R. conceived the design of the study and wrote the manuscript; A.D. and T.F. reviewed the manuscript, all but N.B. participated in the inclusions and management of the patients; N.B. reviewed the microbiology part of the manuscript. All authors have read and agreed to the published version of the manuscript.

Funding: No external funding was received except that tedizolid pills were provided by Merck Sharp and Dohme.

Data Availability Statement: Data are available upon request to Pr Eric Senneville (esenneville@ch-tourcoing.fr); the French authorities do not authorize the sharing of this type of data without prior consent and infor-mation of the patients on their final use.

Acknowledgments: We greatly thank the G. Dron hospital clinical research unit, especially Solange Tréhoux for the technical assistance.

Conflicts of Interest: E.S., A.D., O.R. and T.F. declare congress support, speaker invitation, participation to scientific board with MSD; E.B. and N.B. have nothing to declare in relation with the present study. E.S., A.D., O.R. and T.F. declare congress support, speaker invitation, and participation to scientific board with MSD; E.B. and N.B. have nothing to declare in relation with the present study.

Appendix A

Table A1. Details on tolerance of TZD therapy in 33 patients treated for periprosthetic joint infections.

Pt	Age	Surgery	ASA Score	Type of Infection	Microbiology	Duration of TZD Therapy (Weeks)	Antibiotic Associated with TZD	Premature Discontinuation of TZD (Origin)	No Adverse Events without Premature Discontinuation of TZD
1	88	DAIR	2	Chronic	EC, SB	6	RIF	No	anaemia, asthenia
2	74	1-SR	2	Chronic	SE*	6	None	No	thrush
3	66	DAIR	2	EPO	EF	12	RIF	No	leukopenia
4	62	1-SR	3	Chronic	CA	1	None	Yes (anaemia due to gastric haemorrhage)	
5	80	DAIR	3	Chronic	EF, SA, PM	7	RIF, LEV	No	thrombocytopenia
6	80	1-SR	2	Chronic	SE*	6	None	No	
7	64	2-SR	2	AH	CS, EF, EC	11	None	No	thrombocytopenia
8	73	1-SR	3	AH	SA, SE*	6	DALB	No	anaemia
9	71	2-SR	2	Chronic	SA*	11	None	No	intermittent blurred vision
10	80	DAIR	1	EPO	SE*	11	RIF	No	
11	75	DAIR	2	EPO	CS	11	RIF	No	leukopenia
12	88	DAIR	3	EPO	EF, SE*	12	RIF	No	
13	67	DAIR	1	EPO	EF, SE	6	DOX	Yes (arthralgia)	
14	79	2-SR	2	Chronic	SE*	11	None	No	xerosis, pruritus
15	75	1-SR	2	Chronic	SA	6	None	Yes (vomiting)	headache, dysgeusia
16	78	2-SR	3	Chronic	EF, SA	5	None	Yes (early failure)	
17	77	1-SR	2	Chronic	SE*	11	None	No	abdominal pain, headache, vertigo
18	45	2-SR	1	Chronic	Sterile	10	None	No	pruritus

Table A1. Cont.

Pt	Age	Surgery	ASA Score	Type of Infection	Microbiology	Duration of TZD Therapy (Weeks)	Antibiotic Associated with TZD	Premature Discontinuation of TZD (Origin)	No Adverse Events without Premature Discontinuation of TZD
19	86	DAIR	3	EPO	SA*	6	None	No	
20	70	1-SR	1	Chronic	KP, SA, SE*	6	RIF, LEV	No	tinnitus, insomnia nausea pruritus
21	55	1-SR	1	Chronic	EG	6	None	No	
22	79	DAIR	3	EPO	SA*	6	RIF	No	vomiting
23	83	1-SR	3	Chronic	SE*	7	RIF	No	insomnia
24	78	1-SR	3	Chronic	SE*	6	RIF	No	pruritus
25	67	1-SR	2	Chronic	CS, SA, SE*	6	RIF	No	
26	81	DAIR	2	Chronic	CA, SB	6	None	No	
27	45	DAIR	1	AH	SA, SE	9	None	No	
28	87	1-SR	2	EPO	SA*, CA, EF, PA	1	RIF	Yes (anaemia due to a haematoma at the operated site)	
29	74	1-SR	1	Chronic	SA*	12	RIF	No	
30	76	1-SR	1	Chronic	SE	11	RIF, CIP	No	
31	66	1-SR	2	EPO	SE*	9	RIF	Yes (early failure)	
32	69	1-SR	2	Chronic	SA*	8	RIF	No	epistaxis
33	82	1-SR	3	Chronic	SC*	12	None	No	

Pt: patient; ASA: American Society of Anaesthesiologists, TZD: TZD; DAIR: debridement antibiotic and implant retention, 1-SR: one stage replacement, 2-SR two-stage replacement, EPO: early postoperative, AH: acute haematogenous, RIF: rifampicin, LEV: levofloxacin, DALB: dalbavancin, DOX: doxycycline, CIP: ciprofloxacin, EC: Escherichia coli, SB: group B streptococci, SA: Staphylococcus aureus, SE: Staphylococcus epidermidis, EF: Enterococcus faecalis, CA: Cutibacterium acnes, PM: Pasteurella multocida, CS: Corynebacterium striatum, KP: Klebsiella pneumoniae, EG: Enterococcus gallinarum, PA: Pseudomonas aeruginosa, CA: Staphylococcus caprae, *: methicillin-resistant.

References

1. Li, C.; Renz, N. Management of Periprosthetic Joint Infection. *Hip. Pelvis.* **2018**, *30*, 138–146. [CrossRef] [PubMed]
2. Rabini, A.; Boccia, G. Effects of focal muscle vibration on physical functioning in patients with knee osteoarthritis: A randomized controlled trial. *Eur. J. Phys. Rehabil. Med.* **2015**, *51*, 513–520. [PubMed]
3. De Sire, A.; Stagno, D. Long-term effects of intra-articular oxygen-ozone therapy versus hyaluronic acid in older people affected by knee osteoarthritis: A randomized single-blind extension study. *J. Back Musculoskelet Rehabil* **2020**, *33*, 347–354. [CrossRef] [PubMed]
4. McAlindon, T.E.; Bannuru, R.R. OARSI guidelines for the non-surgical management of knee osteoarthritis. *Osteoarthr. Cartil.* **2014**, *22*, 363–388. [CrossRef]
5. Migliore, A.; Paoletta, M. The perspectives of intra-articular therapy in the management of osteoarthritis. *Expert Opin. Drug Deliv.* **2020**, *17*, 1213–1226. [CrossRef]
6. Del Pozo, J.L.; Patel, R. Clinical practice. Infection associated with prosthetic joints. *N. Engl. J. Med.* **2009**, *361*, 787–794. [CrossRef]
7. Zimmerli, W.; Trampuz, A. Prosthetic-joint infections. *N. Engl. J. Med.* **2004**, *351*, 1645–1654. [CrossRef]
8. Titécat, M.; Senneville, E. Bacterial epidemiology of osteoarticular infections in a referent center: 10-year study. *Orthop. Traumatol. Surg. Res.* **2013**, *99*, 653–658. [CrossRef]
9. Soriano, A.; Gomez, J. Efficacy and tolerability of prolonged linezolid therapy in the treatment of orthopedic implant infections. *Eur. J. Clin. Microbiol. Infect. Dis.* **2007**, *26*, 353–356. [CrossRef]
10. Senneville, E.; Legout, L. Risk factors for anaemia in patients on prolonged linezolid therapy for chronic osteomyelitis: A case-control study. *J. Antimicrob. Chemother.* **2004**, *54*, 798–802. [CrossRef]
11. Bassetti, M.; Vitale, F. Linezolid in the treatment of Gram-positive prosthetic joint infections. *J. Antimicrob. Chemother.* **2005**, *55*, 387–390. [CrossRef] [PubMed]
12. Ruiz-Ripa, L.; Feßler, A.T. Mechanisms of Linezolid Resistance Among Clinical Staphylococcus sin Spain: Spread of Methicillin- and Linezolid-Resistant, S. epidermidis ST2. *Microb. Drug Resist.* **2020**. [CrossRef] [PubMed]
13. Legout, L.; Valette, M. Tolerability of prolonged linezolid therapy in bone and joint infection: Protective effect of rifampicin on the occurrence of anaemia? *J. Antimicrob. Chemother.* **2010**, *65*, 2224–2230. [CrossRef] [PubMed]
14. Tornero, E.; Morata, L. Importance of selection and duration of antibiotic regimen in prosthetic joint infections treated with debridement and implant retention. *J. Antimicrob. Chemother.* **2016**, *71*, 1395–1401. [CrossRef] [PubMed]
15. Schmidt-Malan, S.M.; Greenwood Quaintance, K.E. In vitro activity of tedizolid against staphylococci isolated from prosthetic joint infections. *Diagn. Microbiol. Infect. Dis.* **2016**, *85*, 77–79. [CrossRef]
16. Littorin, C.; Hellmark, B. In vitro activity of tedizolid and linezolid against Staphylococcus epidermidis isolated from prosthetic joint infections. *Eur. J. Clin. Microbiol. Infect. Dis.* **2017**, *36*, 1549–1552. [CrossRef]
17. Ract, P.; Piau-Couapel, C. In vitro activity of tedizolid and comparator agents against Gram-positive pathogens responsible for bone and joint infections. *J. Med Microbiol.* **2017**, *66*, 1374–1378. [CrossRef]
18. Carvalhaes, C.G.; Sader, H.S. Tedizolid in vitro activity against Gram-positive clinical isolates causing bone and joint infections in hospitals in the USA and Europe (2014-17). *J. Antimicrob. Chemother.* **2019**, *74*, 1928–1933. [CrossRef]
19. Prokocimer, P.; De Anda, C. Tedizolid Phosphate vs Linezolid for Treatment of Acute Bacteria Skin Structure Infections. The ESTABLISH-1 Randomized Trial. *JAMA* **2013**, *309*, 559–569. [CrossRef]
20. Moran, G.J.; Fang, E. Tedizolid for 6 days versus linezolid for 10 days for acute bacterial skin and skin-structure infections (ESTABLISH-2): A randomised, double-blind, phase 3, non-inferiority trial. *Lancet Infect. Dis.* **2014**, *14*, 696–705. [CrossRef]
21. *Sivextro Package Insert*; Merck & Co., Inc.: Kenilworth, NJ, USA, 2016.
22. Lee, L.; Kor Hee, K. Rifampicin Reduces tedizolid Concentrations When Co-Administered in Healthy Volunteers. *Open Forum Infect. Dis.* **2019**, *6*, S576. [CrossRef]
23. Werth, B.J. Exploring the Pharmacodynamic Interactions Between tedizolid and Other Orally Bioavailable Antimicrobials Against Staphylococcus aureus and Staphylococcus epidermidis. *J. Antimicrob. Chemother.* **2017**, *72*, 1410–1414. [CrossRef] [PubMed]
24. Park, K.H.; Greenwood-Quaintance, K.E. Activity of tedizolid in Methicillin-Resistant Staphylococcus epidermidis Experimental Foreign Body-Associated Osteomyelitis. *Antimicrob. Agents Chemother.* **2017**, *61*, e01644-16. [CrossRef] [PubMed]
25. Anemüller, R.; Belden, K. Hip and Knee Section, Treatment, Antimicrobials: Proceedings of International Consensus on Orthopedic Infections. *J. Arthroplast.* **2019**, *34* (Suppl. S2), 463–475. [CrossRef]
26. Kim, T.; Wills, A.B. Safety and Tolerability of Long Term Use of tedizolid for Treatment of Nontuberculous Mycobacterial Infections. In *Abstracts of the IDWeek Conference, New Orleans, LA*; Abstract 577; 2016; Available online: www.idweek.org (accessed on 23 December 2020).
27. Khatchatourian, L.; Le Bourgeois, A. Correction of myelotoxicity after switch of linezolid to tedizolid for prolonged treatments. *J. Antimicrob. Chemother.* **2017**, *72*, 2135–2136. [CrossRef]
28. Ferry, T.; Batailler, C. Correction of Linezolid-Induced Myelotoxicity After Switch to tedizolid in a Patient Requiring Suppressive Antimicrobial Therapy for Multidrug-Resistant Staphylococcus epidermidis Prosthetic-Joint Infection. *Open Forum Infect. Dis.* **2018**, *5*. [CrossRef]
29. Lan, S.H.; Lin, W.T. Tedizolid Versus Linezolid for the Treatment of Acute Bacterial Skin and Skin Structure Infection: A Systematic Review and Meta-Analysis. *Antibiotics* **2019**, *8*, 137. [CrossRef]

30. Ferry, T.; Seng, P.; Mainard, D.; Jenny, J.Y.; Laurent, F.; Senneville, E.; Grare, M.; Jolivet-Gougeon, A.; Bernard, L.; Marmor, S. The CRIOAc healthcare network in France: A nationwide Health Ministry program to improve the management of bone and joint infection. *Orthop. Traumatol. Surg. Res.* **2019**, *105*, 185–190. [CrossRef]
31. Parvizi, J.; Tan, T.L. The 2018 Definition of Periprosthetic Hip and Knee Infection: An Evidence-Based and Validated Criteria. *J. Arthroplast.* **2018**, *33*, 1309–1314. [CrossRef]
32. Zimmerli, W.; Sendi, P. Orthopedic-implant associated infections. In *Mandell, Douglas, and Bennett's principles and Practice of Infectious Diseases*, 8th ed.; Bennett, J.E., Dolin, R., Blaser, M., Eds.; Elsevier: Philadelphia, PA, USA, 2014; pp. 1328–1340.

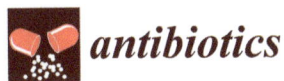

Article

Long-Term Use of Tedizolid in Osteoarticular Infections: Benefits among Oxazolidinone Drugs

Eva Benavent [1,2], Laura Morata [2,3,4], Francesc Escrihuela-Vidal [1], Esteban Alberto Reynaga [5], Laura Soldevila [1,2], Laia Albiach [3], Maria Luisa Pedro-Botet [5], Ariadna Padullés [6], Alex Soriano [2,3,4] and Oscar Murillo [1,2,4,*]

1. Infectious Diseases Department, Hospital Universitari de Bellvitge—IDIBELL, L'Hospitalet de Llobregat, University of Barcelona, 08907 Barcelona, Spain; eva.benavent@bellvitgehospital.cat (E.B.); fescrihuela@bellvitgehospital.cat (F.E.-V.); laura.soldevila@bellvitgehospital.cat (L.S.)
2. Bone and Joint Infection Study Group of the Spanish Society of Infectious Diseases and Clinical Microbiology (GEIO-SEIMC), 28003 Madrid, Spain; lmorata@clinic.cat (L.M.); asoriano@clinic.cat (A.S.)
3. Infectious Diseases Department, Hospital Clínic-IDIBAPS, University of Barcelona, 08036 Barcelona, Spain; lalbiach@clinic.cat
4. Spanish Network for Research in Infectious Diseases (REIPI RD16/0016/0003), Instituto de Salud Carlos III, 28029 Madrid, Spain
5. Department of Infectious Diseases, Hospital Germans Trias i Pujol, 08916 Barcelona, Spain; ereynaga@hotmail.com (E.A.R.); mlpbotet.germanstrias@gencat.cat (M.L.P.-B.)
6. Department of Pharmacy, Hospital Universitari de Bellvitge—IDIBELL, L'Hospitalet de Llobregat, University of Barcelona, 08907 Barcelona, Spain; apadulles@bellvitgehospital.cat
* Correspondence: omurillo@bellvitgehospital.cat; Tel.: +34-93-260-76-25

Abstract: Background: To evaluate the efficacy and safety of long-term use of tedizolid in osteoarticular infections. Methods: Multicentric retrospective study (January 2017–March 2019) of osteoarticular infection cases treated with tedizolid. Failure: clinical worsening despite antibiotic treatment or the need of suppressive treatment. Results: Cases (n = 51; 59% women, mean age of 65 years) included osteoarthritis (n = 27, 53%), prosthetic joint infection (n = 17, 33.3%), and diabetic foot infections (n = 9, 18%); where, 59% were orthopedic device-related. Most frequent isolates were Staphylococcus spp. (65%, n = 47; S. aureus, 48%). Reasons for choosing tedizolid were potential drug-drug interaction (63%) and cytopenia (55%); median treatment duration was 29 days (interquartile range -IQR- 15–44), 24% received rifampicin (600 mg once daily) concomitantly, and adverse events were scarce (n = 3). Hemoglobin and platelet count stayed stable throughout treatment (from 108.6 g/L to 116.3 g/L, $p = 0.079$; and 240×10^9/L to 239×10^9/L, $p = 0.942$, respectively), also in the subgroup of cases with cytopenia. Among device-related infections, 33% were managed with implant retention. Median follow-up was 630 days and overall cure rate 83%; among failures (n = 8), 63% were device-related infections. Conclusions: Long-term use of tedizolid was effective, showing a better safety profile with less myelotoxicity and lower drug-drug interaction than linezolid. Confirmation of these advantages could make tedizolid the oxazolidinone of choice for most of osteoarticular infections.

Keywords: tedizolid; oxazolidinones; osteoarticular infections; diabetic foot infections; drug-drug interaction

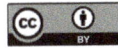

1. Introduction

Oxazolidinones are a young family of antibiotics that have a wide action against Gram-positive bacteria and include the first designed linezolid and the recent tedizolid. In comparison with the former, tedizolid has shown a higher in vitro activity against some microorganisms (four- to eight-fold lower minimum inhibitory concentration (MIC) values), and its pharmacokinetic/pharmacodynamics parameters allow the once-daily administration, which may improve treatment adherence. Also, tedizolid at approved doses seems to provide a better safety profile and less adverse events than linezolid, especially in relation with myelotoxicity and drug–drug interaction [1–3].

Tedizolid is currently only approved for acute bacterial skin and skin structure infections (ABSSSIs), not including diabetic foot infections [4,5]. However, it seems reasonable that tedizolid can be used in other clinical settings where linezolid has played a relevant role. In this sense, difficult-to-treat osteoarticular infections mainly due to staphylococci constitute a notable scenario where linezolid has provided good efficacy [6–8]. However, adherence to linezolid treatment may involve some difficulties such as (i) the appearance of myelotoxicity at two to four weeks of treatment, since osteoarticular infections usually require longer treatments [8,9]; (ii) the decrease in linezolid serum levels when combined with rifampicin, an anti-staphylococcal agent widely used in device-related infections [10–13]; and (iii) the risk of serotonin syndrome when administered concomitantly with antidepressants broadly used nowadays [14,15].

Despite the potential advantages of tedizolid in osteoarticular infections (higher microbiological activity, advantageous pharmacokinetic/pharmacodynamics parameters, lower myelotoxicity, and drug–drug interactions) [1–3], clinical data on long-term treatment are scarce [16]. Knowledge is limited to a few experimental studies [17–19], case reports [20] and recently some case series in which tedizolid is prescribed for different indication including osteoarticular infections [21,22]. Thus, in the present study, we intend to describe our multicenter experience within the Spanish Network for Research in Infectious Diseases (REIPI) with long-term use of tedizolid in a cohort of patients with osteoarticular and diabetic foot infections and focused on the efficacy and safety in monotherapy or combination.

2. Results

A total of 51 cases were included in our study. Mean age was 64.8 ± 14.3 and 59% ($n = 30$) were women. Median Charlson Index adjusted by age was 4 (IQR 3–7). Obesity was present in 33% ($n = 15$) of the cases; other frequent comorbidities were diabetes mellitus ($n = 21$, 41%), chronic renal disease ($n = 16$, 31%), malignancies ($n = 7$, 14%), and chronic anemia ($n = 4$, 8%).

There were 53% ($n = 27$) diagnosis of osteoarthritis ($n = 17$ cases of peripheral osteomyelitis, $n = 6$ septic arthritis and $n = 4$ vertebral osteomyelitis; of which 1 case presented simultaneously with septic arthritis of the ankle and osteomyelitis of the tibia), 33% ($n = 17$) cases had a prosthetic joint infection ($n = 8$ post-surgical acute, $n = 8$ chronic and 1 case with intraoperative positive cultures), and there were 18% ($n = 9$) cases of diabetic foot infection, one of them presenting also with vertebral osteomyelitis. Thirty cases (59%) were orthopedic device-related infections. Only two cases (4%) had bacteremia (both due to methicillin-susceptible *Staphylococcus aureus*).

Microorganisms responsible for osteoarticular infections were identified in all but two cases. There were 20 cases (39%) of polymicrobial etiology, 11 of them at the expense of different Gram-positive isolates that were all treated with tedizolid, and the remaining cases were mixed with Gram-positive and Gram-negative microorganisms. All Gram-positive microorganisms involved are presented in Table 1.

Tedizolid was administered at a dosage of 200 mg per day orally for a median of 29 days (IQR 15–44); 63% of the cases ($n = 32$) received tedizolid for more than 21 days, and in 70% of the cases ($n = 36$) time under tedizolid treatment represented more than 50% of the whole antibiotic treatment duration. Causes for prescription of tedizolid are presented in Table 2 (in 14 cases there was more than one reason); most common reason for initiate tedizolid was the potential interaction between baseline treatment and linezolid (65%), followed by the presence of anemia and/or thrombocytopenia (37%) and toxicity caused by a previous antibiotic (16%).

Table 1. Gram-positive microorganisms responsible of osteoarticular infections and treated with tedizolid, from the 72 isolates in the whole cohort.

Microorganism	Total	%
Staphylococcus spp	47	65.3%
Staphylococcus aureus	21	29.2%
Methicillin resistant *S. aureus*	10	47.6%
Coagulase negative staphylococci	26	36.1%
Staphylococcus epidermidis	18	25%
Others	8	11.1%
Other gram positives	13	18.1%
Corynebacterium striatum	4	5.6%
Enterococcus spp. [1]	4	5.6%
Streptococcus spp. [2]	3	4.2%
Cutibacterium acnes	1	1.4%
Actinotignum schaali	1	1.4%

[1] *Enterococcus faecium* $n = 3$, *Enterococcus raffinosus* $n = 1$. [2] *Streptococcus pyogenes* $n = 1$, *Streptococcus oralis* $n = 1$, *Streptococcus agalactiae* $n = 1$.

Table 2. Reasons for Tedizolid prescription.

Reasons for Tedizolid prescription	N	%
Potential interaction with Linezolid	33	64.7%
Antidepressants [1]	26	51%
Opioids	12	23.5%
Neuroleptics	4	7.8%
Anticonvulsants	2	4%
Cytopenia	19	37.3%
Anemia	10	19.6%
Thrombocytopenia	1	2%
Both	8	15.7%
Toxicity of previous antibiotic treatment	8	15.7%
Failure of previous antibiotic treatment	3	5.9%
Other [2]	2	3.9%

[1] All cases were under treatment with Serotonin Reuptake Inhibitors (SRIs). [2] Shortage of Linezolid.

Tedizolid was mainly administered as part of sequential switching therapy ($n = 47$, 92%; 3 cases as salvage therapy after failure), and only in 4 cases (8%) was the initial treatment. Tedizolid was given in monotherapy ($n = 27$, 53%) and in combination ($n = 24$, 47%) almost in similar proportion; among combination therapy, in half of the cases ($n = 12$) tedizolid was combined with rifampicin (600 mg once daily) representing 25% of all staphylococci infections. Less usual tedizolid combinations were used to treat polymicrobial infections with participation of Gram-negative bacteria; among them the most frequent drugs were quinolones ($n = 7$, 14%) and carbapenems ($n = 4$, 5%).

Beside therapy with tedizolid, most of the cases were managed surgically ($n = 41$, 80%); among device-related infections, implants were removed in 57% cases. Among cases with an evaluable outcome ($n = 48$; median of follow-up 630 days, IQR 269–818), the overall cure rate was 83% and 8 cases (17%) failed. There were 3 deaths, all of them non-related neither with the infection nor with tedizolid therapy, in which the outcome could not be evaluated due to short follow-up after treatment. The cure and failure rates among each type of osteoarticular infection are presented in Figure 1. Among failures, 4 of them were prosthetic joint infections (3 of them were put on suppressive antibiotic treatment and the remaining one underwent further surgery to cure the infection), 3 cases of osteoarthritis (one case was a device-related infection managed with implant removal), and a case of diabetic foot infection. Among staphylococci infections, there was no difference in outcome when tedizolid was used in monotherapy vs. combination with rifampicin (failure rate of 21% vs. 0%, respectively, $p = 0.118$).

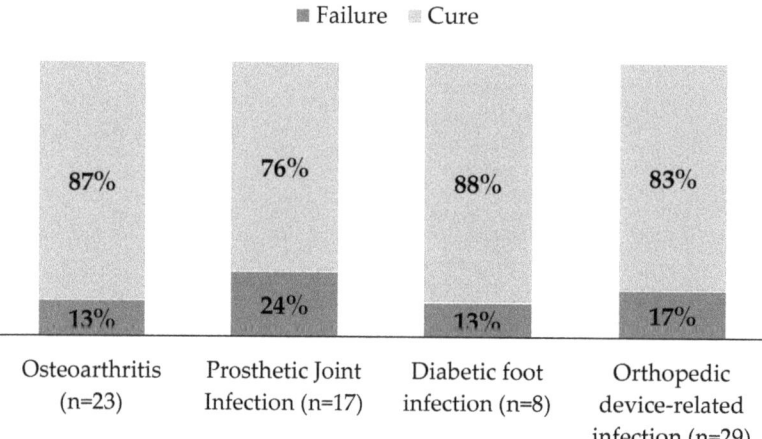

Figure 1. Failure rates among different types of osteoarticular infection.

Therapy with tedizolid was well tolerated; the only adverse effect observed was gastrointestinal disturbances in three cases (6%; nausea and occasional vomiting), but in any case, treatment was withdrawn.

There was no worsening on the hemoglobin or platelet counts in the blood tests between the beginning and the end of treatment with tedizolid neither in the group of patients with cytopenia nor in those without (Table 3) or those where treatment was prolonged for more than 21 days. In three cases, linezolid was switched to tedizolid because myelotoxicity of the former and patients completed treatment without additional worsening. The use of rifampicin in combination with tedizolid did not produce significant differences in the final levels of hemoglobin or platelets in comparison with tedizolid in monotherapy (Figure 2).

Table 3. Analytic values of patients under Tedizolid treatment.

Hematological Parameters	N	At the Beginning of Treatment with Tedizolid (mean, SD)	At the End of Treatment with Tedizolid (mean, SD)	p Value	Use of Rifampicin	Days with Tedizolid (Median, IQR)
Hemoglobin (g/L)	45	108.6 ± 20.3	116.3 ± 18.4	0.079	-	29 (15–44)
No anemia *	10	137.5 ± 15.5	141.5 ± 11.8	0.596	30%	29 (17–42)
Mild anemia *	10	114.2 ± 4.4	116.4 ± 11.9	0.586	10%	20.5 (15–29)
Moderate and severe anemia *	25	94.7 ± 2	105.4 ± 3.2	0.004	28%	31 (14–44)
Platelet count ($\times 10^9$/L)	45	240.6 ± 114.6	238.9 ± 92.3	0.942	-	29 (15–44)
>150 × 10^9/L	33	290.7 ± 15.6	252 ± 20.7	0.134	30.3%	29 (17–42)
<150 × 10^9/L	12	102.7 ± 8.3	196.5 ± 17.5	0.001	8.3%	37 (9–100)
Leucocytes($\times 10^9$/L)	45	6.42	6.51	0.887	-	29 (15–44)

* In accordance with definition in Section 4.2. No anemia was considered when; Hb > 130 g/L for men and Hb > 120 g/L for women. Mild anemia; Hb 110–129 g/L for men and Hb 110–119 g/L for women. Moderate anemia considered Hb < 109 g/L and severe anemia Hb < 80 g/L for men and women in both cases.

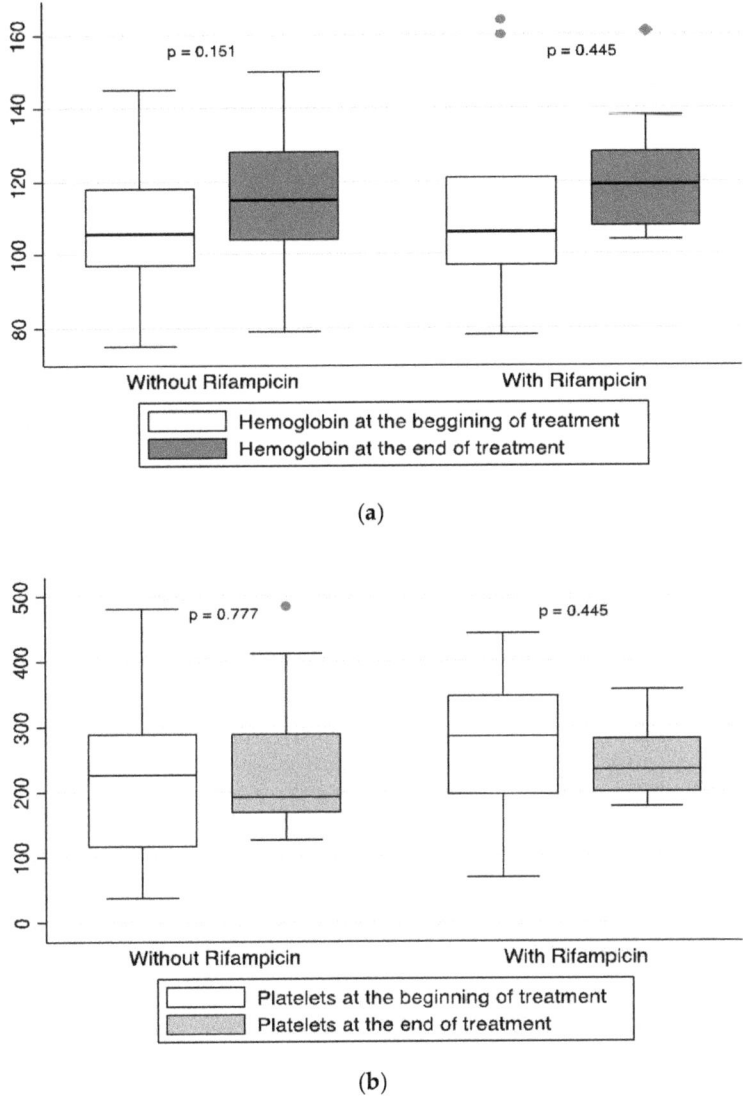

Figure 2. Mean comparison of hemoglobin values and platelet count at the beginning and the end of treatment for those cases receiving Tedizolid in monotherapy (**a**) or combination with Rifampicin (**b**).

Finally, among cases treated with tedizolid because of potential interaction between linezolid and baseline treatment ($n = 33$), they were treated for a median of 34 days (IQR 17–51) and we did not observe adverse events (i.e., serotonin syndrome) or alteration of basal disease (i.e., depressive syndrome) either during therapy with tedizolid or after it was stopped.

3. Discussion

Tedizolid is recommended for the treatment of ABSSSIs for six days and still, there is limited information in other settings or prolonged treatments. In the present study, we provide data about efficacy, the safety of long-term use (median of 29 days), and benefits of tedizolid in a large cohort of patients with osteoarticular and diabetic foot infections.

Linezolid, the first approved oxazolidinone drug, has provided good outcomes in osteoarticular infections [6–8,12]; however, there are still some concerns for its long-term use regarding adverse events and drug–drug interactions. Comparing with linezolid, tedizolid shows a better microbiological activity and more favorable pharmacokinetic/pharmacodynamics parameters when used at the recommended dose of 200 mg daily. In our experience, tedizolid both in monotherapy or combination provide good efficacy in this field (cure rate 83%), comparable to that of linezolid. These results are difficult to compare with previous work, because to our knowledge, there are no studies focused on tedizolid efficacy in diabetic foot infections and only a recent experience of tedizolid for more than six days in different types of infections, including some osteoarticular infection cases [22]. Thus, larger experience in this setting is needed, but our results seem to be in the line of considering tedizolid a good therapeutic alternative.

Among adverse events observed when using linezolid, anemia and/or thrombocytopenia is common when its use is prolonged beyond two weeks [9,12,23]. It requires monitoring patients, especially those with previous cytopenia or particular risk factors. Tedizolid can also cause dose-related myelotoxicity [16], but at a lower rate than linezolid [24]. Safety of long-term use of tedizolid was evaluated in healthy volunteers for 21 days [16], while most of the information in patients is limited to six days of treatment in ABSSSIs [4,5,21], and there is little information with longer therapies where the appearance of thrombocytopenia and anemia was observed in 7.4 and 1.2%, respectively [22]. In our experience, tedizolid was administered a median of 29 days and was well tolerated without relevant hematologic adverse events appearing or need for withdrawn, even in cases with moderate/severe cytopenia at the start of therapy or those that were switched to tedizolid after developing linezolid myelotoxicity [25].

Among the most relevant drug–drug interactions of linezolid, its use with rifampicin should be emphasized since it is a major anti-staphylococcal agent broadly used in osteoarticular infections always in combination. Previous studies confirmed the interaction between both drugs [3,13,26], as a result, serum linezolid levels decrease [10,11]. Interestingly, this effect between tedizolid and rifampicin was not found in preclinical studies [3,17]; however, well-designed clinical and pharmacokinetic studies are not available. In our experience, despite not determining the comparative serum levels of tedizolid when monotherapy or combination with rifampicin was used, we did not observe differences in the clinical outcome or the impact on hemoglobin or platelet counts in both groups. If the absence of interaction between rifampicin and tedizolid is confirmed, the latter could displace the use of linezolid in those patients who require it in a rifampicin combination.

Finally, treatment with linezolid can also be challenging when given concomitantly with monoamine oxidase inhibitors and other antidepressants due to the risk of serotonin syndrome, a rare but serious complication [14,15]. Tedizolid exhibits a weak reversible monoamine oxidase inhibition in vitro effect, so drug–drug interaction is lower [27]. The potential drug–drug interaction was the main reason (62.8%) for choosing tedizolid in our cohort, and none of the patients interrupted their baseline treatment and no adverse event was observed.

Our study has several limitations inherent to its retrospective nature, as well as the heterogeneity between the different osteoarticular infections, and the limited number of cases. As a result, the inference of our results in particular scenarios should be taken with caution while waiting for wider experience. Also, the different surgical approaches, which are a cornerstone of the treatment of osteoarticular infections, and the use of other antibiotics before tedizolid or in combination (mainly with rifampicin), may have played a role in the overall outcome. Furthermore, to assess the suitability of the rifampicintedizolid combination or the use of tedizolid concomitantly with antidepressants, further specific studies are needed. However, to our knowledge this is the first study assessing long-term use of tedizolid specifically in osteoarticular infections and carried out by specialists in the field and, therefore, the information provided in terms of efficacy and safety is of interest.

4. Materials and Methods

4.1. Study Population and Settings

We conducted a retrospective multicenter study in three Spanish hospitals of the REIPI-GEIO Network (January 2017 to March 2019). We included adult patients attended for osteoarticular and diabetic foot infections caused by Gram-positive bacteria who had received as part of their antibiotic treatment tedizolid at a regimen dose of 200 mg daily for at least 7 days. Polymicrobial infections with the participation of Gram-negative microorganisms were also included, whenever they received tedizolid in combination for their treatment. Those cases where Gram-positive bacteria were involved after a different primary infection (superinfection) were excluded.

We aimed to evaluate the efficacy and safety of cases treated with tedizolid for a long-term period. Additionally, we aimed to evaluate the potential drug–drug interaction between tedizolid and rifampicin or antidepressants.

4.2. Definitions and Data Collection

Osteoarticular infections were classified into 3 groups: osteoarthritis (including cases with peripheral or vertebral osteomyelitis and septic arthritis), prosthetic joint infections, and diabetic foot infections. All cases met the main diagnostic criteria [28–30] and management was carried out according to the attending medical team, in all cases, antibiotic treatment was tailored by infectious diseases specialists.

Presence of anemia was classified in mild anemia when hemoglobin concentration was between 110–129 g/L for men and 110–119 g/L for women, moderate anemia when hemoglobin was below 109 g/L, and severe when it was below 80 g/L. Thrombocytopenia was considered when platelet count was below 150×10^9/L.

Demographic data and baseline characteristics were collected. The presence of depressive syndrome was specifically registered and the use of drugs with potential major interaction with oxazolidinones such as mono-amino oxidase inhibitors, selective serotonin reuptake inhibitors, opioids, and anticonvulsant drugs. The presence or absence of orthopedic devices was documented and also the need for debridement surgery and removal or exchange of orthopedic devices when necessary. Antibiotic treatment previous and concomitant with tedizolid was also recorded. Microbiologic data were obtained from intraoperative cultures, joint fluid samples, or targeted biopsies.

Written informed consent was considered not necessary for the study, as it was a retrospective analysis of our clinical practice. Data of patients were anonymized for the purposes of this analysis. Confidential information of patients was protected according the Declaration of Helsinki. This manuscript was revised for its publication by Research Ethics Committee of Bellvitge University Hospital (PR459/20).

4.3. Follow Up and Outcome

To monitor possible hematologic toxicity, we documented laboratory data at the beginning of treatment with tedizolid, during treatment, and at the end of the antibiotic treatment. The patients also underwent clinical follow-up to detect the presence of other adverse events; gastrointestinal or neuropathic toxicity (optical and peripheral).

Cases were considered cured when there was no clinical evidence of infection and no other need for antibiotic or surgical treatment once treatment with tedizolid was concluded. Failure was considered when reappearance of infection signs once treatment was already concluded, in cases of none improvement despite active treatment with tedizolid, the need of suppressive antibiotic therapy to control the infection or death related with the infection.

4.4. Statistical Analysis

Data were analyzed with Stata 14.2 (Stata Corporation, Texas 77845, USA). Categorical variables were described by counts and percentages, while mean and standard deviation or median and interquartile range (IQR) were used to summarize continuous variables. Comparisons between groups were performed with either the chi-square test or Fisher exact test for categorical variables, and the *t*-test or Mann-Whitney U test was used for continuous variables.

5. Conclusions

In conclusion, tedizolid was effective and safe providing a valid therapeutic alternative for osteoarticular infections. Its higher microbiological activity and better pharmacokinetic/pharmacodynamics parameters comparing with linezolid, allow it to be used at doses that show a better safety profile with less myelotoxicity and lower drug-drug interaction including rifampicin and antidepressants. If further studies confirm these advantages, tedizolid may become the oxazolidinone of choice in most patients with osteoarticular infections.

Author Contributions: E.B., L.M., F.E.-V., E.A.R., L.S., L.A., M.L.P.-B., A.P., A.S., O.M. contributed in the supervision of the clinical cases, data collection, and interpretation; F.E.-V., A.P., and O.M. elaborated the study design; E.B. performed the analysis of the data and wrote the first draft of the manuscript. All authors have read and agreed to the published version of the manuscript.

Funding: E.B. was supported with a grant of the Instituto de Salud Carlos III—Ministry of Science and Innovation (FI 16/00397). This research did not receive any specific grant from funding agencies in the public, commercial, or not-for-profit sectors.

Institutional Review Board Statement: The study was conducted according to the guidelines of the Declaration of Helsinki, and approved by the Ethics Committee of Bellvitge University Hospital (protocol code PR459/20).

Informed Consent Statement: Patient consent was waived due to the retrospective nature of the study on the usual clinical practice.

Data Availability Statement: The data presented in this study are available on request from the corresponding author (omurillo@bellvitgehospital.cat).

Acknowledgments: We thank John B. Warren (International House Barcelona) for reviewing the English manuscript. The preliminary results of this study were reported in part at the 30th European Congress of Clinical Microbiology & Infectious Diseases (Paris, France, 2020). We thank CERCA Programme / Generalitat de Catalunya for institutional support.

Conflicts of Interest: O.M. has received honoraria for talks on behalf of Merck Sharp and Dohme and Pfizer. A.S. has received honoraria for lectures and advisory meetings from Pfizer, Merck, Angelini, Shionogi, Menarini, and Gilead. L.M. has received honoraria for talks on behalf of Merck Sharp and Dohme, Pfizer and Angelini. All other others declare no potential conflicts of interest relevant to this article.

References

1. Zhanel, G.G.; Love, R.; Adam, H.; Golden, A.; Zelenitsky, S.; Schweizer, F.; Gorityala, B.; Lagacé-Wiens, P.R.S.; Rubinstein, E.; Walkty, A.; et al. Tedizolid: A novel oxazolidinone with potent activity against multidrug-resistant gram-positive pathogens. *Drugs* **2015**, *75*, 253–270. [CrossRef] [PubMed]
2. Flanagan, S.; Fang, E.; Muñoz, K.A.; Minassian, S.L.; Prokocimer, P.G. Single- and multiple-dose pharmacokinetics and absolute bioavailability of tedizolid. *Pharmacotherapy* **2014**, *34*, 891–900. [CrossRef]
3. Douros, A.; Grabowski, K.; Stahlmann, R. Drug-drug interactions and safety of linezolid, tedizolid, and other oxazolidinones. *Expert Opin. Drug Metab. Toxicol.* **2015**, *11*, 1849–1859. [CrossRef]
4. Prokocimer, P.; De Anda, C.; Fang, E.; Mehra, P.; Das, A. Tedizolid phosphate vs linezolid for treatment of acute bacterial skin and skin structure infections: The ESTABLISH-1 randomized trial. *JAMA* **2013**, *309*, 559–569. [CrossRef] [PubMed]
5. Moran, G.J.; Fang, E.; Corey, G.R.; Das, A.F.; De Anda, C.; Prokocimer, P. Tedizolid for 6 days versus linezolid for 10 days for acute bacterial skin and skin-structure infections (ESTABLISH-2): A randomised, double-blind, phase 3, non-inferiority trial. *Lancet Infect. Dis.* **2014**, *14*, 696–705. [CrossRef]

6. Morata, L.; Tornero, E.; Martínez-Pastor, J.C.; García-Ramiro, S.; Mensa, J.; Soriano, A. Clinical experience with linezolid for the treatment of orthopaedic implant infections. *J. Antimicrob. Chemother.* **2014**, *69*, 47–52. [CrossRef]
7. Senneville, E.; Legout, L.; Valette, M.; Yazdanpanah, Y.; Beltrand, E.; Caillaux, M.; Migaud, H.; Mouton, Y. Effectiveness and tolerability of prolonged linezolid treatment for chronic osteomyelitis: A retrospective study. *Clin. Ther.* **2006**, *28*, 1155–1163. [CrossRef]
8. Cobo, J.; Lora-Tamayo, J.; Euba, G.; Jover-Sáenz, A.; Palomino, J.; Del Toro, M.D.; Rodríguez-Pardo, D.; Riera, M.; Ariza, J. Linezolid in late-chronic prosthetic joint infection caused by gram-positive bacteria. *Diagn. Microbiol. Infect. Dis.* **2013**, *76*, 93–98. [CrossRef] [PubMed]
9. Boak, L.M.; Rayner, C.R.; Grayson, M.L.; Paterson, D.L.; Spelman, D.; Khumra, S.; Capitano, B.; Forrest, A.; Li, J.; Nation, R.L.; et al. Clinical population pharmacokinetics and toxicodynamics of linezolid. *Antimicrob. Agents Chemother.* **2014**, *58*, 2334–2343. [CrossRef] [PubMed]
10. Blassmann, U.; Roehr, A.C.; Frey, O.R.; Koeberer, A.; Briegel, J.; Huge, V.; Vetter-Kerkhoff, C. Decreased Linezolid Serum Concentrations in Three Critically Ill Patients: Clinical Case Studies of a Potential Drug Interaction between Linezolid and Rifampicin. *Pharmacology* **2016**, *98*, 51–55. [CrossRef] [PubMed]
11. Pea, F.; Viale, P.; Cojutti, P.; Del pin, B.; Zamparini, E.; Furlanut, M. Therapeutic drug monitoring may improve safety outcomes of long-term treatment with linezolid in adult patients. *J. Antimicrob. Chemother.* **2012**, *67*, 2034–2042. [CrossRef] [PubMed]
12. Legout, L.; Valette, M.; Dezeque, H.; Nguyen, S.; Lemaire, X.; Loïez, C.; Caillaux, M.; Beltrand, E.; Dubreuil, L.; Yazdanpanah, Y.; et al. Tolerability of prolonged linezolid therapy in bone and joint infection: Protective effect of rifampicin on the occurrence of anaemia? *J. Antimicrob. Chemother.* **2010**, *65*, 2224–2230. [CrossRef]
13. Gandelman, K.; Zhu, T.; Fahmi, O.A.; Glue, P.; Lian, K.; Obach, R.S.; Damle, B. Unexpected effect of rifampin on the pharmacokinetics of linezolid: In silico and in vitro approaches to explain its mechanism. *J. Clin. Pharmacol.* **2011**, *51*, 229–236. [CrossRef]
14. Morales-Molina, J.A.; de Antonio, J.M.; Marín-Casino, M.; Grau, S. Linezolid-associated serotonin syndrome: What we can learn from cases reported so far. *J. Antimicrob. Chemother.* **2005**, *56*, 1176–1178. [CrossRef]
15. Taylor, J.J.; Wilson, J.W.; Estes, L.L. Linezolid and serotonergic drug interactions: A retrospective survey. *Clin. Infect. Dis.* **2006**, *43*, 180–187. [CrossRef] [PubMed]
16. Lodise, T.P.; Bidell, M.R.; Flanagan, S.D.; Zasowski, E.J.; Minassian, S.L.; Prokocimer, P. Characterization of the haematological profile of 21 days of tedizolid in healthy subjects. *J. Antimicrob. Chemother.* **2016**, *71*, 2553–2558. [CrossRef] [PubMed]
17. Park, K.-H.; Greenwood-Quaintance, K.E.; Schuetz, A.N.; Mandrekar, J.N.; Patel, R. Activity of Tedizolid in Methicillin-Resistant Staphylococcus epidermidis Experimental Foreign Body-Associated Osteomyelitis. *Antimicrob. Agents Chemother.* **2017**, *61*, 1–8. [CrossRef] [PubMed]
18. Park, K.-H.; Greenwood-Quaintance, K.E.; Mandrekar, J.; Patel, R. Activity of Tedizolid in Methicillin-Resistant Staphylococcus aureus Experimental Foreign Body-Associated Osteomyelitis. *Antimicrob. Agents Chemother.* **2016**, *60*, 6568–6572. [CrossRef]
19. Carvalhaes, C.G.; Sader, H.S.; Flamm, R.K.; Mendes, R.E. Tedizolid in vitro activity against Gram-positive clinical isolates causing bone and joint infections in hospitals in the USA and Europe (2014–17). *J. Antimicrob. Chemother.* **2019**, *74*, 1928–1933. [CrossRef]
20. Si, S.; Durkin, M.J.; Mercier, M.M.; Yarbrough, M.L.; Liang, S.Y. Successful treatment of prosthetic joint infection due to vancomycin-resistant enterococci with tedizolid. *Infect. Dis. Clin. Pract.* **2017**, *25*, 105–107. [CrossRef]
21. Kullar, R.; Puzniak, L.A.; Swindle, J.P.; Lodise, T. Retrospective Real-World Evaluation of Outcomes in Patients with Skin and Soft Structure Infections Treated with Tedizolid in an Outpatient Setting. *Infect. Dis. Ther.* **2020**, *6*. [CrossRef] [PubMed]
22. Vendrell, M.M.; Pitarch, M.T.; Lletí, M.S.; Muñoz, E.C.; Ruiz, L.M.; Lao, G.C.; Suñé, E.L.; Pueyo, J.M.; Sempere, M.R.O.; Montoya, M.L.P.B.; et al. Safety and tolerability of more than six days of tedizolid treatment. *Antimicrob. Agents Chemother.* **2020**, *64*, 1–9. [CrossRef] [PubMed]
23. Gerson, S.L.; Kaplan, S.L.; Bruss, J.B.; Le, V.; Arellano, F.M.; Hafkin, B.; Kuter, D.J. Hematologic effects of linezolid: Summary of clinical experience. *Antimicrob. Agents Chemother.* **2002**, *46*, 2723–2726. [CrossRef] [PubMed]
24. Flanagan, S.; McKee, E.E.; Das, D.; Tulkens, P.M.; Hosako, H.; Fiedler-Kelly, J.; Passarell, J.; Radovsky, A.; Prokocimer, P. Nonclinical and pharmacokinetic assessments to evaluate the potential of tedizolid and linezolid to affect mitochondrial function. *Antimicrob. Agents Chemother.* **2015**, *59*, 178–185. [CrossRef]
25. Ferry, T.; Batailler, C.; Conrad, A.; Triffault-Fillit, C.; Laurent, F.; Valour, F.; Chidiac, C.; Ferry, T.; Valour, F.; Perpoint, T.; et al. Correction of Linezolid-Induced Myelotoxicity After Switch to Tedizolid in a Patient Requiring Suppressive Antimicrobial Therapy for Multidrug-Resistant Staphylococcus epidermidis Prosthetic-Joint Infection. *Open Forum Infect. Dis.* **2018**, *5*, 1–2. [CrossRef]
26. Egle, H.; Trittler, R.; Kümmerer, K.; Lemmen, S. Linezolid and rifampin: Drug interaction contrary to expectations? *Clin. Pharmacol. Ther.* **2005**, *77*, 451–453. [CrossRef]
27. Flanagan, S.; Bartzial, K.; Minassian, S.L.; Fang, E.; Prokocimer, P. In vitro, In Vivo, and clinical studies of tedizolid to assess the potential for peripheral or central monoamine oxidase interactions. *Antimicrob. Agents Chemother.* **2013**, *57*, 3060–3066. [CrossRef]
28. Osmon, D.R.; Berbari, E.F.; Berendt, A.R.; Lew, D.; Zimmerli, W.; Steckelberg, J.M.; Rao, N.; Hanssen, A.; Wilson, W.R. Diagnosis and Management of Prosthetic Joint Infection: Clinical Practice Guidelines by the Infectious Diseases Society of America. *Clin. Infect. Dis.* **2013**, *56*, e1–e25. [CrossRef]

29. Lew, D.P.; Waldvogel, F.A. Osteomyelitis. *Lancet* **2004**, *364*, 369–379. [CrossRef]
30. Lipsky, B.A.; Senneville, É.; Abbas, Z.G.; Aragón-Sánchez, J.; Diggle, M.; Embil, J.M.; Kono, S.; Lavery, L.A.; Malone, M.; Asten, S.A.; et al. Guidelines on the diagnosis and treatment of foot infection in persons with diabetes (IWGDF 2019 update). *Diabetes Metab. Res. Rev.* **2020**, *36*, 1–24. [CrossRef]

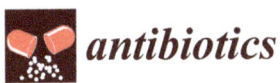

Review

Dalbavancin for the Treatment of Prosthetic Joint Infections: A Narrative Review

Luis Buzón-Martín [1,2,*], Ines Zollner-Schwetz [3], Selma Tobudic [4], Emilia Cercenado [5,6,7] and Jaime Lora-Tamayo [2,8,9]

1. Department of Internal Medicine, Infectious Diseases Division, Hospital Universitario de Burgos, 09006 Burgos, Spain
2. Bone and Joint Infection Study Group of the Spanish Society of Infectious Diseases and Clinical Microbiology (GEIO-SEIMC), 28003 Madrid, Spain; sirsilverdelea@yahoo.com
3. Section of Infectious Diseases and Tropical Medicine, Department of Internal Medicine, Medical University of Graz, 8036 Graz, Austria; ines.schwetz@medunigraz.at
4. Department of Medicine I, Division of Infectious Diseases and Tropical Medicine, Medical University of Vienna, 1090 Wien, Austria; selma.tobudic@meduniwien.ac.at
5. Servicio de Microbiología y Enfermedades Infecciosas, Hospital General Universitario Gregorio Marañón, 28007 Madrid, Spain; emilia.cercenado@salud.madrid.org
6. CIBER Enfermedades Respiratorias-CIBERES (CB06/06/0058), 28029 Madrid, Spain
7. Medicine Department, School of Medicine, Universidad Complutense de Madrid, 28040 Madrid, Spain
8. Department of Internal Medicine, Hospital Universitario 12 de Octubre, Instituto de Investigación Hospital 12 de Octubre i + 12, 28041 Madrid, Spain
9. Red Española de Investigación en Patología Infecciosa (REIPI), 28029 Madrid, Spain
* Correspondence: luisbuzonmartin78@gmail.com

Abstract: Dalbavancin (DAL) is a lipoglycopeptide with bactericidal activity against a very wide range of Gram-positive microorganisms. It also has unique pharmacokinetic properties, namely a prolonged half-life (around 181 h), which allows a convenient weekly dosing regimen, and good diffusion in bone tissue. These features have led to off-label use of dalbavancin in the setting of bone and joint infection, including prosthetic joint infections (PJI). In this narrative review, we go over the pharmacokinetic and pharmacodynamic characteristics of DAL, along with published in vitro and in vivo experimental models evaluating its activity against biofilm-embedded bacteria. We also examine published experience of osteoarticular infection with special attention to DAL and PJI.

Keywords: dalbavancin; prosthetic joint infection; gram-positive

1. Introduction

Total joint arthroplasties are common worldwide, and the incidence of this surgery is expected to increase steadily in the coming years as the population ages [1]. The most feared complication is infection, which is not associated with high mortality rates, but does carry substantial morbidity, may require many surgeries, and the final results in terms of limb functionality and pain resolution are not always satisfactory. At the same time, prosthetic joint infections (PJI) represent a massive economic burden for healthcare systems that continues to rise, and is expected to be around $1.62 billion in USA by 2030 [2].

PJIs are complex infections, in which the formation of biofilm, enabling bacteria to evade the host immune system, is crucial. Biofilm-embedded bacteria can also develop phenotypic changes that ultimately lead to antimicrobial tolerance and infection persistence. Not all antimicrobials perform equally in this scenario, and not all antibiotics are ideal for the treatment of PJI. In this context, the arrival of new antimicrobials is very welcome [3].

DAL is a lipoglycopeptide (Xydalba; https://www.ema.europa.eu (accessed on 27 May 2021)) that is almost universally active against Gram-positive bacteria, which are by far the leading cause of PJIs [4]. A number of clinical trials [4–7] have demonstrated its safety and efficacy for the treatment of skin and soft tissue infections, which stand as the only licensed indication for this antibiotic. However, the wide antimicrobial spectrum of this drug and its unique pharmacokinetic (PK) properties, with a half-life of 181 h [8] and prolonged concentrations in bone tissue [9], along with a good safety profile have led physicians to use it for a number of off-label indications [10,11], which include the treatment of bone and joint infections as well as PJI. In addition, resistance emergence under DAL treatment is, although possible, a very rare phenomenon. In this particular setting, the need for treatment over long periods, coupled with the long half-life of DAL mean that the antibiotic can be used on a convenient weekly basis.

In this narrative review, we assess the role of DAL in the treatment of PJI. We review the drug's PK profile, pharmacodynamic (PD) properties, activity against biofilm-embedded bacteria in in vitro and in vivo experimental models, and finally, we evaluate the available clinical experience in PJI.

2. Search Strategy and Selection Criteria

The PubMed database was screened for any manuscript published at any time addressing the efficacy of DAL in the setting of biofilm-associated infections, bone and joint infections, and especially PJI. The terms "dalbavancin", "prosthetic joint infection", "biofilm", "foreign-body", "arthroplasty", and "osteomyelitis" were combined. Abstracts and relevant full-length articles were reviewed, and a thorough search was made of the references in these papers in order to select other significant studies. Our review is not exhaustive but focuses on relevant articles regarding the efficacy on DAL on the setting of PJI, and it was restricted to articles written in English and Spanish. We directly contacted the corresponding authors of published cases series of PJI treated with DAL in order to obtain further details.

Definitions

MIC_{50}: Minimum inhibitory concentration required to inhibit the growth of 50% of organisms.

MIC_{90}: Minimum inhibitory concentration required to inhibit the growth of 90% of organisms.

MBIC: Minimum biofilm inhibitory concentration. The lowest concentration of an antimicrobial agent required to inhibit the formation of biofilms.

MBBC: Minimum biofilm bactericidal concentration. The lowest concentration of an antimicrobial agent that eradicates 99.9% of biofilm-embedded bacteria.

3. Dalbavancin in Prosthetic Joint Infections

3.1. DAL Pharmacokinetics

The pharmacokinetics of DAL are linear and dose-proportional, with the peak concentration (C_{max}) and area under the curve (AUC) increasing according to the dose administered, while its half-life ($T_{1/2}$) of around 7 days remains essentially unchanged [8]. A high protein-bound fraction (>90%) contributes to this prolonged $T_{1/2}$ [12,13]. It has been proven that serum bactericidal activity remains measurable at 7 days after a dose of 500 mg or higher, which establishes the basis for the weekly based dosing regimen proposed [8,14]. DAL concentrations before the following weekly dose have consistently been shown to range from 33.0 µg/mL to 40.2 µg/mL [12]. For skin and soft tissue infections, the recommended dosage consists of a loading dose of 1000 mg followed by 500 mg seven days later. C_{max} and AUC for doses of 500 and 1000 mg of DAL are 133 µg/mL and 312 µg/mL and 11,393 µg·h/mL and 27,103 µg·h/mL, respectively [8].

Solon et al. studied the diffusion of 20 mg/kg of DAL in bone tissue and periarticular structures by administering radioactive [^{14}C]-DAL to rats. Over a 14-day period, the mean bone-to-plasma concentration ratio was 0.63, and the AUC in bone was 1125 µg eq·h/mL [15]. Later, in a phase-1 trial, Dunne et al. showed that DAL concentrations in cortical bone 12 h and 2 weeks after a single infusion of 1000 mg of DAL were 6.3 µg/g and 4.1 µg/g, respectively. In that study, the bone-to-plasma AUC ratio was determined to be 0.13. Of interest, based on population PK modeling, that study proposed a DAL regimen consisting of two 1500-mg intravenous infusions 1 week apart, which would provide concentrations in bone above the MIC$_{90}$ for staphylococci for at least 8 weeks [9].

There is little information regarding intracellular concentrations of DAL. In macrophages, it has been observed to be higher than vancomycin and teicoplanin [13]. Still, we are not aware of studies on the activity against intracellular bacteria, which may be important reservoirs of infection in the setting of biofilm-associated infections [16].

In contrast with other glycopeptides (i.e., vancomycin, teicoplanin), one-third of the dose of DAL was observed to be excreted unchanged into urine, suggesting that additional non-renal pathways of elimination, probably feces, are important, as demonstrated previously in rat models [17]. Although dose adjustment does not seem necessary for mild renal impairment, patients with creatinine clearance <30 mL/min would need dose adjustment. In contrast, hemodialysis is not an important route of elimination of DAL, so that dose adjustment is not required as described in the summary of product characteristics (Xydalba; https://www.ema.europa.eu (accessed on 27 May 2021)). DAL is neither a substrate, nor an inhibitor or inducer of liver CYP-450. DAL does not require dosage adjustment in patients with hepatic impairment either [18].

3.2. DAL Pharmacodynamics

3.2.1. Mechanism of Action and Determination of In Vitro Activity of Dalbavancin

DAL is a semisynthetic drug, structurally derived from the natural glycopeptide A40926 produced by *Nonomuraea* spp. [19], and its structure is closely related to teicoplanin. DAL inhibits the late stages of peptidoglycan synthesis interrupting bacterial cell wall synthesis by binding to the terminal D-alanyl–D-alanine terminus of pentapeptide peptidoglycan precursors [20].

Determination of DAL minimum inhibitory concentration (MIC) must be made by the standard broth microdilution method in cation-adjusted Mueller–Hinton broth supplemented with 0.002% (v/v) polysorbate-80. In addition, the gradient diffusion method procedure (Etest®) can be used as an alternative that has also demonstrated a high degree of agreement with the standardized broth microdilution method (EUCAST: The European Committee on Antimicrobial Susceptibility Testing. Breakpoint tables for interpretation of MICs and zone diameters. Version 11.0, 2021. http://www.eucast.org (accessed on 27 May 2021) [21]. The disk diffusion method and the agar dilution method are unreliable for the determination of susceptibility to dalbavancin.

The European Committee on Antimicrobial Susceptibility Testing (EUCAST) has defined the breakpoints for interpretation of DAL MICs only against *Staphylococcus* spp., *Streptococcus* groups A, B, C, and G, and *Streptococcus anginosus* group (*S. anginosus, S. intermedius, S. constellatus*), with those isolates with DAL MICs of $\leq$0.125 mg/L being susceptible, and those with dalbavancin MIC values of >0.125 mg/L being resistant. In addition, EUCAST has established DAL PK/PD non-species related breakpoints, with the isolates with DAL MICs of $\leq$0.25 mg/L being susceptible and those with MICs > 0.25 mg/L being resistant.

3.2.2. In Vitro Activity of Dalbavancin against Planktonic Gram-Positive Microorganisms

DAL is bactericidal against most Gram-positive microorganisms commonly involved in the etiology of PJI (essentially *Staphylococcus* spp., *Streptococcus* spp. and *Enterococcus* spp.).

Data from worldwide collections of strains have shown very low DAL MIC values. Of interest, the most recent data on behalf of DAL activity against all these microorganisms, as of January 2021, show that DAL MIC$_{90}$ values have remained stable, being $\leq$0.06 µg/mL against different species [22]. In *S. aureus*, resistance to dalbavancin is exceptional, and the MIC$_{90}$ is 16-fold lower than that of vancomycin (VAN) (0.06 µg/mL vs. 1 µg/mL) [23]. DAL activity has also been observed to be the same irrespective of oxacillin susceptibility [20,24], in contrast to coagulase-negative staphylococci (CoNS), which show a DAL MIC$_{90}$ of 0.06 and 0.12 µg/mL for strains susceptible and resistant to oxacillin, respectively [25]. Since almost all *S. aureus* strains that are vancomycin-susceptible are also DAL-susceptible, vancomycin susceptibility can be considered a surrogate marker of DAL activity. Consequently, vancomycin-resistant *S. aureus* (VRSA) is also resistant to DAL, and its usefulness against heteroresistant vancomycin-intermediate *S. aureus* (hVISA) is currently a matter for debate [26]. The loss of susceptibility against other anti-Gram-positive antibiotics (i.e., teicoplanin, telavancin, daptomycin, and linezolid) does not correlate with a decrease in DAL activity [27]. In the case of CoNS, Cercenado et al. observed that DAL maintained its activity even against teicoplanin-resistant strains, as long as teicoplanin MIC was ≤8 µg/mL. (P1500: XXVII European Congress of Clinical Microbiology and Infectious Diseases; 22–25 April 2017; Vienna, Austria). In summary, according to published data, DAL is very active against *Staphylococcus* spp. with MIC_{90} values below the EUCAST susceptibility breakpoint.

Regarding enterococci, DAL activity against vancomycin-susceptible enterococci is comparable to that of staphylococci, although vancomycin-resistant *Enterococcus* spp. pose a challenge for DAL, as this antimicrobial is not active against isolates exhibiting the VanA phenotype. However, DAL is active against strains displaying the VanB phenotype (vancomycin-resistant, with variable susceptibility to teicoplanin), showing MIC_{90} values around 1 µg/mL, and it is also active against strains of *E. gallinarum* and *E. casseliflavus* that express the VanC phenotype, characterized by intrinsic resistance to vancomycin, but susceptibility to teicoplanin. Overall, it can again be assumed that vancomycin susceptibility is a good surrogate marker of DAL susceptibility in *Enterococcus* spp. and that teicoplanin susceptibility can also be used as a surrogate in vancomycin-resistant strains [23,24].

DAL activity against *Streptococcus* spp. (including penicillin-resistant *viridans* group isolates, penicillin-resistant *S. pneumoniae*, *S. anginosus* group, and ß-haemolytic streptococci) is very high. Resistance to DAL in streptococci is anecdotal, as MIC_{90} values are below 0.3 µg/mL for *S. viridans* and 0.12 µg/mL for *S. agalactiae* [23,28–30]. Finally, DAL has also been found to be active against other Gram-positive microorganisms eventually found to be the cause of PJI. MIC_{90} values for *Corynebacterium* spp. range between <0.03 and 0.5 µg/mL, and DAL also shows bactericidal activity against anaerobic Gram-positive cocci, such as *Peptostreptococcus* spp., *Finegoldia magna*, and *Anaerococcus* spp., with MIC_{90} ranging from 0.12 to 0.5 µg/mL [23,30,31]. Concerning its activity against *Cutibacterium acnes* (formerly *Propionibacterium acnes*), Goldstein et al. [30], in a study including 15 isolates, communicated MICs ranging from 0.03 to 0.5 mg/L, with MIC_{50} and MIC_{90} values of 0.25 and 0.5 mg/L, respectively.

As indicated above, it is important to note that EUCAST (www.eucast.org (accessed on 27 May 27 2021)) has not defined a DAL breakpoint for *Corynebacterium* spp. and for anaerobes and defines a non-species related PK/PD breakpoint for DAL of ≤0.25 µg/mL. In this regard, antimicrobial susceptibility testing should be performed in all of the above-described organisms with MIC_{90} values of 0.5 mg/L.

3.2.3. Activity of DAL against Biofilms of Gram-Positive Microorganisms: In Vitro Experience

A number of studies evaluating the activity of DAL against biofilm formation and eradication are summarized in Table 1 [30–35]. Overall, antimicrobial susceptibility studies on 96-well microtiter plates have shown that very low DAL concentrations are able to inhibit biofilm formation in a very large number of strains of staphylococci (both methicillin-susceptible and methicillin-resistant), streptococci, and enterococci ($MBIC_{90}$ < 1 µg/mL). These values were lower than those observed for other antimicrobials such as vancomycin ($MBIC_{90}$ 2–4 µg/mL), tedizolid, and daptomycin. Concentrations needed to eradicate biofilm are higher, with $MBBC_{90}$ ranging from 1 to 16 µg/mL depending on the species, but they were still much lower relative to other comparators (vancomycin $MBBC_{90}$ > 32–128 µg/mL). The exception were vancomycin-resistant enterococci, which showed very high $MBIC_{90}$ and $MBBC_{90}$ for all the anti-Gram-positive antimicrobials tested, including DAL. Regardless of the vancomycin resistance type (VanA or VanB phenotypes), all vancomycin-resistant enterococci had dalbavancin MICs, MBICs, and MBBCs > 16 µg/mL [33].

Table 1. Summary of in vitro and in vivo pre-clinical models of dalbavancin activity against biofilm-embedded bacteria.

Reference	Microorganisms	Design	Results
Fernández et al., 2016 [32] & Schmidt-Malan et al., 2016 [34]	171 staphylococcal clinical isolates from prosthetic joint infections	Adapted Calgary-device [1]. Biofilms were 6 h mature before confronting antibiotics during 20 h. Comparators: DAL, VAN and TDZ, at increasing concentrations.	DAL: $MBIC_{90}$ 0.12–0.50 µg/mL, $MBBC_{90}$ 2–4 µg/mL VAN: $MBIC_{90}$ 2–4 µg/mL, $MBBC_{90}$ >128 µg/mL TDZ: $MBIC_{90}$ 2–4 µg/mL, $MBBC_{90}$ >32 µg/mL
Knafl et al., 2017 [36]	10 MRSA plus 10 MRSE clinical strains	96-well microtiter plate with a 24 h biofilm, exposed during 24 h to increasing concentrations of DAL. Measure of remaining biofilm was made by CV dying [2]. No comparators.	MRSA: MIC range 0.031–0.064 µg/mL; MBC 1–4 µg/mL MRSE: MIC range 0.023–0.625 µg/mL; MBC 2–16 µg/mL
Neudorfer et al., 2018 [33]	Clinical isolates 58 *E. faecalis* 25 *E. faecium*	Adapted Calgary-device [1]. Biofilms were 6 h mature before confronting antibiotics during 20 h. Comparators: DAP and VAN	DAL: for VSE: $MBIC_{90}$ 0.25 µg/mL, $MBBC_{90}$ 1 µg/mL for VRE: $MBIC_{90}$ > 16 µg/mL, $MBBC_{90}$ >16 µg/mL VAN: $MBIC_{90}$ 2 µg/mL, $MBBC_{90}$ >128 µg/mL for VRE: $MBIC_{90}$ > 128 µg/mL, $MBBC_{90}$ > 128 µg/mL DAP: for VSE: $MBIC_{90}$ 4 µg/mL, $MBBC_{90}$ 128 µg/mL for VRE: $MBIC_{90}$ 4 µg/mL, $MBBC_{90}$ 128 µg/mL
Di Pilato et al., 2020 [35]	9 clinical isolates plus 3 referral isolates (3 MSSA, 3 MRSA, 2 MSSE, 4 MRSE)	Model 1. Adapted Calgary device. Biofilms were 7-days mature before confronting antibiotics during other 7 d. Model 2. Ti and Cr-Co disks cultured during 48 h and then confronted to antibiotics during 7 d. Both experiments used DAL and VAN at doses of 1, 4, and 16 µg/mL	Model 1. Heterogeneous response to antibiotics. Overall, DAL showed a higher and faster reduction of biofilm-embedded bacteria over time as compared with VAN, both at lower and higher dosages. Model 2. Similar effect against biofilm formed over Ti and Cr-Co disks, except for medium dosages (4 µg/mL), where DAL showed higher reductions of biofilm-embedded bacteria
Žiemytė et al., 2020 [37]	Clinical isolates of MSSA, MRSA and MRSE	Experiments of biofilm inhibition and treatment (6–9 h-old biofilms). Measurement of biofilm growing over 20 h by electrical impedance. Treatment with increasing concentrations of DAL, CLX, VAN, LNZ, and RIF	1. Biofilm inhibition. MBIC of DAL ranged 0.5–2 µg/mL. RIF and DAL showed the highest inhibitory efficacy as compared with CLX, VAN and LNZ. 2. Biofilm treatment. DAL stopped or reduced biofilm at 8–32 µg/mL. Comparators had no effect for *S. aureus* biofilm. For *S. epidermidis* biofilm, RIF and CLX were more effective than DAL at lower concentrations.
Darouiche et al., 2005 [38]	*S. aureus* (MIC 0.06 µg/mL)	Rabbit model of infection with catheter tips implanted in subcutaneous pockets. Treatments are administered pre-operatively so to avoid the infection of the foreign material. DAL is given at 10 mg/kg, and VAN at 20 mg/kg (and then again 24 h after surgery)	In animals treated with placebo, only 47% of catheter tips were infected. The rate of infection in the DAL group was 28% (p = 0.2 when compared to placebo), and 53% in the VAN group (p = 0.8). Serum C_{max} of DAL was 80.3 µg/mL, and at day 3 it was 1.3 µg/mL. At day 7 it was only detectable in two rabbits of four (0.4 and 0.6 µg/mL).
Baldoni et al., 2013 [39]	MRSA ATCC 43300 MIC 0.078 µg/mL	Tissue-cage infection model in guinea-pigs. Treatment starts 3 days after inoculation. Three regimes of DAL: 40 mg/kg—C_{max} 44.6 µg/mL, AUC_{0-7d} 3393 µg·h/mL 60 mg/kg—C_{max} 55.6 µg/mL, AUC_{0-7d} 4298 µg·h/mL 80 mg/kg—C_{max} 68.8 µg/mL, AUC_{0-7d} 4464 µg·h/mL [3] $T_{1/2}$ 35.8 to 45.4 h. Other regimes: DAL + RIF, RIF	DAL monotherapies had a discreet killing (inferior to RIF alone) with an infection eradication rate of 0%. The combination of RIF + DAL achieved an eradication rate similar to RIF alone (25–36%). Only high doses of DAL (80 mg/kg) avoided the emergence of rifampin resistance.
Barnea et al., 2016 [40]	MRSA (Clinical strain). MIC 0.06 µg/mL	Rat animal infection model of wound infection and sternal osteomyelitis. Treatment started 24 h after inoculation. DAL was given as an initial bolus of 20 mg/kg followed by 10 mg/kg/d for 7 or 14 days. VAN was given at 50 mg/kg/12 h for 7 or 14 days.	DAL was similar to VAN and better than the absence of treatment. Administration of DAL and VAN avoided systemic dissemination of staphylococcal infection. Concentration of DAL in bone tissue at 4, 6 and 10 days was 9.5 µg/g, 9.2 µg/g, and 10.7 µg/g, respectively

DAL: Dalbavancin. DAP: Daptomycin. VAN: Vancomycin. LNZ: Linezolid. TDZ: Tedizolid. CLX: Cloxacillin. RIF: Rifampin. MRSA: Methicillin-resistant *Staphylococcus aureus*. MSSA: Methicillin-susceptible *S. aureus*. MRSE: Methicillin-resistant *Staphylococcus epidermidis*. MSSE: Methicillin-susceptible *S. epidermidis*. VSE: Vancomycin-susceptible enterococci. VRE: Vancomycin-resistant enterococci. CV: Crystal violet. MIC: Minimal inhibitory concentration. [1] Pegged-lids confronted to 96-well microtiter plates. MBIC (minimal biofilm inhibitory concentration) is determined by turbidity after confronting the pegs with antibiotics. MBBC (minimal biofilm bactericidal concentration) is determined after incubating the pegged-lid in 96-well microtiter plates with fresh media after having confronted the pegs with antibiotics. [2] MBC was defined as a 50%-reduction in the optic density value as compared with positive controls in the 96-well microtiter plate. [3] PK of 80 mg/kg is comparable to data observed in blister of patients after a single dose of DAL 1000 mg (C_{max} 67 µg/mL, and AUC_{0-7d} 6438 µg·h/mL) [41].

Information regarding the anti-biofilm activity of DAL using models with long exposure times was almost non-existent until the end of the last decade, when Di Pilato et al. evaluated the time-kill kinetics of DAL against biofilms of nine clinical strains of *S. aureus* and CoNS, using both a standardized biofilm model and biofilms grown on titanium and cobalt-chrome disks. DAL and vancomycin were used at concentrations of 1, 4, and 16 µg/mL. Against biofilms formed over 7 days on microtiter plates, the response to antibiotics was heterogeneous, although DAL showed faster and greater reduction of biofilm-embedded bacteria in the majority of the strains studied, especially at concentrations of 4 µg/mL and 16 µg/mL. In biofilms formed on Ti and Co-Cr disks, DAL was more active than vancomycin at medium concentrations (4 µg/mL), which may be expected in bone tissue [35].

More recently, Žiemytė et al. proposed a real-time, impedance-based cell analysis in order to facilitate the determination of antimicrobial susceptibility when bacteria grow in biofilms [37]. In this study, DAL ability to prevent *S. aureus* and *S. epidermidis* biofilm formation was compared with that of other antimicrobials commonly used for treating PJI (linezolid, rifampin, vancomycin, cloxacillin). The MBIC of DAL ranged from 0.5 to 2 µg/mL, and in combination with rifampin showed the highest biofilm inhibitory effect. With respect to the eradication of 6- to 9-h biofilm, DAL stopped or reduced biofilm formation at concentrations of 8–32 µg/mL. The other antimicrobials showed no activity against biofilm formed by *S. aureus*. For biofilms of *S. epidermidis*, low concentrations of DAL were active, although less than the combination of cloxacillin plus rifampin.

3.2.4. Activity of DAL against Biofilm of Gram-Positive Microorganisms: Experimental In Vivo Experience

A few in vivo experimental models [37–39,42] have assessed the efficacy of DAL in biofilm prevention and treatment (Table 1). Darouiche et al. compared DAL, vancomycin, and a placebo for preventing colonization of subcutaneously placed devices in a rabbit animal model inoculated with 10^3 colony-forming units of *S. aureus*. Although not statistically significant, there was a trend toward a lower colonization rate in rabbits that received DAL before the procedure [38]. Nevertheless, the rate of foreign body contamination in rabbits receiving placebo was around 50% (lower as compared with other animal models), thus questioning the validity of the model and its discriminatory power for assessing the efficacy of antimicrobials.

In 2013, Baldoni et al. tested the ability of DAL to eliminate methicillin-resistant *S. aureus* (MRSA) biofilms in an animal model of tissue-cage infection. DAL and rifampin were administered intraperitoneally, the former at different doses (20, 40, and 80 mg/kg, which produced AUC_{0-7d} of 3393, 4298, and 4464 µg·h/mL, respectively). In monotherapy, DAL yielded a very modest killing, but in combination with rifampin, eradicated infection in one third of the cages. Of note, only the higher dosage (80 mg/kg) of DAL was able to prevent the development of rifampin resistance [39].

More recently, Barnea et al. studied the efficacy of DAL for the treatment of sternal osteomyelitis and mediastinitis caused by MRSA using a median sternotomy model in Lewis rats. The efficacy of DAL was proven to be similar to that of vancomycin for the treatment of sternal osteomyelitis and superior to placebo, and also reduced systemic dissemination of staphylococcal infection. DAL concentrations in bone tissue after 10 days of administration were 10.7 µg/g [40].

The models of animal infection suggest a role for DAL in the PJI setting, although some concerns arise after a thorough study of their results. First, in contrast to many of the in vitro studies previously reviewed, the dosages of DAL in some of the in vivo models may have provided lower antibiotic exposure compared to human PK. Second, more data on the combination of DAL with rifampin and comparisons with other rifampin-based combinations would be welcome in order to place DAL in the armamentarium of PJI caused by Gram-positive microorganisms.

3.2.5. Clinical Experience with DAL for Treating Prosthetic Joint Infections

As stated above, the broad antimicrobial spectrum of DAL and its PK properties support its use outside its approved indications. DAL is an attractive alternative in scenarios such as bloodstream infections, endocarditis, and osteomyelitis [10,43–46], even though clinical trials exploring these off-label indications of DAL are scarce.

However, in a randomized clinical trial, Rappo et al. explored the efficacy and safety of DAL for the treatment of osteomyelitis known or suspected to be caused by Gram-positive pathogens [46]. In that single-center study conducted in the Ukraine, DAL was compared with the standard of care (vancomycin was the most frequently used comparator) and the primary endpoint was clinical response at day 42. Failure was defined as the requirement of additional antibiotics, new purulence, the need for new surgery, and/or amputation. A clinical cure at day 42 was 97% in the DAL arm compared to 88% in the standard of care. Reported follow up only extends to 1 year. Even though the patients included did not have orthopedic hardware, the results are encouraging for the use of DAL in the treatment of osteitis persisting after prosthesis removal, in other words, in the setting of a two-step exchange procedure.

Meanwhile, scattered cases have been reported [47]. Furthermore, Buzón-Martín et al. reported their experience of 16 cases of PJI treated with DAL, which is so far the largest single-institution report [48]. Brief details of surgical strategies and antimicrobial treatment were provided. Overall, so as to now, 88% of patients had their infection resolved and there were no major adverse events (Buzón-Martín, unpublished data).

In addition, a number of case series with real-world experience with DAL have been published, also including cases of PJI (Table 2) [45,48–52]. Common limitations found in these case series are the inclusion of small sample sizes, patient heterogeneity, aggregate outcomes of patients with PJI along with other orthopedic-related infections, and lack of details about surgical management. In fact, the goals and difficulties of treatment vary considerably depending on the type of PJI (acute vs. chronic) and whether the prosthesis is retained or removed. The main objectives of the treatment of PJI are to eradicate infection and maintain a pain-free prosthetic joint. In this context, one of three major strategies can be chosen when faced with a given PJI: To attempt eradication and cure with prosthesis retention (debridement, antibiotics, and implant retention—DAIR), attempt eradication and cure with prosthesis removal (followed by prosthesis reimplantation in either a one- or two-stage exchange procedure, or else a joint arthrodesis), or prosthesis retention, abandoning the attempt to eradicate the infection in favor of chronic suppressive antimicrobial therapy [53]. Bearing this in mind, a given antibiotic can perform very differently depending on which surgical strategy has been chosen.

Table 2. Clinical series published on the experience with DAL, including cases of bone and joint infection and prosthetic joint infection.

Reference	n	Bone & Joint Infection (Other than PJI)	Episodes of PJI	PJI Outcome (Success, %)
Bouza et al., 2017 [51]	69	13	20	80%
Morata et al., 2019 [50]	64	NP	26	NP
Tobudic et al., 2019 [45]	72	20	8	75%
Wunsch et al., 2019 [49]	101	30	32	94%
Martín et al., 2019 [48]	16	0	16	88%
Dinh et al., 2019 [52]	75	48	NP	NP

NP: not provided. PJI: prosthetic joint infection.

An additional limitation of these studies is the wide heterogeneity in the use of DAL, even within the same institutions. Loading doses on day 1 ranged from 1000 mg to 1500 mg, and following doses at day 7 ranged from 500 to 1500 mg. The number of doses was also very variable, as some patients were treated with just two doses after prosthesis removal and others received more than 20 doses in the setting of a suppressive strategy [45,48,49,54]. Some authors [48] have even suggested that a biweekly administration strategy might be useful in this setting. As mentioned before, Dunne et al. [9] settled the rationale basis for a weekly administration of two doses of 1500 mg of DAL, and Rappo et al. proved its efficacy for treating osteomyelitis [46]. Noteworthily, these two 1500 mg doses on day 1 and day 7 of the scheme were only used in 6 out of 12 cases in the Graz series [49], but were not used in the series of Buzón-Martín, Tobudic, and Morata [45,48,50]. So far, the ideal dosing strategy of DAL for PJI remains unanswered, but perhaps two 1500 mg doses on day 1 and 7 after prosthetic removal is the scheme with a more solid investigational and clinical evidence backup [9,46].

In order to overcome the limitation of the studies heterogeneity, we contacted the authors of three of the above-mentioned case series. Dr. Zollner-Schwetz, Dr. Tobudic, and Dr. Buzón-Martín kindly provided more specific data of 36 patients treated at their institutions (Table 3). The majority of patients had already been given other antimicrobials and undergone previous surgeries, and DAL was used as salvage therapy, thus facing greater challenges. The reported etiologies were also heterogeneous, and half the patients were given DAL in combination. DAIR management was anecdotal in these cases and was only performed in two patients. The majority of infections were treated with prosthesis removal (27/36, 75%), a strategy that led to a success rate of 25/27 (92.6%) after a median follow up of 16 months. Within this group, 20/27 (74%) patients were treated with a two-stage revision procedure, two (7.4%) with single-stage revision, and three (11.1%) patients with resection arthroplasty. Of interest, a number of patients were treated with prosthesis retention plus DAL as suppressive antimicrobial therapy (7/36, 19.4%) with successful retention of the prosthesis in the short term in three cases (42.9%). Although large series of suppressive treatment with DAL for other conditions are lacking, there is some evidence to suggest that DAL can be safely administered as compassionate treatment for several months, or even years for non-surgical prosthetic endocarditis (Dr. Buzón-Martín, unpublished data).

Table 3. Cases of PJI treated with dalbavancin according to the surgical strategy adopted (data from Buzón et al., Tobudic et al., and Wunsch et al.).

	DAIR (n = 2)	Prosthesis Removal (n = 27)	Implant Retention and Suppressive Treatment (n = 7)	All Patients (n = 36)
Sex (female)	1 (50%)	11 (40.7%)	3 (42%)	15 (43%)
Age *,[1] (years)	69 (67–71)	69 (18–87)	62 (15–92)	67 (15–92)
Number of surgeries before DAL	1	2 (1–4)	2.5 (1–3)	1.8 (1–4)
Treatments				
DAL alone	2 (100%)	11 (40.7%)	5 (71%)	18 (50%)
DAL + rifampin	0	7 (26%)	2	9 (25%)
DAL + other treatments	0	9 (30%)	0	9 (25%)
Etiology				
S. aureus [2]	0	5 (18.5%)	1 (14%)	6 (17%)
CoN staphylococci	2 (100%)	6 (22.2%)	2 (29%)	10 (28%)
Enterococcus spp [3]	0	4 (14.8%)	1 (14%)	5 (14%)
Anaerobic GP	0	1 (3.7%)	0	1 (3%)
Other GP	0	0	2 (29%)	2 (6%)
Mixed GP	0	10 (37%)		10 (28%)
Unknown etiology	0		1 (14%)	1 (3%)
Outcome (Success)	1 (50%)	25 (93%)	4 (57%) [4]	29 (81%)
Follow up (months) *,[1]	4 (2–6)	16 (3–40)	6 (3–14)	14 (2–40)

* Continuous variables are expressed as median and (range). [1] Data available for 20 patients. [2] There were 4 methicillin-susceptible strains (3 managed with prosthesis removal and 1 by suppressive antimicrobial therapy), and 2 methicillin-resistant strains (both managed by prosthesis removal). [3] There were 4 *E. faecium* (all treated with prosthesis removal) and 1 *E. faecalis* (treated with suppressive antimicrobial treatment). [4] One patient died to unrelated causes after three months with no clinical or biochemical signs of failure. Abbreviations: DAL: dalbavancin. CoN: coagulase-negative. GP: Gram-positives. DAIR: debridement, antibiotics, and implant retention.

Overall, these revisited cases suggest that there is still insufficient experience with the use of DAL in the setting of DAIR, but that good results can be expected in the case of prosthesis removal. The use of DAL as chronic suppressive therapy could be considered in very carefully selected situations when other alternatives are lacking, although we still need more experience and information regarding the most suitable and sustainable dosage. Finally, as expected, we still need to find out which is the best DAL dosing schedule for treating PJI.

3.3. DAL as a Cost-Saving Strategy

Cost-saving is an additional issue, which probably justifies the use of DAL in patients with PJI. In the DALBUSE study, Bouza et al. found DAL to be cost-saving [51], and Buzón-Martín et al. observed that the use of DAL allowed an early discharge of most patients, with a presumably relevant impact in terms of healthcare costs. Applying the same cost analysis previously reported by Bouza et al. in the DALBUSE study, an estimated 571 days of hospitalization were avoided and a total of US $264,769 saved [48].

Several other reports position DAL as a cost-saving alternative [55,56], although, in a recent study, the results of González et al. pointed in the opposite direction [57], finding DAL to be more expensive than the standard of care for the treatment of skin and soft tissue infections. Nevertheless, in the same journal, Bookstaver et al. replied with more specific considerations other than cost and calling for other issues to be taken into account when thinking about antimicrobial stewardship [58]. It is also important to state that cost-saving analyses are quite difficult to extrapolate from the USA to other health systems in Europe, mainly those that are 100% public.

4. Conclusions

DAL's unique PK properties and high bactericidal activity are attractive characteristics for the treatment of bone and joint infections, including PJI. The possibility of using DAL in an outpatient setting, with the associated cost-saving impact, as well as the obvious improvement in therapeutical adherence compared with oral treatments, increases its value in infections where long treatments are necessary.

With regard to this, although the specific DAL concentrations used in pre-clinical models are not always consistent with human PK, and there is very scarce information on intracellular activity, the results of DAL against biofilm-embedded bacteria are encouraging. In addition, a randomized clinical trial states that DAL is non-inferior to the standard of care in bone infections with no orthopedic hardware. The reported clinical experiences of use of DAL in PJI are scarce and heterogeneous, but its use in the setting of prosthesis removal seems reasonable and effective. We still need more data regarding its use in the setting of prosthesis retention, and also in combination with established antimicrobials such as rifampin.

Author Contributions: Conceptualization, L.B.-M. and J.L.-T.; methodology, L.B.-M., I.Z.-S., S.T., E.C. and J.L.-T.; software, L.B.-M. and J.L.-T.; validation, L.B.-M., I.Z.-S., S.T., E.C. and J.L.-T.; formal analysis, L.B.-M.; investigation, L.B.-M., I.Z.-S., S.T., E.C. and J.L.-T.; resources, L.B.-M., I.Z.-S., S.T., E.C. and J.L.-T.; data curation, L.B.-M., I.Z.-S., S.T. and J.L.-T.; writing—original draft preparation, L.B.-M.; writing—review and editing, L.B.-M. and J.L.-T.; visualization, L.B.-M., E.C. and J.L.-T.; supervision, L.B.-M. and J.L.-T.; project administration, L.B.-M. All authors have read and agreed to the published version of the manuscript.

Funding: This research received no external funding.

Institutional Review Board Statement: Ethical review and approval were waived for this study, as this is a review of previously published studies.

Informed Consent Statement: Not applicable.

Data Availability Statement: Not applicable.

Acknowledgments: We thank Janet Dawson for reviewing the English Manuscript. We are also indebted to Florian Thalhammer for his collaboration.

Conflicts of Interest: J.L.-T. and L.B.-M have received conference grants from Angelini. I.Z.-S. received conference grants from Angelini and served on an advisory board for Angelini.

References

1. Kurtz, S.; Ong, K.; Lau, E.; Mowat, F.; Halpern, M. Projections of primary and revision hip and knee arthroplasty in the United States from 2005 to 2030. *J. Bone Jt. Surg. Ser. A* **2007**, *89*, 780–785. [CrossRef]
2. Kurtz, S.M.; Lau, E.; Watson, H.; Schmier, J.K.; Parvizi, J. Economic burden of periprosthetic joint infection in the United States. *J. Arthroplast.* **2012**, *27*, 61–65. [CrossRef]
3. Beam, E.; Osmon, D. Prosthetic joint infection update. *Infect. Dis. Clin.* **2018**, *32*, 843–859. [CrossRef]
4. Tande, A.J.; Patel, R. Prosthetic joint infection. *Clin. Microbiol. Rev.* **2014**, *27*, 302–345. [CrossRef]
5. Dunne, M.W.; Puttagunta, S.; Giordano, P.; Krievins, D.; Zelasky, M.; Baldassarre, J. A randomized clinical trial of single-dose versus weekly dalbavancin for treatment of acute bacterial skin and skin structure infection. *Clin. Infect. Dis.* **2016**, *62*, 545–551. [CrossRef] [PubMed]
6. Jauregui, L.E.; Babazadeh, S.; Seltzer, E.; Goldberg, L.; Krievins, D.; Frederick, M.; Krause, D.; Satilovs, I.; Endzinas, Z.; Breaux, J.; et al. Randomized, double-blind comparison of once-weekly dalbavancin versus twice-daily linezolid therapy for the treatment of complicated skin and skin structure infections. *Clin. Infect. Dis.* **2005**, *41*, 1407–1415. [CrossRef] [PubMed]
7. Boucher, H.W.; Wilcox, M.; Talbot, G.H.; Puttagunta, S.; Das, A.F.; Dunne, M.W. Once-weekly dalbavancin *versus* daily conventional therapy for skin infection. *N. Engl. J. Med.* **2014**, *370*, 2169–2179. [CrossRef]
8. Leighton, A.; Gottlieb, A.B.; Dorr, M.B.; Jabes, D.; Mosconi, G.; VanSaders, C.; Mroszczak, E.J.; Campbell, K.C.M.; Kelly, E. Tolerability, pharmacokinetics, and serum bactericidal activity of intravenous dalbavancin in healthy volunteers. *Antimicrob. Agents Chemother.* **2004**, *48*, 1043–1046. [CrossRef] [PubMed]
9. Dunne, M.W.; Puttagunta, S.; Sprenger, C.R.; Rubino, C.; Van Wart, S.; Baldassarre, J. Extended-duration dosing and distribution of dalbavancin into bone and articular tissue. *Antimicrob. Agents Chemother.* **2015**, *59*, 1849–1855. [CrossRef]
10. Hidalgo-Tenorio, C.; Vinuesa, D.; Plata, A.; Dávila, P.M.; Iftimie, S.; Sequera, S.; Loeches, B.; Lopez-Cortés, L.E.; Fariñas, M.C.; Fernández-Roldan, C.; et al. DALBACEN cohort: Dalbavancin as consolidation therapy in patients with endocarditis and/or bloodstream infection produced by gram-positive cocci. *Ann. Clin. Microbiol. Antimicrob.* **2019**, *18*, 1–10. [CrossRef] [PubMed]
11. Hitzenbichler, F.; Mohr, A.; Camboni, D.; Simon, M.; Salzberger, B.; Hanses, F. Dalbavancin as long-term suppressive therapy for patients with Gram-positive bacteremia due to an intravascular source—A series of four cases. *Infection* **2021**, *49*, 181–186. [CrossRef]
12. Andes, D.; Craig, W.A. In Vivo Pharmacodynamic activity of the glycopeptide dalbavancin. *Antimicrob. Agents Chemother.* **2007**, *51*, 1633–1642. [CrossRef]
13. Monogue, M.; Nicolau, D.P. *Kucers the Use of Antibiotics*; CRC Press: Boca Raton, FL, USA, 2018; pp. 917–929.
14. Dorr, M.B.; Jabes, D.; Cavaleri, M.; Dowell, J.; Mosconi, G.; Malabarba, A.; White, R.J.; Henkel, T.J. Human pharmacokinetics and rationale for once-weekly dosing of dalbavacin, a semi-synthetic glycopeptide. *J. Antimicrob. Chemother.* **2005**, *55* (Suppl. S2), ii25–ii30. [CrossRef]
15. Solon, E.G.; Dowell, J.A.; Lee, J.; King, S.P.; Damle, B.D. Distribution of radioactivity in bone and related structures following administration of [14C]Dalbavancin to New Zealand white rabbits. *Antimicrob. Agents Chemother.* **2007**, *51*, 3008–3010. [CrossRef] [PubMed]
16. Murillo, O.; Pachón, M.E.; Euba, G.; Verdaguer, R.; Carreras, M.; Cabellos, C.; Cabo, J.; Gudiol, F.; Ariza, J. Intracellular antimicrobial activity appearing as a relevant factor in antibiotic efficacy against an experimental foreign-body infection caused by Staphylococcus aureus. *J. Antimicrob. Chemother.* **2009**, *64*, 1062–1066. [CrossRef]
17. Cavaleri, M.; Riva, S.; Valagussa, A.; Guanci, M.; Colombo, L.; Dowell, J.; Stogniew, M. Pharmacokinetics and excretion of dalbavancin in the rat. *J. Antimicrob. Chemother.* **2005**, *55*, ii31–ii35. [CrossRef] [PubMed]
18. Marbury, T.; Dowell, J.A.; Seltzer, E.; Buckwalter, M. Pharmacokinetics of dalbavancin in patients with renal or hepatic impairment. *J. Clin. Pharmacol.* **2009**, *49*, 465–476. [CrossRef]
19. Malabarba, A.; Goldstein, B.P. Origin, structure, and activity in vitro and in vivo of dalbavancin. *J. Antimicrob. Chemother.* **2005**, *55*, ii15–ii20. [CrossRef]
20. McCurdy, S.P.; Jones, R.N.; Mendes, R.; Puttagunta, S.; Dunne, M.W. In vitro activity of dalbavancin against drug-resistant *Staphylococcus aureus* Isolates from a global surveillance program. *Antimicrob. Agents Chemother.* **2015**, *59*, 5007–5009. [CrossRef] [PubMed]
21. Fritsche, T.R.; Rennie, R.P.; Goldstein, B.P.; Jones, R.N. Comparison of dalbavancin MIC values determined by Etest (AB BIODISK) and reference dilution methods using Gram-positive organisms. *J. Clin. Microbiol.* **2006**, *44*, 2988–2990. [CrossRef]
22. Sader, H.S.; Streit, J.M.; Mendes, R.E. Update on the in vitro activity of dalbavancin against indicated species (*Staphylococcus aureus*, *Enterococcus faecalis*, β-hemolytic streptococci, and *Streptococcus anginosus* group) collected from United States hospitals in 2017–2019. *Diagn. Microbiol. Infect. Dis.* **2021**, *99*, 115195. [CrossRef] [PubMed]
23. Cercenado, E. Espectro antimicrobiano de dalbavancina. Mecanismo de acción y actividad in vitro frente a microorganismos Gram positivos. *Enferm. Infecc. Microbiol. Clin.* **2017**, *35*, 9–14. [CrossRef]
24. Biedenbach, D.J.; Bell, J.M.; Sader, H.S.; Turnidge, J.D.; Jones, R.N. Activities of dalbavancin against a worldwide collection of 81,673 Gram-positive bacterial isolates. *Antimicrob. Agents Chemother.* **2009**, *53*, 1260–1263. [CrossRef]

25. Jones, R.N.; Flamm, R.K.; Sader, H.S. Surveillance of dalbavancin potency and spectrum in the United States (2012). *Diagn. Microbiol. Infect. Dis.* **2013**, *76*, 122–123. [CrossRef] [PubMed]
26. Bongiorno, D.; Lazzaro, L.M.; Stefani, S.; Campanile, F. In vitro activity of dalbavancin against refractory multidrug-resistant (MDR) *Staphylococcus aureus* isolates. *Antibiotics* **2020**, *9*, 865. [CrossRef]
27. Sader, H.S.; Mendes, R.; Duncan, L.R.; Pfaller, M.; Flamm, R.K. Antimicrobial activity of dalbavancin against *Staphylococcus aureus* with decreased susceptibility to glycopeptides, daptomycin, and/or linezolid from U.S. medical centers. *Antimicrob. Agents Chemother.* **2017**, *62*. [CrossRef]
28. Jones, R.N.; Sader, H.S.; Flamm, R.K. Update of dalbavancin spectrum and potency in the USA: Report from the SENTRY Antimicrobial Surveillance Program (2011). *Diagn. Microbiol. Infect. Dis.* **2013**, *75*, 304–307. [CrossRef]
29. Streit, J.M.; Fritsche, T.R.; Sader, H.S.; Jones, R.N. Worldwide assessment of dalbavancin activity and spectrum against over 6000 clinical isolates. *Diagn. Microbiol. Infect. Dis.* **2004**, *48*, 137–143. [CrossRef]
30. Goldstein, E.J.C.; Citron, D.M.; Warren, Y.A.; Tyrrell, K.L.; Merriam, C.V.; Fernandez, H.T. In vitro activities of dalbavancin and 12 other agents against 329 aerobic and anaerobic Gram-positive isolates recovered from diabetic foot infections. *Antimicrob. Agents Chemother.* **2006**, *50*, 2875–2879. [CrossRef]
31. Goldstein, E.J.C.; Citron, D.M.; Merriam, C.V.; Warren, Y.; Tyrrell, K.; Fernandez, H.T. In vitro activities of dalbavancin and nine comparator agents against anaerobic Gram-positive species and corynebacteria. *Antimicrob. Agents Chemother.* **2003**, *47*, 1968–1971. [CrossRef]
32. Fernández, J.; Greenwood-Quaintance, K.E.; Patel, R. In vitro activity of dalbavancin against biofilms of staphylococci isolated from prosthetic joint infections. *Diagn. Microbiol. Infect. Dis.* **2016**, *85*, 449–451. [CrossRef]
33. Neudorfer, K.; Schmidt-Malan, S.M.; Patel, R. Dalbavancin is active *in vitro* against biofilms formed by dalbavancin-susceptible enterococci. *Diagn. Microbiol. Infect. Dis.* **2018**, *90*, 58–63. [CrossRef] [PubMed]
34. Schmidt-Malan, S.M.; Quaintance, K.E.G.; Karau, M.J.; Patel, R. *In vitro* activity of tedizolid against staphylococci isolated from prosthetic joint infections. *Diagn. Microbiol. Infect. Dis.* **2016**, *85*, 77–79. [CrossRef] [PubMed]
35. Di Pilato, V.; Ceccherini, F.; Sennati, S.; D'Agostino, F.; Arena, F.; D'Atanasio, N.; Di Giorgio, F.P.; Tongiani, S.; Pallecchi, L.; Rossolini, G.M. In vitro time-kill kinetics of dalbavancin against *Staphylococcus* spp. biofilms over prolonged exposure times. *Diagn. Microbiol. Infect. Dis.* **2020**, *96*, 114901. [CrossRef] [PubMed]
36. Knafl, D.; Tobudic, S.; Cheng, S.C.; Bellamy, D.R.; Thalhammer, F. Dalbavancin reduces biofilms of methicillin-resistant *Staphylococcus aureus* (MRSA) and methicillin-resistant *Staphylococcus epidermidis* (MRSE). *Eur. J. Clin. Microbiol. Infect. Dis.* **2017**, *36*, 677–680. [CrossRef]
37. Žiemytė, M.; Rodríguez-Díaz, J.C.; Ventero, M.P.; Mira, A.; Ferrer, M.D. Effect of dalbavancin on staphylococcal biofilms when administered alone or in combination with biofilm-detaching compounds. *Front. Microbiol.* **2020**, *11*, 553. [CrossRef]
38. Darouiche, R.; Mansouri, M. Dalbavancin compared with vancomycin for prevention of *Staphylococcus aureus* colonization of devices in vivo. *J. Infect.* **2005**, *50*, 206–209. [CrossRef]
39. Baldoni, D.; Tafin, U.F.; Aeppli, S.; Angevaare, E.; Oliva, A.; Haschke, M.; Zimmerli, W.; Trampuz, A. Activity of dalbavancin, alone and in combination with rifampicin, against meticillin-resistant *Staphylococcus aureus* in a foreign-body infection model. *Int. J. Antimicrob. Agents* **2013**, *42*, 220–225. [CrossRef]
40. Barnea, Y.; Lerner, A.; Aizic, A.; Navon-Venezia, S.; Rachi, E.; Dunne, M.W.; Puttagunta, S.; Carmeli, Y. Efficacy of dalbavancin in the treatment of MRSA rat sternal osteomyelitis with mediastinitis. *J. Antimicrob. Chemother.* **2015**, *71*, 460–463. [CrossRef]
41. Nicolau, D.P.; Sun, H.K.; Seltzer, E.; Buckwalter, M.; Dowell, J.A. Pharmacokinetics of dalbavancin in plasma and skin blister fluir. *J. Antimicrob. Chemother.* **2007**, *60*, 681–684. [CrossRef]
42. Ferrer, M.; Rodriguez, J.; Álvarez, L.; Artacho, A.; Royo, G.; Mira, A. Effect of antibiotics on biofilm inhibition and induction measured by real-time cell analysis. *J. Appl. Microbiol.* **2017**, *122*, 640–650. [CrossRef] [PubMed]
43. Lampejo, T. Dalbavancin and telavancin in the treatment of infective endocarditis: A literature review. *Int. J. Antimicrob. Agents* **2020**, *56*, 106072. [CrossRef] [PubMed]
44. Ajaka, L.; Heil, E.; Schmalzle, S. Dalbavancin in the treatment of bacteremia and endocarditis in people with barriers to standard care. *Antibiotics* **2020**, *9*, 700. [CrossRef]
45. Tobudic, S.; Forstner, C.; Burgmann, H.; Lagler, H.; Ramharter, M.; Steininger, C.; Vossen, M.G.; Winkler, S.; Thalhammer, F. Dalbavancin as primary and sequential treatment for Gram-positive infective endocarditis: 2-year experience at the General Hospital of Vienna. *Clin. Infect. Dis.* **2018**, *67*, 795–798. [CrossRef] [PubMed]
46. Rappo, U.; Puttagunta, S.; Shevchenko, V.; Shevchenko, A.; Jandourek, A.; Gonzalez, P.L.; Suen, A.; Casullo, V.M.; Melnick, D.; Miceli, R.; et al. Dalbavancin for the treatment of osteomyelitis in adult patients: A randomized clinical trial of efficacy and safety. *Open Forum Infect. Dis.* **2019**, *6*, ofy331. [CrossRef]
47. Ramírez Hidalgo, M.; Jover-Sáenz, A.; García-González, M.; Barcenilla-Gaite, F. Dalbavancin treatment of prosthetic knee infection due to oxacillin-resistant *Staphylococcus epidermidis*. *Enferm. Infecc. Microbiol. Clin.* **2018**, *36*, 142–143. [CrossRef]
48. Martín, L.B.; Fernández, M.M.; Ruiz, J.M.; Lafont, M.O.; Paredes, L.Á.; Rodríguez, M.Á.; Regueras, M.F.; Morón, M.Á.; Lobón, G.M. Dalbavancin for treating prosthetic joint infections caused by Gram-positive bacteria: A proposal for a low dose strategy. A retrospective cohort study. *Rev. Esp. Quimioter.* **2019**, *32*, 532–538.

49. Wunsch, S.; Krause, R.; Valentin, T.; Prattes, J.; Janata, O.; Lenger, A.; Bellmann-Weiler, R.; Weiss, G.; Zollner-Schwetz, I. Multicenter clinical experience of real life dalbavancin use in gram-positive infections. *Int. J. Infect. Dis.* **2019**, *81*, 210–214. [CrossRef] [PubMed]
50. Morata, L.; Cobo, J.; Fernández-Sampedro, M.; Vasco, P.G.; Ruano, E.; Lora-Tamayo, J.; Somolinos, M.S.; Ruano, P.G.; Nieto, A.R.; Arnaiz, A.; et al. Safety and efficacy of prolonged use of dalbavancin in bone and joint infections. *Antimicrob. Agents Chemother.* **2019**, *63*. [CrossRef]
51. Bouza, E.; Valerio, M.; Soriano, A.; Morata, L.; Carus, E.G.; Rodríguez-González, M.C.; Hidalgo-Tenorio, C.; Plata, A.; Muñoz, P.; Vena, A.; et al. Dalbavancin in the treatment of different gram-positive infections: A real-life experience. *Int. J. Antimicrob. Agents* **2018**, *51*, 571–577. [CrossRef]
52. Dinh, A.; Duran, C.; Pavese, P.; Khatchatourian, L.; Monnin, B.; Bleibtreu, A.; Denis, E.; Etienne, C.; Rouanes, N.; Mahieu, R.; et al. French national cohort of first use of dalbavancin: A high proportion of off-label use. *Int. J. Antimicrob. Agents* **2019**, *54*, 668–672. [CrossRef]
53. Ariza, J.; Cobo, J.; Baraia-Etxaburu, J.; de Benito, N.; Bori, G.; Cabo, J.; Corona, P.; Esteban, J.; Horcajada, J.P.; Lora-Tamayo, J.; et al. Executive summary of management of prosthetic joint infections. Clinical practice guidelines by the Spanish Society of Infectious Diseases and Clinical Microbiology (SEIMC). *Enferm. Infecc. Microbiol. Clin.* **2017**, *35*, 189–195. [CrossRef]
54. Barbero Allende, J.M.; García Sánchez, M.; Culebras López, A.M.; Agudo Alonso, R. Suppressive antibiotic treatment with dalbavancin. A case report. *Rev. Esp. Quimioter.* **2021**, *34*, 151–153. [CrossRef]
55. Streifel, A.C.; Sikka, M.K.; Bowen, C.D.; Lewis, J.S. Dalbavancin use in an academic medical centre and associated cost savings. *Int. J. Antimicrob. Agents* **2019**, *54*, 652–654. [CrossRef] [PubMed]
56. Pizzuti, A.G.; Murray, E.Y.; Wagner, J.L.; Gaul, D.A.; Bland, C.M.; Jones, B.M. Financial analysis of dalbavancin for acute bacterial skin and skin structure infections for self-pay patients. *Infect. Dis. Ther.* **2020**, *9*, 1043–1053. [CrossRef]
57. Gonzalez, J.; Andrade, D.C.; Niu, J. Cost-consequence analysis of single-dose dalbavancin versus standard of care for the treatment of acute bacterial skin and skin structure infections in a multi-site healthcare system. *Clin. Infect. Dis.* **2020**. [CrossRef] [PubMed]
58. Bookstaver, P.B.; Milgrom, A. Stewarding the costly antibiotic: Considerations for dalbavancin. *Clin. Infect. Dis.* **2020**. [CrossRef] [PubMed]

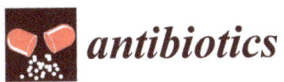

Communication

Risk Factors of Daptomycin-Induced Eosinophilic Pneumonia in a Population with Osteoarticular Infection

Laura Soldevila-Boixader [1,2], Bernat Villanueva [1], Marta Ulldemolins [1], Eva Benavent [1,2], Ariadna Padulles [3], Alba Ribera [1,2], Irene Borras [1], Javier Ariza [1,2,4] and Oscar Murillo [1,2,4,*]

1. Infectious Diseases Service, IDIBELL-Hospital Universitari Bellvitge, Feixa Llarga s/n, Hospitalet de Llobregat, 08907 Barcelona, Spain; laura.soldevila@bellvitgehospital.cat (L.S.-B.); bvillanueva@bellvitgehospital.cat (B.V.); mulldemolins@bellvitgehospital.cat (M.U.); eva.benavent@bellvitgehospital.cat (E.B.); ARibera@scias.com (A.R.); Iborras@scias.com (I.B.); jariza@bellvitgehospital.cat (J.A.)
2. Bone and Joint Infection Study Group of the Spanish Society of Clinical Microbiology and Infectious Diseases (GEIO-SEIMC), 28003 Madrid, Spain
3. Pharmacy Department, IDIBELL-Hospital Universitari Bellvitge, Feixa Llarga s/n, Hospitalet de Llobregat, 08907 Barcelona, Spain; apadulles@bellvitgehospital.cat
4. Spanish Network for Research in Infectious Diseases (REIPI RD16/0016/0003), Instituto de Salud Carlos III, 28029 Madrid, Spain
* Correspondence: omurillo@bellvitgehospital.cat; Tel.: +34-93-260-7625

Abstract: Background: Daptomycin-induced eosinophilic pneumonia (DEP) is a rare but severe adverse effect and the risk factors are unknown. The aim of this study was to determine risk factors for DEP. Methods: A retrospective cohort study was performed at the Bone and Joint Infection Unit of the Hospital Universitari Bellvitge (January 2014–December 2018). To identify risk factors for DEP, cases were divided into two groups: those who developed DEP and those without DEP. Results: Among the whole cohort (n = 229) we identified 11 DEP cases (4.8%) and this percentage almost doubled in the subgroup of patients ≥70 years (8.1%). The risk factors for DEP were age ≥70 years (HR 10.19, 95%CI 1.28–80.93), therapy >14 days (7.71, 1.98–30.09) and total cumulative dose of daptomycin ≥10 g (5.30, 1.14–24.66). Conclusions: Clinicians should monitor cumulative daptomycin dosage to minimize DEP risk, and be cautious particularly in older patients when the total dose of daptomycin exceeds 10 g.

Keywords: daptomycin; eosinophilic pneumonia; risk factors

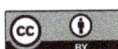

1. Introduction

Daptomycin is a cyclic lipopeptide antibiotic approved for use against complicated skin and soft tissue infection, *Staphylococcus aureus* bacteremia and right-sided infective endocarditis. However, daptomycin has become widely used also in staphylococcal osteoarticular infections because of its remarkable anti-biofilm activity. Indeed, current guidelines advise for its use mainly as an initial induction course of intravenous antimicrobial therapy and often in combination with other antibiotics to avoid the appearance of resistance [1,2]. In this setting, the use of daptomycin for prolonged periods should be balanced between the potential benefits in the outcome and the risk of adverse events [3–5].

Although daptomycin has proven safety, daptomycin-induced eosinophilic pneumonia (DEP) is a rare but severe adverse effect [6,7]. This toxicity is partially related to the usual daptomycin uptake by pulmonary surfactant in the alveoli, which may lead to concentrations high enough to cause injury but also to impair its efficacy; in fact, daptomycin is not recommended to treat pulmonary infections. Despite the fact that the pathophysiology is not totally clear, it seems that DEP is an antigen-mediated process in which alveolar macrophages and T-cells may be activated, which then release interleukin-5 that causes eosinophil production and migration to the lungs. Additionally, alveolar macrophages can also excrete cytokines that selectively recruits eosinophils, which may promote further eosinophil accumulation into the lungs [8,9].

Since the introduction of daptomycin, while some cases of DEP have been reported, these have only described the most common clinical manifestations and outcome [10–13]. To date, therefore, we do not know which factors are associated with DEP and thus, in the present study we aimed to determine the risk factors for developing DEP.

2. Results

In total, 229 cases received at least one dose of daptomycin and among them, 11 (4.8%) had DEP; a comparison of both groups in regard with main clinical and analytical characteristics is presented in Table 1. All DEP cases underwent a chest X-ray while on daptomycin therapy, which showed peripheral lung infiltrates (alveolar or interstitial), and only one patient had a CT scan that showed radiological findings of organizing pneumonia. In contrast, only 26% cases (57/218) of the remaining cohort underwent a chest X-ray, which was considered similar to the baseline one. Of interest, the performance of a chest X-ray significantly increased in accordance with the length of daptomycin therapy, ranging from 21% in cases treated less than 7 days to 42% in those treated more than 14 days ($p = 0.005$). With regard to the age of patients, cases aged ≥ 70 years underwent a chest X-ray during daptomycin therapy in greater proportion than younger patients (31% vs. 24%, respectively).

Table 1. Analysis of risk factors for daptomycin-induced eosinophilic pneumonia (DEP).

	Cases with DEP $n = 11$	Cases without DEP $n = 218$	HR (95% CI)	p-Value
Age (median, IQR)	77.4 (71.3–85.5)	69.7 (55.6–78.1)	1.06 (1.01–1.12)	0.042
<70 years			1	
≥70 years	10 (91)	108 (50)	10.19 (1.28–80.93)	0.028
Female	5 (45)	104 (48)	0.91 (0.27–3.08)	0.884
Comorbidities				
Charlson score (median, IQR)	5 (4–7)	4 (2–5)	1.31 (1.03–1.67)	0.031
Chronic heart disease	3 (30)	27 (12)	2.65 (0.66–10.62)	0.168
Chronic pulmonary disease	3 (30)	20 (9)	3.71 (0.91–15.12)	0.067
Chronic kidney disease	2 (20)	56 (26)	0.64 (0.13–3.07)	0.579
Analytical data (baseline)				
Creatinine (µmol/L)	62 (49–70)	72 (57–105)	0.98 (0.960–1.005)	0.134
Leucocytes ($\times 10^9$ cells/L)	10.1 (7.3–11)	9.4 (7.2–12.3)	0.965 (0.829–1.122)	0.640
Eosinophils (cells/µL; median, IQR)	130 (30–230)	100 (30–240)	0.99 (0.996–1.003)	0.709
Analytical data (end of treatment)				
[2]Creatine kinase (mkat/L)	0.68 (0.31–0.89)	0.87 (0.54–1.85)	0.81 (0.498–1.316)	0.395
C-reactive protein (mg/L)	223 (120–315)	36 (17–83)	1.01 (1.007–1.018)	<0.001
Leucocytes ($\times 10^9$ cells/L)	12.9 (9.5–15.4)	7.8 (6–9.8)	1.14 (1.035–1.258)	0.008
Eosinophils (cells/µL)	650 (520–1410)	220 (100–400)	1.01 (1.002–1.004)	<0.001
Daptomycin therapy				
Daily dose (mg; median, IQR)	700 (700–700)	700 (600–800)	1 (0.99–1.01)	0.719
Length (days; median, IQR)	19 (12–25)	7 (4–15)	1.08 (1.03–1.14)	0.005
≤14 days	3 (27)	162 (74)	1	
>14 days	8 (73)	56 (26)	7.71 (1.98–30.09)	0.003
[1]TCDD (g; median, IQR)	13.2 (8.4–17.5)	5.1 (2.4–11.2)	1.11 (1.03–1.19)	0.004
<10 g	3 (27)	155 (71)	1	
10–15 g	4 (36)	39 (18)	5.30 (1.14–24.66)	0.034
>15 g	4 (36)	24 (11)	8.61 (1.81–40.87)	0.007
Repeated exposure	2 (20)	23 (10)	1.88 (0.38–9.26)	0.435

Analytical data is presented as median, IQR. The remaining data are presented as n (%) unless otherwise noted. [1] TCDD (Total Cumulative Dose of Daptomycin; daily dose X days of treatment; The result was expressed in grams-g-) [2] Cases without DEP in which creatine kinase values were analyzed had a median of 12 days (IQR 6–19.5) of daptomycin therapy.

All DEP cases were treated with daptomycin withdrawal and seven (64%) with corticosteroid therapy. One patient, who had a delay in diagnosis of DEP and therapy, died because of respiratory failure.

In the univariate analysis (Table 1), factors associated with DEP were advanced age, the presence of comorbidities measured by Charlson score, long treatment with daptomycin and high values of TCDD. Concisely, daptomycin therapy for two weeks or longer was associated with high risk of DEP (HR 7.71, 95%CI 1.98–30.09), as well as TCDD values $\geq$10 g (HR 5.30, 95%CI 1.14–24.66). The presence of blood eosinophilia at the end of daptomycin treatment was significantly higher in DEP cases than in controls (82% and 16%, respectively; $p < 0.001$), as well as leucocyte counts and C-reactive protein values were also higher in DEP cases.

We noted that among older patients aged $\geq$70 years ($n = 123$), the percentage with DEP (8.1%; 10/123) almost doubled the value of the whole cohort. Also, the percentage of cases with DEP increased significantly among cases aged $\geq$70 years in comparison with the whole cohort either in cases treated for >14 days or in those with high values of TCDD (Figure 1).

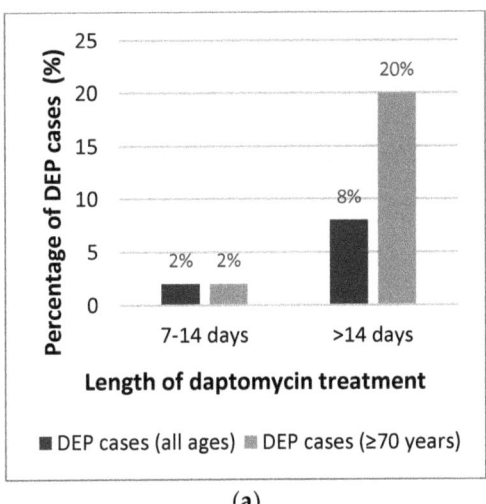

(a)

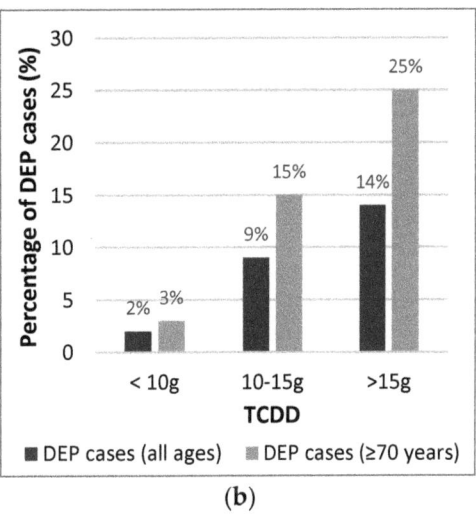

(b)

Figure 1. Percentage of Daptomycin-induced eosinophilic pneumonia (DEP) cases in the whole cohort and in those aged $\geq$70 years by (**a**) Length of therapy and by (**b**) The total cumulative dose of daptomycin (TCDD).

Finally, 25 cases had a re-challenge to daptomycin therapy, and two of these presented promptly with DEP (8%) by 4 and 8 days after the re-challenge (3 and 5 months after the first exposure, respectively). Both cases presented blood eosinophilia after the first course of treatment, having received >11 g over >14 days. By contrast, among the remaining patients re-challenged with daptomycin, the eosinophilia was only observed at the prior exposure for four patients (17%).

3. Discussion

In the present study we reported the main risk factors for developing DEP in a population with osteoarticular infections, providing important new information that may be helpful to clinicians.

Daptomycin has been reported as the leading cause of drug-induced eosinophilic pneumonia [14], and clinicians should maintain a high index of suspicion for DEP because of its potential severity. Although most of cases in our series were resolved by daptomycin withdrawal and corticosteroid therapy, one patient died, which illustrates the inherent risk of failing to identify DEP promptly.

Daptomycin use for the treatment of osteoarticular infection is currently recommended mainly against staphylococcal infections and as initial induction antimicrobial therapy [1,2]. In contrast with the high activity of daptomycin in animal and in vitro studies, its clinical efficacy reported from non-comparative studies appeared to be quite similar to other therapies [5,15,16]. However, prolonged therapy at higher doses than usual seems to be increased in recent years. Our cases were treated with daptomycin for a median of 19 days and resulted in DEP proportions of 4.8% overall and 8.1% among those aged $\geq$70 years. This data may seem high compared with previous experiences and without placing it in context. Thus, populations with 102 cases of infective endocarditis and 43 cases of complex osteoarticular infections that received high doses of daptomycin (median 8.2 mg/kg/d) for long periods (20–80 days), the authors showed 3% and 4.6% developed DEP, respectively [17,18]. These are consistent with our results given that the populations in both studies were younger (mean age 61.5 years) than in the present study.

Taking all the previous into account, the prolonged therapy with daptomycin against osteoarticular infections or the use of higher doses than usual should be considered on the basis of a list of pros and cons. Probably, the efficacy of daptomycin therapy is related with its anti-biofilm activity and can be benefited through an initial intensive phase of treatment (i.e., 7–14 days). Further therapy should be balanced with inconveniences derived from its use; indeed, monitoring for daptomycin toxicity appears crucial in long therapies and includes not only the risk for DEP but also other adverse events such as rhabdomyolysis. In our experience, performance of chest-X ray was useful to identify DEP and thus, it appears as valid screening to be interpreted together with other clinical signs and analytical parameters.

To our knowledge, no previous studies had been performed to analyze the risk factors of developing DEP. We identified advanced age, high values of Charlson comorbidity index, length of daptomycin therapy and TCDD as the main risk factors for DEP. Of interest, we show that patients older than 70 years, which commonly have more underlying diseases, are at higher risk of DEP; however, further research is needed to evaluate the importance of particular comorbidities in increasing the risk of DEP.

Regarding cumulative dosages of daptomycin and long therapies, our results seem to be consistent with previous works. Hirai et al. [19] reported 40 cases of DEP, 73% of them received a daptomycin dosage >6 mg/kg/d for a median of 14.8 days, whereas the remaining cases were treated with daptomycin at $\leq$6 mg/kg/d for a median of 23 days. In a systematic review of DEP cases the mean length of daptomycin therapy was 2.8 weeks and main indication for treatment was osteoarticular infection [20]. Overall, it seems that higher risk of DEP is not only dose dependent but also time-dependent. We therefore recommend monitoring the cumulative dose of daptomycin, which is a product of the dosage and length of therapy, rather than considering either variable separately. In our experience, clinicians should be cautious when the TCDD is $\geq$10 g, and particularly if it increases to $\geq$15 g, which can be easily attained after 2 weeks of treatment in patients receiving high doses.

Cases with DEP at the end of therapy had higher blood eosinophil counts and more often eosinophilia than controls, a fact that has been mainly reported previously [20,21]. Of interest, we noted a scenario in which severe DEP occurred shortly after a re-challenge with daptomycin, indicating that a drug hypersensitivity mechanism may be play. These cases presented with eosinophilia at the end of their previous course of daptomycin, a finding that was rarely observed in patients given a rechallenge without developing DEP. This clinical situation has been poorly reported to date [22], but it seems that eosinophilia during daptomycin therapy should prompt clinicians to consider avoiding further drug exposure.

The main limitations of the study are those inherent to the retrospective design. Generalizability is affected because patients were recruited from a single center and because the cohort mostly comprised elderly people with heterogeneous clinical presentations of osteoarticular infections. Also, unfortunately, our sample size of DEP cases was small to allow subgroup analyses or to design other comparative study. These factors must be factored when considering other heterogeneous populations. Irrespective of these shortcomings, however, we believe that our results provide information that can be led to improved management of daptomycin therapy.

4. Materials and Methods

4.1. Study Design, Setting, and Inclusion/Exclusion Criteria

This retrospective cohort study was performed at the Bone and Joint Infection Unit of the Hospital Universitari Bellvitge between January 2014 and December 2018. We included all patients with osteoarticular infection (prosthetic joint infection, septic arthritis and osteomyelitis), aged ≥ 18 years, and treated at least with one dose of daptomycin because of empirical treatment or guided therapy addressed to Gram-positive microorganisms. Polymicrobial osteoarticular infections treated with daptomycin in combination with other antibiotics were also included. We excluded cases attended in our Bone and Joint Infection Unit that received daptomycin due to causes different than osteoarticular infections (i.e., catheter-related sepsis).

To identify risk factors for DEP, cases were divided into two groups: Those who developed DEP and those without DEP.

Written informed consent was considered unnecessary for the study, as it was a retrospective analysis of our clinical practice. Data of patients were anonymized for the purposes of this analysis. Confidential information of patients was protected according National and European normative. This manuscript has been revised for its publication by Research Ethics Committee of Bellvitge University Hospital (PR097/21).

4.2. Definitions and Clinical Data

All cases fulfilled the main diagnostic criteria for each osteoarticular infection, including those with prosthetic joint infection or osteoarthritis, with or without an orthopedic device.

The modified diagnostic criteria established by Philips et al. were used to define DEP [23], which required exposure to daptomycin with the following features: fever, dyspnea with increased oxygen requirement or requiring mechanical ventilation, new infiltrates on chest X-ray or computed tomography, and clinical improvement following daptomycin withdrawal. In accordance with these criteria, we did not require the previous pre-requisite of a bronchoalveolar lavage with >25% eosinophils.

Demographic, clinical, radiological and analytical data were collected for the included cases. Chronic heart failure, chronic pulmonary disease and chronic kidney disease were defined according to accepted criteria. The total cumulative dose of daptomycin (TCDD) was defined as daily dose of daptomycin $\times$ days of treatment; the result was expressed in grams (g).

4.3. Statistical Analysis

Data were analyzed using Stata software (version 16.0, Stata Corporation, College Station, TX, USA). Categorical variables are described by counts and percentages, while medians and interquartile ranges (IQRs) are used to summarize continuous variables.

Univariate analysis was performed to screen the risk factors for DEP, and logistic regression models were built to estimate unadjusted hazard ratios (HR). In all situations, p-values of <0.05 were considered to be statistically significant.

5. Conclusions

In conclusion, main factors associated with DEP were advanced age, high values of Charlson score, longer treatments and high total cumulative doses of daptomycin. Particularly, clinicians should take care in cases with cumulative doses greater than 10 g, which can be achieved after 2 weeks of daptomycin therapy. In this high risk population and after the beginning of treatment, performing a chest-X ray is useful to identify DEP.

Where eosinophilia has previously occurred with daptomycin exposure, further drug challenges should be considered with great care to minimize the risk of DEP.

Author Contributions: L.S.-B., B.V., M.U., E.B., A.P., A.R., I.B., J.A. and O.M. contributed in the supervision of the clinical cases, data collection, and interpretation; L.S.-B. and O.M. elaborated the study design; L.S.-B. performed the analysis of the data and wrote the first draft of the manuscript. All authors have read and agreed to the published version of the manuscript.

Funding: L.S-B. was supported with a grant of the Ministerio de Ciencia, Innovación y Universidades (FPU (18/02768). This research did not receive any specific grant from funding agencies in the public, commercial, or not-for-profit sectors. This research received no external funding.

Institutional Review Board Statement: The study was conducted according to the guidelines of the Declaration of Helsinki, and approved by the Ethics Committee of Bellvitge University Hospital (protocol code PR097/21).

Informed Consent Statement: Patient consent was waived due to the retrospective nature of the study on the usual clinical practice.

Data Availability Statement: The data presented in this study are available on request from the corresponding author (omurillo@bellvitgehospital.cat).

Acknowledgments: We thank Dolors Rodriguez-Pardo from Hospital Vall d'Hebron, Isabel Mur from Hospital de la Santa Creu i Sant Pau and Rosa Escudero from Hospital Ramon y Cajal for their collaboration with the manuscript. We thank Michael Maudsley for revising the English manuscript. We thank CERCA Program/Generalitat de Catalunya for institutional support. The preliminary results of this study were reported in part at the 30th European Congress of Clinical Microbiology & Infectious Diseases (Paris, France, 2020).

Conflicts of Interest: The authors declare no conflict of interest.

References

1. Osmon, D.R.; Berbari, E.F.; Berendt, A.R.; Lew, D.; Zimmerli, W.; Steckelberg, J.M.; Rao, N.; Hanssen, A.; Wilson, W.R. Diagnosis and management of prosthetic joint infection: Clinical practice guidelines by the infectious diseases Society of America. *Clin. Infect. Dis.* **2013**, *56*, 1–25. [CrossRef]
2. Ariza, J.; Cobo, J.R.; Artetxe, J.B.-E.; de Benito Hernandez, N.; Tuneu, G.B.; Cabo, J.; Perez-Cardona, P.C.; Moreno, J.E.; Horcajada Gallego, J.P.; Lora-Tamayo, J.; et al. Management of Prosthetic Joint Infections. Clinical Practice Guidelines by the Spanish Society of Infectious Diseases and Clinical Microbiology (SEIMC). Available online: https://seimc.org/contenidos/gruposdeestudio/geio/dcientificos/documentos/geio-dc-2017-Guia_IPAS_EIMC.pdf (accessed on 1 April 2021).
3. Falagas, M.E.; Giannopoulou, K.P.; Ntziora, F.; Papagelopoulos, P.J. Daptomycin for treatment of patients with bone and joint infections: A systematic review of the clinical evidence. *Int. J. Antimicrob. Agents* **2007**, *30*, 202–209. [CrossRef] [PubMed]
4. Chang, Y.-J.; Lee, M.S.; Lee, C.-H.; Lin, P.-C.; Kuo, F.-C. Daptomycin treatment in patients with resistant staphylococcal periprosthetic joint infection. *BMC Infect. Dis.* **2017**, *17*, 736. [CrossRef] [PubMed]
5. Lora-Tamayo, J.; Parra-Ruiz, J.; Rodríguez-Pardo, D.; Barberán, J.; Ribera, A.; Tornero, E.; Pigrau, C.; Mensa, J.; Ariza, J.; Soriano, A. High doses of daptomycin (10 mg/kg/d) plus rifampin for the treatment of staphylococcal prosthetic joint infection managed with implant retention: A comparative study. *Diagn. Microbiol. Infect. Dis.* **2014**, *80*, 66–71. [CrossRef] [PubMed]
6. He, W.; Zhang, Y.; Chen, H.; Zhao, C.; Wang, H. Efficacy and safety of daptomycin for the treatment of infectious disease: A meta-analysis based on randomized controlled trials. *J. Antimicrob. Chemother.* **2014**, *69*, 3181–3189. [CrossRef] [PubMed]
7. Benvenuto, M.; Benziger, D.P.; Yankelev, S.; Vigliani, G. Pharmacokinetics and Tolerability of Daptomycin at Doses up to 12 Milligrams per Kilogram of Body Weight Once Daily in Healthy Volunteers. *Antimicrob. Agents Chemother.* **2006**, *50*, 3245–3249. [CrossRef]
8. Silverman, J.A.; Mortin, L.I.; VanPraagh, A.D.G.; Li, T.; Alder, J. Inhibition of Daptomycin by Pulmonary Surfactant: In Vitro Modeling and Clinical Impact. *J. Infect. Dis.* **2005**, *191*, 2149–2152. [CrossRef] [PubMed]
9. Allen, J.N. Drug-induced eosinophilic lung disease. *Clin. Chest Med.* **2004**, *25*, 77–88. [CrossRef]
10. Hayes, D.; Anstead, M.I.; Kuhn, R.J. Eosinophilic pneumonia induced by daptomycin. *J. Infect.* **2007**, *54*, e211–e213. [CrossRef]
11. Cobb, E.; Kimbrough, R.C.; Nugent, K.M.; Phy, M.P. Organizing Pneumonia and Pulmonary Eosinophilic Infiltration Associated with Daptomycin. *Ann. Pharm.* **2007**, *41*, 696–701. [CrossRef]
12. Lal, Y.; Assimacopoulos, A.P. Two cases of daptomycin-induced eosinophilic pneumonia and chronic pneumonitis. *Clin. Infect. Dis.* **2010**, *50*, 737–740. [CrossRef] [PubMed]
13. Miller, B.A.; Gray, A.; LeBlanc, T.W.; Sexton, D.J.; Martin, A.R.; Slama, T.G. Acute Eosinophilic Pneumonia Secondary to Daptomycin: A Report of Three Cases. *Clin. Infect. Dis.* **2010**, *50*, e63–e68. [CrossRef] [PubMed]
14. Bartal, C.; Sagy, I.; Barski, L. Drug-induced eosinophilic pneumonia. *Medicine* **2018**, *97*, e9688. [CrossRef] [PubMed]

15. Saleh-Mghir, A.; Muller-Serieys, C.; Dinh, A.; Massias, L.; Crémieux, A.-C. Adjunctive Rifampin Is Crucial to Optimizing Daptomycin Efficacy against Rabbit Prosthetic Joint Infection Due to Methicillin-Resistant Staphylococcus aureus. *Antimicrob. Agents Chemother.* **2011**, *55*, 4589–4593. [CrossRef] [PubMed]
16. John, A.-K.; Baldoni, D.; Haschke, M.; Rentsch, K.; Schaerli, P.; Zimmerli, W.; Trampuz, A. Efficacy of Daptomycin in Implant-Associated Infection Due to Methicillin-Resistant Staphylococcus aureus: Importance of Combination with Rifampin. *Antimicrob. Agents Chemother.* **2009**, *53*, 2719–2724. [CrossRef] [PubMed]
17. Durante-Mangoni, E.; Andini, R.; Parrella, A.; Mattucci, I.; Cavezza, G.; Senese, A.; Trojaniello, C.; Caprioli, R.; Diana, M.V.; Utili, R. Safety of treatment with high-dose daptomycin in 102 patients with infective endocarditis. *Int. J. Antimicrob. Agents* **2016**, *48*, 61–68. [CrossRef] [PubMed]
18. Roux, S.; Valour, F.; Karsenty, J.; Gagnieu, M.-C.; Perpoint, T.; Lustig, S.; Ader, F.; Martha, B.; Laurent, F.; Chidiac, C.; et al. Daptomycin >6 mg/kg/day as salvage therapy in patients with complex bone and joint infection: Cohort study in a regional reference center. *BMC Infect. Dis.* **2016**, *16*, 83. [CrossRef]
19. Hirai, J.; Hagihara, M.; Haranaga, S.; Kinjo, T.; Hashioka, H.; Kato, H.; Sakanashi, D.; Yamagishi, Y.; Mikamo, H.; Fujita, J. Eosinophilic pneumonia caused by daptomycin: Six cases from two institutions and a review of the literature. *J. Infect. Chemother.* **2017**, *23*, 245–249. [CrossRef]
20. Uppal, P.; LaPlante, K.L.; Gaitanis, M.M.; Jankowich, M.D.; Ward, K.E. Daptomycin-induced eosinophilic pneumonia-a systematic review. *Antimicrob. Resist. Infect. Control* **2016**, *5*, 55. [CrossRef] [PubMed]
21. Higashi, Y.; Nakamura, S.; Tsuji, Y.; Ogami, C.; Matsumoto, K.; Kawago, K.; Tokui, K.; Hayashi, R.; Sakamaki, I.; Yamamoto, Y. Daptomycin-induced eosinophilic pneumonia and a review of the published literature. *Intern. Med.* **2018**, *57*, 253–258. [CrossRef]
22. Nickerson, M.; Bhargava, A.; Kale-Pradhan, P. Daptomycin-associated eosinophilic pneumonia with rechallenge: A case report. *Int. J. Clin. Pharm.* **2017**, *55*, 521–524. [CrossRef] [PubMed]
23. Phillips, J.; Cardile, A.P.; Patterson, T.F.; Lewis, J.S. Daptomycin-induced acute eosinophilic pneumonia: Analysis of the current data and illustrative case reports. *Scand. J. Infect. Dis.* **2013**, *45*, 804–808. [CrossRef] [PubMed]

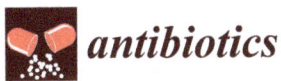

Review

Suppressive Antibiotic Treatment in Prosthetic Joint Infections: A Perspective

Javier Cobo and Rosa Escudero-Sanchez *

Infectious Disease Department, Hospital Ramón y Cajal, IRYCIS, Ctra. Colmenar Viejo, 28034 Madrid, Spain; javier.cobo@salud.madrid.org
* Correspondence: rosa.escudero0@gmail.com

Abstract: The treatment of prosthetic joint infections (PJIs) is a complex matter in which surgical, microbiological and pharmacological aspects must be integrated and, above all, placed in the context of each patient to make the best decision. Sometimes it is not possible to offer curative treatment of the infection, and in other cases, the probability that the surgery performed will be successful is considered very low. Therefore, indefinite administration of antibiotics with the intention of "suppressing" the course of the infection becomes useful. For decades, we had little information about suppressive antibiotic treatment (SAT). However, due to the longer life expectancy and increase in orthopaedic surgeries, an increasing number of patients with infected joint prostheses experience complex situations in which SAT should be considered as an alternative. In the last 5 years, several studies attempting to answer the many questions that arise on this issue have been published. The aim of this publication is to review the latest published evidence on SAT.

Keywords: suppressive antibiotic treatment; prosthetic joint infection; prolonged antibiotic

1. Therapeutic Options for Prosthetic Joint Infections

The goal of treating a prosthetic joint infection (PJI) is to eradicate the infection and to maintain or regain implant function. This often involves the replacement of the prostheses, although in some cases (acute infections), the original implant can be salvaged through extensive debridement and prolonged antibiotic therapy, which is referred to as DAIR (debridement, antibiotics and implant retention) [1]. In the remaining situations, the cure can be obtained only by removing the implant, followed by the placement of a new prosthesis, either during the same surgical procedure (one-stage revision) or after a period with antibiotics (two-stage revision) [2]. However, reimplantation is sometimes not possible after removal (resection arthroplasty), and in rare situations, amputation may be necessary. Eventually, due to the patient's conditions or the anticipated sequelae of the intervention, a potentially curative surgical intervention is waived. In this scenario, orthopaedic surgeons turn their gaze to infectious disease (ID) consultants. Can antibiotic treatment help the patient?

2. Concept and Definition of Suppressive Antibiotic Treatment (SAT)

The term "suppressive antibiotic treatment" (SAT) refers to the administration of antibiotics in the long term or indefinitely over time. In the area of PJI, SAT is considered a "noncurative" strategy, in which antimicrobials are administered with the aim of reducing symptoms and delaying or preventing the progression of PJI that needs a surgical procedure to be cured that, for some reason, will not be performed (at least for a prolonged period of time). SAT can also be used in situations in which adequate surgical treatment is performed and the probability of cure is considered very low.

3. SAT Indications

SAT appears to be an infrequent therapeutic option in a series (5–14%) that reports the approach of patients with PJI [3–5]. However, in those patients over 80 years of age, the percentage treated by SAT can reach 36.5% [6].

SAT is intended to reduce local symptoms (presence of a sinus tract, inflammation, pain, etc.) and thus delay or elude a surgical intervention that has been rejected or is intended to be avoided. It is possible that SAT may delay or prevent prosthetic loosening by reducing the local peri-implant inflammatory process, although no studies have evaluated this potential effect. Additionally, SAT can be considered a general benefit for the patient's health as a result of the reduction in persistent chronic inflammation [7].

In summary, SAT can be considered for patients with acute PJI for whom conservative treatment (DAIR) has failed, or for patients with chronic-late PJI whose implants are not going to be removed or replaced due to any of the following circumstances:

- Unacceptable anticipated functional results.
- Surgical sequelae (or risks) disproportionate to the symptoms.
- Presence of another disease or condition that makes it advisable to substantially delay the intervention.
- Short life expectancy.
- Major surgical contraindication.
- Patient's refusal of the intervention.

These situations would therefore be considered PJI with "certain" treatment failure. This would mean that there is evidence of PJI with no curative treatment planned.

There are other situations in which the probability of failure of surgical-medical treatment can be anticipated to be high, although not certain [8,9]. Here, we would cite the following scenarios:

- Chronic PJI managed with partial replacement of components.
- Early PJI managed with DAIR and high risk of failure (or potential serious consequences thereof), such as immunosuppressed patients on chemotherapy, patients managed by arthroscopic debridement and/or without replacement of modular components, and cases with suboptimal antimicrobial therapy (multidrug-resistant organisms).
- Multiple previous failures of treatment of PJI

Once the indications are established, certain conditions are required to be able to carry out SAT:

- Known aetiology (not essential but lack of knowledge clearly hinders decision-making).
- Possibility of monitoring and clinical control of adherence and toxicity.
- Availability of orally active antibiotics against the causal aetiological agent (although, as we will see later, there may be alternatives).

4. Evidence on SAT Efficacy

4.1. Does SAT Truly Work? What Results Does It Offer?

Evidence of the efficacy of SAT is scarce. A cohort study in which patients with stable PJI (69% with implants for <90 days) were managed with implant retention and prolonged antibiotic therapy for more than 1 year showed that the failure rate (recurrence of infection or need for surgical revision) was four times higher in patients who discontinued antibiotic treatment [10]. Interestingly, most of the patients with discontinued treatment did not exhibit treatment failure, suggesting that many were actually cured. However, the higher rate of treatment failure in patients who stopped taking antibiotics indicates that, in this series, a proportion of patients not cured by DAIR benefited from continuing antibiotic treatment, via delayed or avoidance of failure, which occurred mostly in the first four months. Further arguments in favour of SAT efficacy are provided by the cases that were "rescued" through SAT after the failure of other strategies [10–12], as well as by the observation that some SAT failures were temporarily related to the suspension of antibiotic treatment [13].

The interpretation of SAT efficacy is very difficult for three reasons: the absence of controlled studies, the inclusion of patients with acute infections who would be cured by DAIR, and differences in the criteria for evaluating efficacy in published series (Table 1). For example, for some authors, the efficacy criterion was to avoid surgery (even if infection was not controlled) [3], while others required, in addition, control of the symptoms [4,9,11,14]. Success rates varied in the different series from 23% to 84%. However, the series with the highest success rates included patients with early PJI [4,9,14], many of whom would have had the same outcome with much shorter treatments.

Table 1. Published Series on SAT in PJI.

Reference	Number of Patients	Type of Infection	Aetiology (%)	Follow-Up (Months)	Criteria for Success	Success Rate	Toxicity
Goulet, 1988 [3]	19	90% chronic 10% acute	S. aureus (21%), CoNS (21%), Streptococcus spp. (32%)	49.2	Retention of the implant	63%	No data
Tsukayama, 1991 [15]	13	100% chronic	S. aureus, (54%), CoNS (46%)	37.2	Retention of the implant	23%	38% antibiotic needed to be changed
Segreti, 1998 [4]	18	50% chronic 50% acute	S. aureus (44%), CoNS (44%)	48	Remained asymptomatic and functional prosthesis	83%	22% CDI
Rao, 2003 [14]	36	53% chronic 47% acute	S. aureus (26%), CoNS (50%)	60	Remained asymptomatic and functional prosthesis	86%	8% diarrhoea
Marculescu, 2006 [13]	88	No data	S. aureus (32%), CoNS (23%)	23.3	Absence of the following: Relapse, reinfection, presence of acute inflammation in the periprosthetic tissue or at any subsequent surgery on the joint, development of a sinus tract, death from prosthesis-related infection, or indeterminate clinical failure	57%	3% diarrhoea, 11% hyper-sensitivity, one case of CDI
Byren, 2009 [9]	112	31% chronic 69% acute	S. aureus (40%), CoNS (23%)	27.6	Absence of the following: Recurrence, wound or sinus drainage recurring or persisting for 3 months beyond the index debridement procedure or requirement for revision surgery (irrespective of the indication)	82%	No data
Prendki, 2014 [6]	38	61% chronic 39% acute	S. aureus (39%), Streptococcus spp. (18%), Gram-negative bacilli (17%)	24	Absence of the following: Persisting infection, relapse, new infection, treatment discontinuation because of severe adverse events, or related or unrelated death	60%	1 case of recurrent CDI.

Table 1. Cont.

Reference	Number of Patients	Type of Infection	Aetiology (%)	Follow-Up (Months)	Criteria for Success	Success Rate	Toxicity
Siqueira, 2015 [16]	92	61% chronic 39% acute	S. aureus (48%), CoNS (35%)	69.1	Absence of the following: Subsequent surgical intervention for infection after the index procedure, persistent sinus tract, drainage, or joint pain at the last follow-up visit, or death related to the PJI	69%	No data
Prendki, 2017 [10]	136	No data	S. aureus (62%), CoNS (21%)	24	Absence of the following: Local or systemic progression of the infection, death, or discontinuation because an adverse drug reaction	61%	18.4% discontinued antibiotics, but in half of cases, the antibiotic could be replaced by another.
Pradier, 2017 [8]	39	61% delayed or late 39% acute	S. aureus (79%), CoNS (10%)	24	Absence of the following: Signs of infection assessed ≥24 months after the end of the curative treatment and then at the last contact with the patient, or death related to the PJI	74%	15% (phototoxicity and gastrointestinal intolerance)
Wouthuyzen-Bakker, 2017 [17]	21	62% late or delayed 38% early	S. aureus (33%), CoNS (38%)	21	Absence of the following: Pain during follow-up, surgical intervention is needed to control the infection, or death related to PJI	67%	43% reported side effects and needed change or adjustment of the dosage.
Pradier, 2018 [18]	78	60% delayed or late 40% early	S. aureus (40%), CoNS (32%)	34	Absence of the following: Signs of infection assessed ≥24 months after the end of the curative treatment and then at the last contact with the patient, or death related to the PJI	72%	18% phototoxicity and gastrointestinal disturbance
Escudero-Sánchez, 2019 [19]	302	73% chronic 11% haematogenous 16% early postoperative	S. aureus (31%), CoNS (33%)	36.5	Absence of the following: Appearance or persistence of a sinus tract, need for debridement or replacement of the prosthesis due to persistence of the infection, or the presence of uncontrolled symptoms, death related to PJI	59%	17% gastrointestinal 5% cutaneous

Table 1. Cont.

Reference	Number of Patients	Type of Infection	Aetiology (%)	Follow-Up (Months)	Criteria for Success	Success Rate	Toxicity
Leijtens, 2019 [20]	23	30% early 70% late or delayed	S. aureus (2%), CoNS (61%)	33	Absence of the following: Reoperation for PJI or death related to PJI	56.5	24% needed change or dosage modifications.
Sandiford, 2019 [5]	24	No data	S. aureus (25%), CoNS (21%)	38.4	Absence of the following: Sepsis arising from the affected joint, no progression to further surgery, or death related to PJI.	83	4.2% rash 4.2% rifampicin interaction

CDI: Clostridioides difficile infection; CoNS: coagulase-negative staphylococci.

We found only one controlled study where patients with PJI at high risk of failure after surgery (DAIR or replacement) managed with SAT were compared with patients in the same conditions who were not managed with SAT. The cases were "matched" using a propensity score. Patients who received SAT had a better outcome at 5 years (68.5% free of infection) than those who did not receive SAT (41.1%) [16]. In a recent multicentre cohort that represents the largest series published to date, we estimated that SAT was effective (control of symptoms and no reintervention) in approximately 75% of the patients after two years and in 50% of patients at 5 years of follow-up [19]. Only patients with persistent infection from whom the implant was not removed were included in this cohort.

4.2. What Factors Are Associated with SAT Failure?

Few studies have analysed the factors associated with SAT failure. The failure rate seems higher among patients with a sinus tract and in those with infections caused by S. aureus [13,20–22].

In the multicentre study mentioned above, we investigated predictors of failure (defined as the persistence of uncontrolled symptoms of PJI, including sinus tract, or the need for further surgery for debridement or removal of the prosthesis due to infection) [19]. A multivariate analysis showed that the factors associated with failure were the following:

- Aetiology of infection other than Gram-positive cocci (essentially Gram-negative rods, fungi, or negative cultures). This could be explained because, in general, we have fewer orally active antimicrobials for Gram-negative bacilli.
- Location of the prosthesis in the upper limbs. It is difficult to explain this finding. In any case, the number of PJIs in the upper limbs was very low.
- Age less than 70 years. It seems paradoxical, but perhaps younger patients managed by SAT could be more often immunosuppressed or have "tumoural" prostheses, which has been associated with the worst prognosis [17].

In our opinion, at this moment, there are no firm or clear predictors of failure, which means that SAT should not be excluded if the patient meets the conditions mentioned above.

4.3. Why Could SAT Stop Working? Is the Development of Resistance Frequent?

In our previously cited cohort study, the coinvestigators were unable to attribute the failure to any specific cause in 52% of the cases. Among the known or attributable causes, the most frequent was the abandonment of treatment or poor adherence (24% of all failures). The development of resistance was not a common cause, as it could only be invoked as a cause of failure in 12% of the cases. This observation has also been made by other authors [18]. In another 11% of patients, the cause of failure was the existence of a previously unsuspected pathogen in cultures that was not covered by the prescribed SAT [19].

5. Practical Aspects of SAT

5.1. Is a Debridement Mandatory before Starting SAT?

It seems reasonable to think that the reduction in the inoculum and the debridement of infected tissues favours the success of SAT. In most of the series, patients undergo debridement surgery before starting SAT [21]. The difficulty arises in stable patients who present few symptoms, especially if the surgical risks are high. Thus, in the series of SAT in elderly patients, only 24% were operated on [10].

In our analysis, the failure of the SAT was not associated with the absence of a previous debridement [19]. However, surgical debridement makes it possible to obtain valuable samples for microbiological culture, which is a relevant advantage since culture from sinus tracts is not usually representative of the actual aetiology [23].

5.2. What Are the Most Suitable Antibiotics for SAT? Is a Combination of Antibiotics Necessary?

From the analysis of the data available in the literature, it is not possible to infer recommendations. The most widely used antibiotic regimens in published series have been the combination of tetracyclines and rifampicin (the last cannot be used alone because of development of resistance) or monotherapy with a beta-lactam or tetracycline antibiotic [3,4,10,14]. In a recent survey of orthopaedists and ID consultants who prescribed SAT, 74% stated that they did not use rifampicin [24].

Since SAT is intended to reduce symptoms and local inflammation, which can be achieved by reducing the bacterial load, antibiotics with activity against stationary growing bacteria are probably not indispensable. In fact, monotherapy with beta-lactams was associated with better outcomes in a large series [10]. It seems reasonable to prioritize tolerability and therapeutic compliance, and for this, it is easier to use monotherapy. In the vast majority of cases, SAT is carried out with orally administered antibiotics. However, there are some recent experiences with intravenous dalbavancin, which have taken advantage of the fact that this drug can be administered once per week or even every two weeks [25], and with the use of beta-lactams such as ceftriaxone or ertapenem subcutaneously [26].

There are no studies on the optimal dosage of antibiotics in SAT. In general, low doses should not be used initially, at least until a reduction in inoculum has been achieved. However, the risks of each antibiotic–bacteria pair must be taken into account. For example, a low dosage of quinolones poses a risk of resistance selection in both staphylococci and Gram-negative bacilli; however, beta-lactam susceptible staphylococci should not develop resistance to a low dose of oral cephalosporins.

5.3. Is Intravenous Treatment Necessary at the Beginning of SAT?

Similarly, published studies do not provide an answer to this question. In almost all published series, patients receive several weeks of initial intravenous treatment, but in the aforementioned survey, most of the respondents stated that they do so only occasionally [24].

5.4. Can There Be Periods Without Treatment?

The series in the literature reviewed do not include antibiotic treatment-free periods in their protocols. In fact, in some series, failures are reported coinciding with the interruption of treatment, which, in general, appears in the first 4 months after suspension [9].

6. Safety of SAT

Information on the safety of prolonged antibiotic treatments can be obtained, not only from studies on SAT in PJI or other osteoarticular infections but also from other areas, such as antibiotic prophylaxis in immunosuppressed patients, the management of specific infections that require very long treatments (multidrug-resistant tuberculosis, actinomycosis, mycobacteriosis, Coxiella endocarditis, etc.) or entities in which infection and bacterial colonization play a relevant role in the natural history of the disease (cystic fibrosis, acne, suppurative hidradenitis, etc.), for which long-term treatments have been tried.

In SAT series, adverse effects are not uncommon, but they rarely require discontinuation of treatment [19,21,22]. In addition, in many cases, poorly tolerated antibiotics can be substituted for another [10,17]. Data collection on adverse effects has not been systematized in any of the published studies and it was always retrospective. Gastrointestinal disturbances and skin reactions appear to be the most common reported adverse events. It should be borne in mind that in most series, ID consultants with extensive experience in the management of antimicrobials are those who prescribe and monitor treatments. Surprisingly, *C. difficile* infection is an infrequent event despite very long treatments that last many years [19,21].

In a preliminary study including several patients on SAT, colonization by multidrug-resistant bacteria was not common. However, the patients who developed infections did so due to bacterial resistance to the antibiotic that they received for SAT [27].

7. Reflections and Conclusions

The information on SAT is fragmentary, heterogeneous and of low evidence. Despite this, the analysis of the available series suggests that SAT may represent an option with acceptable efficacy for selected cases in which potentially curative surgery cannot be performed or where the probabilities of success of the treatment are low. It is possible to administer antibiotics safely in the long term, provided that the clinician has the appropriate knowledge and experience. More studies are needed to answer the many questions that remain unanswered. To form useful conclusions in future investigations, it would be desirable to establish pragmatic criteria for efficacy, as well as to separate the cases in which SAT is indicated as an alternative to surgical treatment from those where it is indicated due to a high risk of failure of the surgical treatment used.

Author Contributions: J.C. and R.E.-S. review of the available information, draft of the manuscript preparation and approve the final version of the manuscript.

Funding: This research received no external funding.

Institutional Review Board Statement: Not applicable.

Informed Consent Statement: Not applicable.

Data Availability Statement: The data presented in this study are available on request from the corresponding author. The data are not publicly available due to the fact that it is a multicenter study and the complexity of the clinical history in some centers.

Conflicts of Interest: The authors declare no conflict of interest.

References

1. Tsang, S.-T.J.; Ting, J.; Simpson, A.H.R.W.; Gaston, P. Outcomes following debridement, antibiotics and implant retention in the management of periprosthetic infections of the hip: A review of cohort studies. *Bone Jt. J.* **2017**, *99-B*, 1458–1466. [CrossRef]
2. Zimmerli, W.; Ochsner, P.E. Management of infection associated with prosthetic joints. *Infection* **2003**, *31*, 99–108. [CrossRef]
3. Goulet, J.A.; Pellicci, P.M.; Brause, B.D.; Salvati, E.M. Prolonged suppression of infection in total hip arthroplasty. *J. Arthroplast.* **1988**, *3*, 109–116. [CrossRef]
4. Segreti, J.; Nelson, J.A.; Trenholme, G.M. Prolonged suppressive antibiotic therapy for infected orthopedic prostheses. *Clin. Infect. Dis.* **1998**, *27*, 711–713. [CrossRef] [PubMed]
5. Sandiford, N.A.; Hutt, J.R.; Kendoff, D.O.; Mitchell, P.A.; Citak, M.; Granger, L. Prolonged suppressive antibiotic therapy is successful in the management of prosthetic joint infection. *Eur. J. Orthop. Surg. Traumatol.* **2020**, *30*, 313–321. [CrossRef] [PubMed]
6. Prendki, V.; Zeller, V.; Passeron, D.; Desplaces, N.; Mamoudy, P.; Stirnemann, J.; Marmor, S.; Ziza, J.-M. Outcome of patients over 80 years of age on prolonged suppressive antibiotic therapy for at least 6 months for prosthetic joint infection. *Int. J. Infect. Dis.* **2014**, *29*, 184–189. [CrossRef] [PubMed]
7. Furman, D.; Campisi, J.; Verdin, E.; Carrera-Bastos, P.; Targ, S.; Franceschi, C.; Ferrucci, L.; Gilroy, D.W.; Fasano, A.; Miller, G.W.; et al. Chronic inflammation in the etiology of disease across the life span. *Nat. Med.* **2019**, *25*, 1822–1832. [CrossRef]

8. Pradier, M.; Nguyen, S.; Robineau, O.; Titecat, M.; Blondiaux, N.; Valette, M.; Loïez, C.; Beltrand, E.; Dézeque, H.; Migaud, H.; et al. Suppressive antibiotic therapy with oral doxycycline for Staphylococcus aureus prosthetic joint infection: A retrospective study of 39 patients. *Int. J. Antimicrob. Agents* **2017**, *50*, 447–452. [CrossRef] [PubMed]
9. Byren, I.; Bejon, P.; Atkins, B.L.; Angus, B.; Masters, S.; McLardy-Smith, P.; Gundle, R.; Berendt, A. One hundred and twelve infected arthroplasties treated with "DAIR" (debridement, antibiotics and implant retention): Antibiotic duration and outcome. *J. Antimicrob. Chemother.* **2009**, *63*, 1264–1271. [CrossRef]
10. Prendki, V.; Sergent, P.; Barrelet, A.; Oziol, E.; Beretti, E.; Berlioz-Thibal, M.; Bouchand, F.; Dauchy, F.-A.; Forestier, E.; Gavazzi, G.; et al. Efficacy of indefinite chronic oral antimicrobial suppression for prosthetic joint infection in the elderly: A comparative study. *Int. J. Infect. Dis.* **2017**, *60*, 57–60. [CrossRef] [PubMed]
11. Pavoni, G.L.; Giannella, M.; Falcone, M.; Scorzolini, L.; Liberatore, M.; Carlesimo, B.; Serra, P.; Venditti, M. Conservative medical therapy of prosthetic joint infections: Retrospective analysis of an 8-year experience. *Clin. Microbiol. Infect.* **2004**, *10*, 831–837. [CrossRef]
12. Cobo, J.; Miguel, L.G.S.; Euba, G.; Rodríguez, D.; García-Lechuz, J.M.; Riera, M.; Falgueras, L.; Palomino, J.; Benito, N.; del Toro, M.D.; et al. Early prosthetic joint infection: Outcomes with debridement and implant retention followed by antibiotic therapy. *Clin. Microbiol. Infect.* **2011**, *17*, 1632–1637. [CrossRef]
13. Marculescu, C.E.; Berbari, E.F.; Hanssen, A.D.; Steckelberg, J.M.; Harmsen, S.W.; Mandrekar, J.N.; Osmon, D.R. Outcome of prosthetic joint infections treated with debridement and retention of components. *Clin. Infect. Dis.* **2006**, *42*, 471–478. [CrossRef]
14. Rao, N.; Crossett, L.S.; Sinha, R.K.; Le Frock, J.L. Long-term suppression of infection in total joint arthroplasty. *Clin. Orthop. Relat. Res.* **2003**, *414*, 55–60. [CrossRef]
15. Tsukayama, D.T.; Wicklund, B.; Gustilo, R.B. Suppressive antibiotic therapy in chronic prosthetic joint infections. *Orthopedics* **1991**, *14*, 841–844. [CrossRef]
16. Siqueira, M.B.P.; Saleh, A.; Klika, A.K.; O'Rourke, C.; Schmitt, S.; Higuera, C.A.; Barsoum, W.K. Chronic Suppression of Periprosthetic Joint Infections with Oral Antibiotics Increases Infection-Free Survivorship. *J. Bone Jt. Surg. Am.* **2015**, *97*, 1220–1232. [CrossRef]
17. Wouthuyzen-Bakker, M.; Nijman, J.M.; Kampinga, G.A.; van Assen, S.; Jutte, P.C. Efficacy of Antibiotic Suppressive Therapy in Patients with a Prosthetic Joint Infection. *J. Bone Jt. Infect.* **2017**, *2*, 77–83. [CrossRef]
18. Pradier, M.; Robineau, O.; Boucher, A.; Titecat, M.; Blondiaux, N.; Valette, M.; Loïez, C.; Beltrand, E.; Nguyen, S.; Dézeque, H.; et al. Suppressive antibiotic therapy with oral tetracyclines for prosthetic joint infections: A retrospective study of 78 patients. *Infection* **2018**, *46*, 39–47. [CrossRef] [PubMed]
19. Escudero-Sanchez, R.; Senneville, E.; Digumber, M.; Soriano, A.; del Toro, M.D.; Bahamonde, A.; del Pozo, J.L.; Guio, L.; Murillo, O.; Rico, A.; et al. Suppressive antibiotic therapy in prosthetic joint infections: A multicentre cohort study. *Clin. Microbiol. Infect.* **2020**, *26*, 499–505. [CrossRef] [PubMed]
20. Leijtens, B.; Weerwag, L.; Schreurs, B.W.; Kullberg, B.-J.; Rijnen, W. Clinical Outcome of Antibiotic Suppressive Therapy in Patients with a Prosthetic Joint Infection after Hip Replacement. *J. Bone Jt. Infect.* **2019**, *4*, 268–276. [CrossRef] [PubMed]
21. Malahias, M.A.; Gu, A.; Harris, E.C.; Adriani, M.; Miller, A.O.; Westrich, G.H.; Sculco, P.K. The Role of Long-Term Antibiotic Suppression in the Management of Peri-Prosthetic Joint Infections Treated With Debridement, Antibiotics, and Implant Retention: A Systematic Review. *J. Arthroplast.* **2020**, *35*, 1154–1160. [CrossRef]
22. Rao, K.; Young, V.B. Fecal Microbiota Transplantation for the Management of Clostridium difficile Infection. *Infect. Dis. Clin. N. Am.* **2015**, *29*, 109–122. [CrossRef]
23. Akinyoola, A.L.; Adegbehingbe, O.O.; Aboderin, A.O. Therapeutic decision in chronic osteomyelitis: Sinus track culture versus intraoperative bone culture. *Arch. Orthop. Trauma Surg.* **2009**, *129*, 449–453. [CrossRef] [PubMed]
24. Lensen, K.-J.; Escudero-Sanchez, R.; Cobo, J.; Soriano, A.; Wouthuyzen-Bakker, M. Chronic prosthetic joint infections with a draining sinus. Who should receive suppressive antibiotic treatment? *J. Bone Jt. Infect.* **2020**, *6*, 43–45. [CrossRef]
25. Dinh, A.; Duran, C.; Pavese, P.; Khatchatourian, L.; Monnin, B.; Bleibtreu, A.; Denis, E.; Etienne, C.; Rouanes, N.; Mahieu, R.; et al. French national cohort of first use of dalbavancin: A high proportion of off-label use. *Int. J. Antimicrob. Agents* **2019**, *54*, 668–672. [CrossRef]
26. Pouderoux, C.; Becker, A.; Goutelle, S.; Lustig, S.; Triffault-Fillit, C.; Daoud, F.; Fessy, M.H.; Cohen, S.; Laurent, F.; Chidiac, C.; et al. Lyon Bone and Joint Infection Study Group Subcutaneous suppressive antibiotic therapy for bone and joint infections: Safety and outcome in a cohort of 10 patients. *J. Antimicrob. Chemother.* **2019**, *74*, 2060–2064. [CrossRef] [PubMed]
27. Escudero-Sanchez, R.; Ponce-Alonso, M.; Barragán-Prada, H.; Morosini, M.-I.; Cantón, R.; Cobo, J.; Del Campo, R. Long-Term Impact of Suppressive Antibiotic Therapy on Intestinal Microbiota. *Genes* **2020**, *12*, 41. [CrossRef] [PubMed]

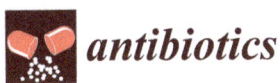

Article

Implant Removal in the Management of Prosthetic Joint Infection by *Staphylococcus aureus*: Outcome and Predictors of Failure in a Large Retrospective Multicenter Study

Joan Gómez-Junyent [1], Jaime Lora-Tamayo [2], Josu Baraia-Etxaburu [3], Mar Sánchez-Somolinos [4], Jose Antonio Iribarren [5,6], Dolors Rodriguez-Pardo [7], Julia Praena-Segovia [8], Luisa Sorlí [9], Alberto Bahamonde [10], Melchor Riera [11], Alicia Rico [12], Mª Dolores del Toro [13], Laura Morata [14], Javier Cobo [15], Luis Falgueras [16], Natividad Benito [17,18], Elena Muñez [19], Alfredo Jover-Sáenz [20], Carles Pigrau [7], Javier Ariza [1,21] and Oscar Murillo [1,21,*] on behalf of the Bone and Joint Infection Study Group of the Spanish Society of Infectious Diseases and Clinical Microbiology (GEIO-SEIMC) and the Spanish Network for Research in Infectious Diseases (REIPI)

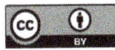

Citation: Gómez-Junyent, J.; Lora-Tamayo, J.; Baraia-Etxaburu, J.; Sánchez-Somolinos, M.; Iribarren, J.A.; Rodriguez-Pardo, D.; Praena-Segovia, J.; Sorlí, L.; Bahamonde, A.; Riera, M.; et al. Implant Removal in the Management of Prosthetic Joint Infection by *Staphylococcus aureus*: Outcome and Predictors of Failure in a Large Retrospective Multicenter Study. *Antibiotics* **2021**, *10*, 118. https://doi.org/10.3390/antibiotics10020118

Academic Editor: Nicholas Dixon
Received: 30 December 2020
Accepted: 22 January 2021
Published: 26 January 2021

Publisher's Note: MDPI stays neutral with regard to jurisdictional claims in published maps and institutional affiliations.

Copyright: © 2021 by the authors. Licensee MDPI, Basel, Switzerland. This article is an open access article distributed under the terms and conditions of the Creative Commons Attribution (CC BY) license (https://creativecommons.org/licenses/by/4.0/).

1. Department of Infectious Diseases, Hospital Universitari de Bellvitge, IDIBELL, Universitat de Barcelona, 08907 L'Hospitalet de Llobregat, Spain; gjunyent@hotmail.com (J.G.-J.); jariza@bellvitgehospital.cat (J.A.)
2. Department of Internal Medicine, Hospital Universitario 12 de Octubre, 28041 Madrid, Spain; sirsilverdelea@yahoo.com
3. Department of Infectious Diseases, Hospital Universitario de Basurto, 48013 Bilbao, Spain; baraiajosu@gmail.com
4. Department of Microbiology and Infectious Diseases, Hospital General Universitario Gregorio Marañón, 28009 Madrid, Spain; msanchezs35@yahoo.es
5. Department of Infectious Diseases, Hospital Universitario Donostia, Universidad del País Vasco (EHU/UPV), 20014 San Sebastián, Spain; joseantonio.iribarrenloyarte@osakidetza.eus
6. IIS BioDonostia, 20014 San Sebastián, Spain
7. Infectious Diseases Department, Hospital Universitari Vall d'Hebron, Universitat Autònoma de Barcelona, 08035 Barcelona, Spain; dolorodriguez@vhebron.net (D.R.-P.); cpigrau@vhebron.net (C.P.)
8. Clinical Unit of Infectious Diseases, Microbiology and Preventive Medicine, Hospital Universitario Virgen del Rocío, 41013 Seville, Spain; juliapraena@gmail.com
9. Department of Infectious Diseases, Hospital del Mar, Institut Hospital del Mar d'Investigacions Mèdiques (IMIM), 08003 Barcelona, Spain; lsorli@parcdesalutmar.cat
10. Department of Internal Medicine, Hospital El Bierzo, 24411 Ponferrada, Spain; med007783@me.com
11. Fundació Institut d'Investigació Sanitària Illes Balears, Hospital Universitario Son Espases, 07120 Palma, Spain; melchor.riera@ssib.es
12. Unit of Infectious Diseases and Clinical Microbiology, Hospital Universitario La Paz, 28046 Madrid, Spain; alicia.rico@salud.madrid.org
13. Clinical Unit of Infectious Diseases, Microbiology and Preventive Medicine, Hospital Universitario Virgen Macarena, Department of Medicine, Universidad de Sevilla, Instituto de Biomedicina de Sevilla (IBiS), 41009 Seville, Spain; mdeltoro@us.es
14. Department of Infectious Diseases, Hospital Clínic de Barcelona, Universitat de Barcelona, IDIBAPS, 08036 Barcelona, Spain; lmorata@clinic.cat
15. Department of Infectious Diseases, Hospital Universitario Ramón y Cajal, 28034 Madrid, Spain; javier.cobo@salud.madrid.org
16. Department of Infectious Diseases, Hospital Universitario Parc Taulí, 08208 Sabadell, Spain; lfalgueras@tauli.cat
17. Infectious Diseases Unit, Hospital de la Santa Creu i Sant Pau- Institut d'Investigació Biomèdica Sant Pau, 08025 Barcelona, Spain; nbenito@santpau.cat
18. Department of Medicine, Universitat Autònoma de Barcelona, 08025 Barcelona, Spain
19. Unit of Infectious Diseases, Department of Internal Medicine, Hospital Universitario Puerta de Hierro, 28220 Madrid, Spain; elmuru@gmail.com
20. Territorial Unit of Nosocomial Infections, Hospital Universitari Arnau de Vilanova, 25198 Lleida, Spain; ajover.lleida.ics@gencat.cat
21. Spanish Network for Research in Infectious Diseases (REIPI RD16/0016/0005), 41071 Sevilla, Spain
* Correspondence: omurillo@bellvitgehospital.cat; Tel.: +34-93-260-76-25

Abstract: Objectives: To compare the characteristics and outcomes of cases with acute prosthetic joint infection (PJI; early post-surgical or hematogenous) by *Staphylococcus aureus* managed with implant removal (IRm) or debridement and retention (DAIR). To analyze the outcomes of all cases managed with IRm (initially or after DAIR failure). Methods: Retrospective, multicenter, cohort study of PJI by *S. aureus* (2003–2010). Overall failure included mortality within 60 days since surgery and local failure due to staphylococcal persistence/relapse. Results: 499 cases, 338 initially managed with DAIR, 161 with IRm. Mortality was higher in acute PJI managed initially with IRm compared to DAIR, but not associated with the surgical procedure, after propensity score matching. Underlying conditions, hemiarthroplasty, and methicillin-resistant *S. aureus* were risk factors for mortality. Finally, 249 cases underwent IRm (88 after DAIR failure); overall failure was 15.6%. Local failure (9.3%) was slightly higher in cases with several comorbidities, but independent of previous DAIR, type of IRm, and rifampin treatment. Conclusions: In a large multicenter study of *S. aureus* PJI managed with IRm, failure was low, but mortality significant, especially in cases with acute PJI and underlying conditions, but not associated with the IRm itself. Rifampin efficacy was limited in this setting.

Keywords: *Staphylococcus aureus*; prosthetic joint infection; implant removal; outcome; rifampin

1. Introduction

Prosthetic joint infection (PJI) is a serious complication after joint replacement [1]. *Staphylococcus aureus* represents almost a third of all episodes [2], mostly associated with acute PJI (early post-surgical and hematogenous infections) [3], but also with chronic post-surgical infections.

Surgery is central for the optimal management of PJI by *S. aureus*, with two main strategies: debridement, antibiotics, and implant retention (DAIR), or implant removal (IRm) [3,4]. Observational studies have analyzed the outcome of DAIR [5–9], but the prognosis of IRm, generally performed in chronic PJI or after DAIR failure, has not been extensively evaluated [10,11]. Some authors have suggested that IRm as salvage therapy may lead to poorer outcomes compared with an initial management with IRm [12,13]. The role of rifampin is not formally established, contrasting with its benefits in DAIR [8,14].

Previously, the prognosis of the largest case-series of staphylococcal PJI managed with DAIR was analyzed [8]. However, the characteristics and outcome of cases treated with IRm were not reported in that analysis.

Therefore, our aim was to revise this large multicenter study with the objectives of (i) analyzing the subcohort of cases with acute PJI to compare the characteristics and outcomes of those initially managed with IRm or DAIR; and (ii) evaluating the outcomes of the subgroup of all cases managed with IRm, initially or as salvage therapy after DAIR failure including the role of rifampin.

2. Results

During the study period, 561 cases were initially identified to have PJI by *S. aureus*, but 62 cases had exclusion criteria. Thus, 499 cases were finally included: 325 (65.1%) with early post-surgical (EA) PJI, 75 (15.0%) with hematogenous PJI, and 99 (19.8%) with chronic post-surgical PJI.

Follow-up data (median 781 days, interquartile range [IQR] 355-1375) and/or known outcomes were available for 478 cases. Figure 1 shows the percentage of cases with overall failure (local failure plus mortality), local failure, and mortality in all cases and according to the type of PJI.

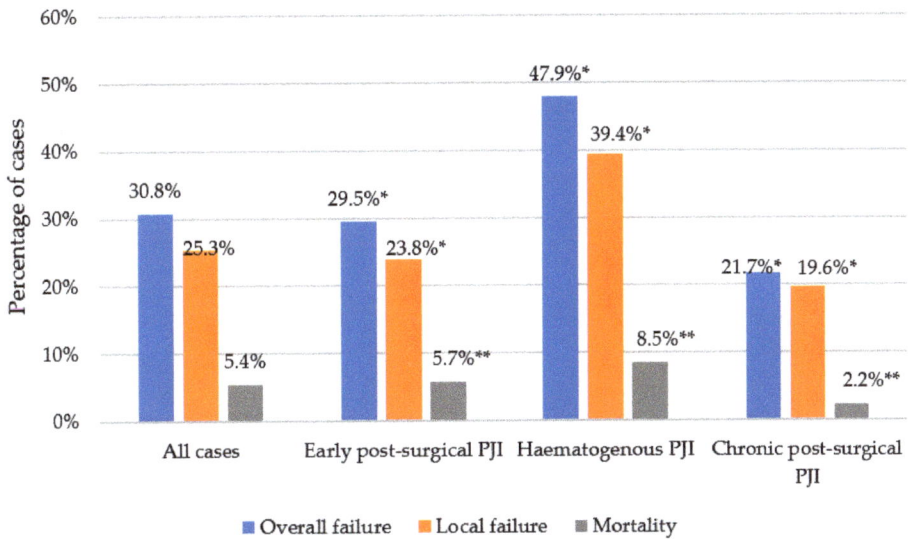

Figure 1. Outcomes of cases with prosthetic joint infection (PJI) by *Staphylococcus aureus* according to the type of infection. * p value < 0.01 in overall and local failure between hematogenous, early post-surgical, and chronic post-surgical PJI; ** p value = 0.201 in mortality between hematogenous, early post-surgical, and chronic post-surgical PJI.

2.1. Implant Removal as the Initial Surgical Strategy in the Cohort of Acute Prosthetic Joint Infection (PJI)

Similar differences in characteristics between cases managed with IRm and DAIR were found in EA and hematogenous PJI, which were therefore analyzed together as acute PJI (n = 400, Table 1). Cases with acute PJI managed with IRm were more likely to have a hemiarthroplasty or hematogenous PJI, but also other factors such as abnormal radiography, symptoms duration >21 days, poor condition of soft tissues, or infection by MRSA.

Table 1. Characteristics, adjusted odds ratios of implant removal and outcome of 400 cases of acute prosthetic joint infection (early post-surgical and hematogenous) by *Staphylococcus aureus*, according to their initial surgical management.

Characteristic	Acute PJI Managed with DAIR (n = 311)	Acute PJI Managed with Implant Removal (n = 89)	p Value	Adjusted OR of Implant Removal (95% CI) *	p Value
PATIENT CHARACTERISTICS					
Female sex	184 (59.2)	59 (66.3)	0.225		
Age (years) [1]	72 (64–78)	74 (68–78)	0.168	1.01 (0.99–1.04)	0.294
Two or more comorbidities [2]	60 (19.3)	17 (19.1)	0.968		
Chronic kidney disease	16 (5.1)	8 (9.0)	0.178		
PROSTHESIS CHARACTERISTICS					
Total hip arthroplasty	109 (35.1)	27 (30.3)	0.408		
Total knee arthroplasty	174 (56.0)	45 (50.6)	0.368		
Hemiarthroplasty	24 (7.7)	14 (15.7)	0.023	3.73 (1.60–8.68)	0.003
Revision prosthesis	53 (17.0)	14 (15.7)	0.770		

Table 1. Cont.

Characteristic	Acute PJI Managed with DAIR (n = 311)	Acute PJI Managed with Implant Removal (n = 89)	p Value	Adjusted OR of Implant Removal (95% CI) *	p Value
CLINICAL AND ANALYTICAL DATA					
Hematogenous PJI	49 (15.8)	26 (29.2)	0.004	3.34 (1.72–6.46)	<0.001
Leukocytosis [3]	157 (50.5)	52 (58.4)	0.186		
CRP (mg/L)	109 (28–120)	100 (30–107)	0.415		
Abnormal radiography [4]	27 (8.7)	26 (29.2)	<0.001	3.70 (1.85–7.43)	<0.001
Duration of symptoms >21 days	33 (10.6)	37 (41.6)	<0.001	7.69 (4.03–14.68)	<0.001
Poor condition of soft tissues	37 (11.9)	19 (21.4)	0.023	1.50 (0.72–3.12)	0.282
Infection by MRSA	75 (24.1)	34 (38.2)	0.008	1.42 (0.95–3.19)	0.074
Bacteremia	57 (18.3)	17 (19.1)	0.868		
Polymicrobial infection	58 (18.7)	19 (21.4)	0.569		
OUTCOME [5]					
Overall failure	107 (35.7)	20 (23.3)	0.031		
Local failure	94 (31.3)	9 (10.5)	<0.001		
Mortality <60 days	13 (4.3)	11 (12.8)	0.004		

Categorical variables expressed in absolute number and (percentage); continuous variables expressed in median and (interquartile range). PJI: Prosthetic joint infection. DAIR: Debridement, antibiotics and implant retention. OR: Odds ratio. 95%CI: 95% Confidence Interval. IQR: Interquartile range. MRSA: Methicillin-resistant *S. aureus*. * Refers to a multivariate analysis of factors associated with implant removal in patients with acute PJI (n = 400). [1] Odds ratio expressed as per year. [2] These include severe comorbidities (diabetes, liver cirrhosis, chronic kidney disease, immunosuppressive treatment, rheumatoid arthritis, malignancy, chronic lung, and heart diseases) present in the McPherson Staging System [15]. [3] Leukocytosis is defined as baseline leukocyte count above $10 \times 10^9/L$. [4] Abnormal radiography is defined according to radiologic signs of infection (loosening, periprosthetic osteolysis, migration, subperiostic reaction). [5] Calculated among 300 patients with acute PJI managed with DAIR and 86 patients with acute PJI managed with implant removal.

Mortality was greater in acute PJI managed initially with IRm compared to DAIR. However, after performing propensity score matching including several pre-surgical variables (age, number of comorbidities, hemiarthroplasty, hematogenous PJI, abnormal radiography, symptoms duration, condition of soft tissues, infection by MRSA and hospital), mortality was not associated with the IRm procedure itself (OR 1.55; 95%CI 0.47–4.56; p = 0.387) (Figure S1A).

Among cases with acute PJI initially managed with IRm (Figure 2), mortality was greater if they had two or more comorbidities (7/16 [43.8%] vs. 4/70 [5.7%]; p < 0.001), especially rheumatoid arthritis (3/7 [42.9%] vs. 8/79 [10.1%]; p = 0.042) and immunosuppressive treatment (4/7 [57.1%] vs. 7/79 [8.9%]; p = 0.004). Mortality was also higher if they had a hemiarthroplasty (5/14 [35.7%] vs. 6/72 [8.3%]; p = 0.015), bacteremia (5/9 [55.6%] vs 6/77 [7.8%]; p = 0.001), and infection by MRSA (8/32 [25.0%] vs. 3/54 [5.6%]; p = 0.016).

2.2. Cohort of All Cases Managed with Implant Removal (Initially or Salvage Therapy)

Together with 161 cases managed initially with IRm (63, 26, and 72 with EA, hematogenous and chronic post-surgical PJI, respectively), there were 88 cases (78 with acute and 10 with chronic post-surgical PJI) who finally underwent IRm as salvage therapy. Thus, this procedure was performed in 249 cases (Table 2): two-stage exchange (188, 75.5%), hip resection arthroplasty (44, 17.7%), and one-stage exchange (17, 6.8%). No significant differences were found in surgical strategies between clinical groups (p = 0.440). There were 52 cases (27.7%) under the two-stage scheme without a second stage performed; thus, 96 cases (38.6%) finally had resection arthroplasty, who more often had two or more comorbidities (26.0% vs. 16.3%; p = 0.063).

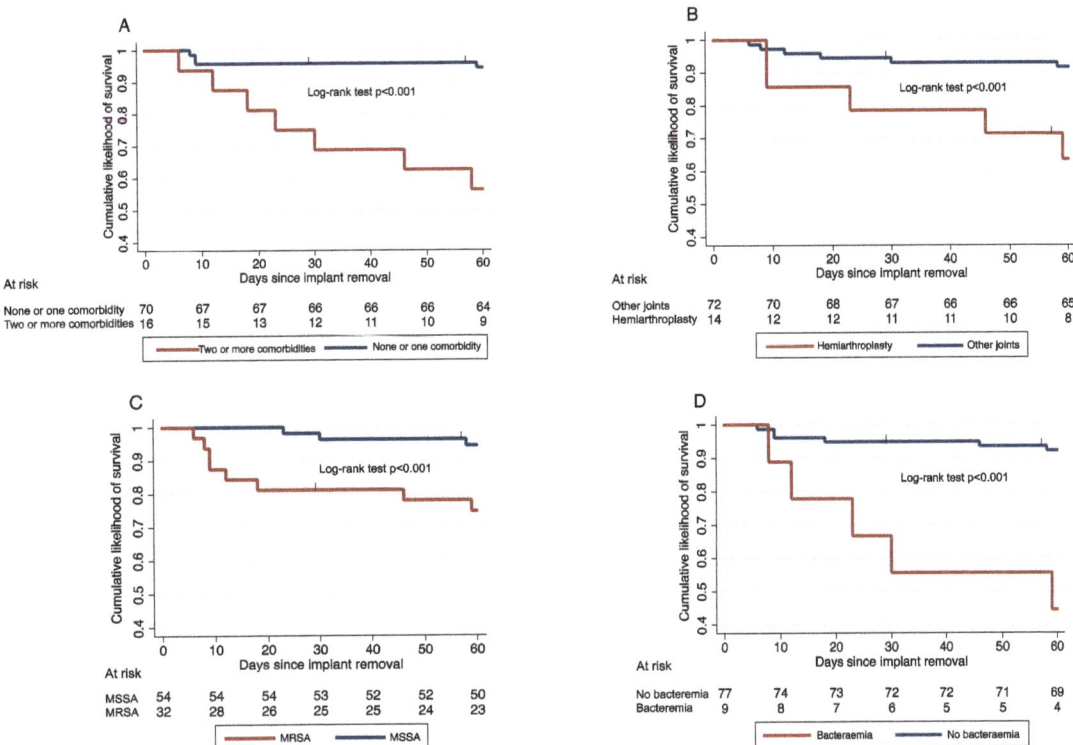

Figure 2. Kaplan–Meier curves of mortality of cases with acute prosthetic joint infection by *Staphylococcus aureus* managed initially with implant removal. (**A**) Patients with and without two or more comorbidities. (**B**) Patients with and without hemiarthroplasty. (**C**) Patients with infection by methicillin-resistant (MRSA) or methicillin-susceptible *S. aureus* (MSSA). (**D**) Patients with and without bacteremia.

Table 2. Characteristics and outcome of the subcohort of cases of prosthetic joint infection by *Staphylococcus aureus* managed with implant removal (*n* = 249), according to their type of infection.

Characteristic	Acute PJI (Early Post-Surgical and Hematogenous)			Chronic Post-Surgical PJI		
	IRm as Initial Strategy (*n* = 89)	IRm as Salvage Therapy (*n* = 78)	*p* Value *	IRm as Initial Strategy (*n* = 72)	IRm as Salvage Therapy (*n* = 10)	*p* Value **
Female sex	59 (66.3)	52 (66.7)	0.959	46 (63.9)	7 (70.0)	0.705
Age (years)	74 (68–78)	72 (60–79)	0.470	74 (64–79)	68 (57–76)	0.082
Two or more comorbidities [1]	17 (19.1)	16 (20.5)	0.819	13 (18.1)	4 (40.0)	0.109
Chronic kidney disease	8 (9.0)	6 (7.7)	0.763	8 (11.1)	0	0.267
Hemiarthroplasty	14 (15.7)	3 (3.9)	0.011	3 (4.2)	0	0.511
Revision prosthesis	14 (15.7)	18 (23.1)	0.229	15 (20.8)	5 (50.0)	0.044
Infection by MRSA	34 (38.2)	16 (20.5)	0.013	12 (16.7)	3 (30.0)	0.307
Bacteremia	9 (10.1)	4 (5.1)	0.230	1 (1.4)	0	0.708
Polymicrobial infection	19 (21.4)	20 (25.6)	0.513	20 (27.8)	2 (20.0)	0.603

Table 2. Cont.

Characteristic	Acute PJI (Early Post-Surgical and Hematogenous)			Chronic Post-Surgical PJI		
	IRm as Initial Strategy (n = 89)	IRm as Salvage Therapy (n = 78)	p Value *	IRm as Initial Strategy (n = 72)	IRm as Salvage Therapy (n = 10)	p Value **
OUTCOME [2]						
Overall failure	20 (23.3)	9 (12.0)	0.064	6 (9.0)	2 (22.2)	0.223
Local failure	9 (10.5)	7 (9.3)	0.811	4 (6.0)	2 (22.2)	0.090
Mortality < 60 days	11 (12.8)	2 (2.7)	0.019	2 (3.0)	0	0.599

Categorical variables expressed in absolute number and (percentage); continuous variables expressed in median and (interquartile range). IRm as salvage therapy refer to cases who failed after an initial management with DAIR (Debridement, antibiotics, and implant retention). PJI: Prosthetic joint infection. IRm: Implant removal. MRSA: Methicillin-resistant *S. aureus*. * Comparison between acute PJI. ** Comparison between chronic PJI. [1] These include severe comorbidities (diabetes, liver cirrhosis, chronic kidney disease, immunosuppressive treatment, rheumatoid arthritis, malignancy, chronic lung and heart diseases) present in the McPherson Staging System [15]. [2] Calculated among 86 patients with acute PJI initially managed with implant removal, 75 patients with acute PJI initially managed with DAIR, 67 patients with chronic PJI initially managed with implant removal, and nine patients with chronic PJI initially managed with DAIR.

The median length of antimicrobial therapy was 59 days (IQR 43–92). There were 119 cases (55.4%) who received rifampin in combination during ≥21 days in the first 42 days after IRm. Other antibiotics commonly given, either alone or in combination with rifampin, were quinolones (43.3%), beta-lactams (28.8%), cotrimoxazole (16.3%), and glycopeptides (11.6%).

Overall, 237 cases had outcome data, of whom 37 (15.6%; 95%CI 11.2–20.9) presented overall failure, 22 (9.3%; 95%CI 5.9–13.7) local failure, and 15 patients died (6.3%; 95%CI 3.6–10.2). Mortality occurred to 11 patients (12.8%) with acute PJI initially managed with IRm, two (2.7%) with acute PJI requiring IRm as salvage therapy and two (3.0%) with chronic post-surgical PJI initially managed with IRm.

Local failure was similar in all IRm strategies, but slightly higher (22.2%) in those with chronic PJI initially managed with DAIR (Table 2). In an analysis of predictive factors of local failure (Table 3), having two or more comorbidities showed a trend toward greater local failure, whereas cases requiring IRm as salvage therapy after DAIR failure did not present worse outcomes. Cases receiving rifampin for 21 days or longer within the first 42 days did not present lower rates of local failure (10.1% vs. 7.3%; $p = 0.473$). Similar results (HR 0.82; 95%CI 0.39–1.70; $p = 0.590$) were found when estimating the effect of rifampin ≥ 21 days after propensity score matching (including age, number of comorbidities, liver cirrhosis, type of infection, infection by MRSA, previous DAIR, type of IRm, and hospital; Figure S1B).

Table 3. Predictive factors of local failure among 237 cases of prosthetic joint infection by *Staphylococcus aureus* managed with implant removal (22 cases failed).

Characteristic		Failed/Total (%)	Crude HR (95%CI)	p Value	Adjusted HR (95% CI)	p Value
Age	<75 years	15/127 (11.8)	1		1	
	≥75 years	7/110 (6.4)	0.59 (0.24–1.44)	0.234	0.59 (0.24–1.44)	0.231
Sex	Male	9/80 (11.3)	1			
	Female	13/157 (8.3)	0.67 (0.29–1.57)	0.364		
Two or more comorbidities [1]	No	15/192 (7.8)	1		1	
	Yes	7/45 (15.6)	2.44 (0.99–5.99)	0.051	2.46 (1.00–6.09)	0.051
Hemiarthroplasty	No	21/218 (9.6)	1			
	Yes	1/19 (5.3)	0.87 (0.12–6.50)	0.891		
Revision prosthesis	No	15/185 (8.1)	1			
	Yes	7/52 (13.5)	1.77 (0.72–4.37)	0.232		

Table 3. Cont.

Characteristic		Failed/Total (%)	Crude HR (95%CI)	p Value	Adjusted HR (95% CI)	p Value
Hematogenous PJI	No	18/193 (9.3)	1			
	Yes	4/44 (9.1)	0.93 (0.31–2.75)	0.891		
Infection by MRSA	No	18/179 (10.1)	1			
	Yes	4/58 (6.9)	0.87 (0.29–2.57)	0.798		
Bacteremia	No	21/223 (9.4)	1			
	Yes	1/14 (7.1)	1.76 (0.23–13.32)	0.613		
Polymicrobial infection	No	19/178 (10.7)	1			
	Yes	3/59 (5.1)	0.51 (0.15–1.71)	0.236		
Initially managed with DAIR	No	13/153 (8.5)	1		1	
	Yes	9/84 (10.7)	1.06 (0.45–2.49)	0.886	0.94 (0.40–2.23)	0.897
Surgical management	One-stage exchange	2/16 (12.5)	1			
	Two-stage exchange	16/182 (8.8)	0.60 (0.14–2.62)			
	Hip resection arthroplasty	4/39 (10.3)	0.84 (0.15–4.61)	0.720		
Rifampin [2]	No	7/96 (7.3)	1			
	Yes	12/119 (10.1)	1.01 (0.37–2.73)	0.989		

HR: Hazard ratio. 95% CI: 95% Confidence interval. PJI: Prosthetic joint infection. MRSA: Methicillin-resistant *S. aureus*. DAIR: Debridement, antibiotics, and implant retention. [1] These include severe comorbidities (diabetes, liver cirrhosis, chronic kidney disease, immunosuppressive treatment, rheumatoid arthritis, malignancy, chronic lung and heart diseases) present in the McPherson Staging System [15]. [2] Among those treated with rifampin for 21 days or longer in the initial 42 days since implant removal.

Among the cases with local failure, nine presented symptomatic persistence of infection, eight relapsed, and five presented positive cultures in a second-stage exchange. There were 16 cases with positive staphylococcal cultures upon failure, but none were rifampin-resistant. Long-term follow-up was available in 19/22 cases; four needed long-term SAT, while the rest eventually were considered cured after further treatment.

3. Discussion

PJI by *S. aureus* represents a therapeutic challenge for physicians. While most of the knowledge on its outcome involves patients managed with DAIR [5–9], IRm has received scarce attention in the literature [10,11]. To the best of our knowledge, the present study includes the largest series of cases with *S. aureus* PJI managed with IRm.

The selection of patients with acute PJI (early post-surgical or hematogenous PJI) to be managed either with DAIR or IRm usually follows well-known algorithms such as the standardized Zimmerli criteria [3], which do not include host conditions but factors related to symptom duration, the condition of the implant and soft tissues, and anti-biofilm antimicrobial susceptibility. Additionally, there is still controversy whether DAIR should be performed in infections within 30–90 days since arthroplasty. In this study, among cases with acute PJI, those with hemiarthroplasty, hematogenous PJI, and/or infection by MRSA were more likely to be managed with IRm.

In this line, previous studies found higher failure rates in patients managed with DAIR who presented these characteristics [8,16] as well as those with particular comorbidities, suggesting that Zimmerli criteria may be revisited. Some authors have attempted to build scores such as the KLIC score [16,17], which may provide guidance in selecting the optimal surgical management for patients with acute PJI. Similarly, the McPherson staging system [15], which includes host factors, has been correlated with the outcome of acute and chronic PJI [18,19] and may define the optimal surgical strategy for each patient [20]. However, these scores were built from studies that include heterogeneous patients with diverse causative microorganisms and have shown poor prediction in staphylococcal PJI. Overall, it seems plausible that future research should address the development of specific scores for *S. aureus* PJI. Additionally, the surgeon's and/or patient's preferences should also be considered.

Mortality was higher in patients with acute PJI managed with IRm compared to those undergoing DAIR. Importantly, the surgical procedure was not associated with the higher mortality observed after propensity score matching. Interestingly, the same characteristics (hemiarthroplasty, MRSA) that were driving IRm in acute PJI were also associated with a greater probability of mortality. While some characteristics such as hemiarthroplasty and/or MRSA have been previously recognized as risk factors for mortality [21,22], the results suggest that patients with several underlying conditions also have greater likelihood of mortality, especially if bacteremic [23]. Importantly, these factors may present together [22] and, therefore, physicians should rapidly identify and provide accurate care of older patients, with hemiarthroplasties and/or infections by MRSA when managing acute staphylococcal PJI.

IRm was associated with low local failure. Obviously, the physical removal of biofilm facilitates the activity of antimicrobials, resulting in a greater chance of cure, compared to DAIR [24,25]. However, even in this favorable situation, some patients failed. Salvage therapy eventually cured most patients, suggesting a good overall prognosis when a first procedure is unsuccessful.

Most factors associated with mortality did not influence the likelihood of local failure, but cases with several comorbidities had slightly higher local failure [15]. Interestingly, the outcome was not worse in patients who needed IRm as salvage therapy, suggesting that DAIR can be attempted without affecting the prospects for a future removal surgery, if needed. This study, though, could not evaluate whether an initial DAIR might affect the functional outcome of patients needing IRm, which has aroused some controversy in the literature [12]. Failure rates were similar according to IRm strategies including one-stage exchange, as reported also by Senneville et al. [11]. However, since the vast majority of our patients were managed with two-stage exchange, more data are needed to evaluate the outcome of other strategies with larger sample sizes.

The role of rifampin following IRm is not well established, in contrast with staphylococcal PJI managed with DAIR. In a short series evaluating cases managed with DAIR or IRm [11], Senneville et al. reported better results in patients receiving rifampin, but unfortunately, the authors did not provide a thorough analysis of cases managed with IRm. In this study, a better outcome in patients treated with rifampin during more than 21 days could not be proven. The design of this study did not allow us to draw definitive conclusions on the benefits of rifampin in this setting and further research should address this clinical question.

Several limitations are inherent to the observational retrospective study design, despite being multicentric and its large sample size. Patients included were potentially heterogeneous in their characteristics, presentations, and management, which may have underpowered some analyses. Matching and multivariate analyses have been performed to adjust for this variability, but possible biases and imbalances may still have occurred. Local failure was evaluated based solely on persistence/relapse of *S. aureus*; thus, higher failure rates may have been found if other criteria such as superinfections or orthopedic problems had been included. Finally, not only monomicrobial PJIs by *S. aureus* were included, but also polymicrobial infections. However, we believe that the present data offer an overall perspective of the prognosis of PJI by *S. aureus*.

4. Materials and Methods

4.1. Design, Setting, and Patients

This was a retrospective, multicenter cohort study performed in 17 hospitals in Spain, in the framework of the Spanish Network for Research in Infectious Diseases (REIPI) during 2003–2010, which included all consecutive cases of PJI caused by *S. aureus* identified from previously registered databases or from the general archives in each hospital. Two cohorts were analyzed: (i) the subcohort of acute PJI was used to compare the characteristics and outcomes of cases managed initially with IRm or DAIR; and (ii) the subcohort of all cases managed with IRm, either initially or as salvage therapy after DAIR failure, was used to investigate their outcome (mortality and factors predicting failure).

Cases of PJI caused by *S. aureus*, monomicrobial or polymicrobial, managed with DAIR or IRm were included. Cases where *S. aureus* did not cause the original PJI, but participated later as a superinfecting microorganism, those requiring amputation as the initial surgical procedure for IRm, and those catalogued as positive intraoperative cultures according to Tsukayama's criteria [26] were excluded. Patient consent was not required, given the retrospective design; data were anonymized, without sensitive information that may enable the participant's identification.

4.2. Definitions

PJI was defined according to Infectious Diseases Society of America guidelines and microorganisms were identified according to standard criteria [3,4,8,27]. In accordance with the most commonly used classifications of types of PJI, these were categorized into early post-surgical (EA), chronic post-surgical, and acute hematogenous. The latter included cases with ≤3 weeks of symptoms duration appearing three months after surgery in the setting of microbiologically confirmed or clinically suspected staphylococcal bacteremia. Regarding EA and chronic post-surgical PJI, there is still controversy on definitions based on time from arthroplasty and accordingly, EA-PJI may include cases that present within one month or three months [3,4,26,28,29], and these time cut-offs are usually employed in selecting patients to be managed successfully with DAIR. Thus, for the purpose of this study, PJI occurring within three months after prosthesis placement were classified as EA, whereas defined as chronic post-surgical, if these started thereafter [3,4]. When analyzing the subcohort of acute PJI, EA and acute hematogenous PJI were included.

Baseline characteristics were recorded and included severe comorbidities (diabetes, liver cirrhosis, chronic kidney disease (CKD), immunosuppressive treatment, rheumatoid arthritis, malignancy, chronic lung, and heart diseases) present in the McPherson Staging System [15].

4.3. Clinical and Surgical Management

The decision to manage patients with DAIR or IRm was taken by the attending medical team, commonly following Zimmerli's criteria [3]; patients with duration of symptoms ≤21 days, a stable implant, and appropriate soft tissues condition usually qualify for DAIR. Regarding the controversies in definitions of EA PJI above-mentioned, infections occurring within 30–90 days since prosthesis placement were usually considered for IRm, but might have also been managed with DAIR.

DAIR management, which was performed only as an initial strategy, has been described elsewhere [7,8]. IRm was performed as an initial strategy or after DAIR in patients who failed. IRm was classified into three surgical approaches [30]: (a) two-stage exchange; (b) one-stage exchange; and (c) hip resection arthroplasty. Cases were considered under the two-stage exchange scheme if the intention was to implant a new prosthesis or arthrodesis, irrespective of whether this second stage was finally performed.

In most hospitals, the usual perioperative antimicrobial prophylaxis for arthroplasties consists of intravenous cefazolin 2 g. After the surgical procedure for PJI, intravenous antibiotics of wide antimicrobial-spectrum are administered. Once the antimicrobial susceptibility is available, antibiotics are adjusted according to current guidelines. However, the ultimate choice of the antimicrobial treatment is at the discretion of the medical team. The intravenous route is maintained for a variable period depending on each hospital protocol, usually followed by oral antibiotics, also for a variable time.

4.4. Outcomes and Follow-Up

Patients were followed until death, failure, or loss to follow-up. Overall failure was defined as a composite endpoint consisting of local failure and/or mortality due to any cause occurring within 60 days since surgery (cut-off selected to reflect mortality potentially linked to the PJI process).

In cases managed with DAIR, local failure has been defined elsewhere [8], but only considered if related to staphylococcal persistence/relapse. In cases managed with IRm, it was defined also only if staphylococcal persistence/relapse as: (a) symptom persistence beginning within 30 days after IRm, leading to long-term suppressive antimicrobial therapy (SAT) and/or new surgeries, irrespective of when these were performed; (b) relapsing symptoms in asymptomatic patients initially considered cured after IRm; and (c) positive *S. aureus* cultures in asymptomatic patients undergoing a second-stage surgery.

4.5. Statistical Analysis

Data were analyzed with Stata 13.1 (Stata Corporation, USA). Categorical and continuous variables were described by counts and percentages, and median and interquartile range (IQR), respectively. Comparisons between groups were performed with the chi-square test or Fisher exact test for categorical variables and the t-test or Mann–Whitney test for continuous variables.

Multivariate logistic regression was used to analyze factors associated with initial management with IRm in acute PJI including the commonly used Zimmerli's criteria [3]. Kaplan–Meier survival curves were used to evaluate the probability of success during follow-up and the log-rank test analyzed differences between groups, censoring cases lost to follow-up. Multivariate Cox regression was performed to estimate factors associated with local failure, censoring death as a competing event.

To evaluate the impact of interventions (surgical procedure [DAIR vs. IRm] and rifampin) on mortality and local failure, respectively, propensity score matching analyses were performed. Clinically relevant variables were introduced in the propensity model, together with baseline characteristics found to have a univariate association with the intervention ($p < 0.1$). The adequacy of the models was assessed with calibration plots and the Hosmer–Lemeshow test. Nearest neighbor matching with replacement was performed with 0.1 calipers. Mean standardized differences for covariates between matched groups were checked prior to treatment effects estimation.

The length of antibiotic therapy could be shortened in cases failing prematurely and would not actually be the cause of failure but its consequence. Thus, in order to avoid survivor's bias, the influence of rifampin on local failure was only analyzed in cases treated for ≥ 21 days and not requiring salvage surgeries within the first 42 days after IRm.

5. Conclusions

In conclusion, while mortality was significant in acute PJI by *S. aureus* managed with IRm, there was no evident association with the surgical approach itself. Additionally, we identified factors related to the patient's condition that were associated with a greater probability of death among these cases. Local failure was low, but a previous DAIR strategy did not worsen the outcome of cases. Despite the limited efficacy found in this study, further research should confirm whether rifampin may still offer a potential benefit in the treatment of patients with staphylococcal PJI managed with IRm.

Supplementary Materials: The following are available online at https://www.mdpi.com/2079-6382/10/2/118/s1, Figure S1: Standardized bias for covariates before and after propensity score matching for the evaluation of implant removal on mortality in cases with acute prosthetic joint infection by *Staphylococcus aureus* (A) and the role of rifampin on local failure in all cases managed with implant removal (B).

Author Contributions: All authors contributed to the supervision of clinical cases, data collection, and interpretation. J.G.-J., J.L-T., J.A., and O.M. conceptualized and designed the study. J.G.-J. analyzed the data and wrote a first draft of the manuscript. The manuscript was further reviewed and rewritten by J.G-J., J.L.-T., J.A., and O.M. All authors have read and agreed to the published version of the manuscript.

Funding: This study was supported by Plan Nacional I+D+I 2013–2016 and Instituto de Salud Carlos III, Subdirección General de Redes y Centros de Investigación Cooperativa, Ministerio de Economía, Industria y Competitividad, Spanish Network for Research in Infectious Diseases (REIPI RD16/0016/0005), co-financed by the European Development Regional Fund "A way to achieve Europe", Operative program Intelligent Growth 2004–2020. J. G-J was supported by a grant from the Spanish Ministry of Education (FPU 14/03124).

Institutional Review Board Statement: Ethical review and approval were waived for this study, due to the retrospective observational design based on clinical routine data.

Informed Consent Statement: Patient consent was not required, given the retrospective design.

Data Availability Statement: The data presented in this study are available upon request from the corresponding author.

Acknowledgments: We thank John B. Warren (International House Barcelona) for revising the English manuscript. We thank CERCA Program/Generalitat de Catalunya for institutional support. The preliminary results were presented in part at the 29th European Congress of Clinical Microbiology and Infectious Diseases, Amsterdam, Netherlands, 13–16 April 2019. Collaborators of the GEIO-SEIMC and REIPI also include Xavier Cabo and Eva Benavent (Hospital Universitari de Bellvitge, Barcelona, Spain); Fernando Chaves and Mikel Mancheño (Hospital Universitario 12 de Octubre, Madrid, Spain); Iñigo Lopez Azkarreta and Mireia De la Peña Trigueros (Hospital Universitario de Basurto, Bilbao, Spain); Mercedes Marín Arriaza (Hospital General Universitario Gregorio Marañón, Madrid, Spain); Juan Manuel García-Lechuz (Hospital Universitario Miguel Servet, Zaragoza, Spain); Miguel Angel Goenaga and Gaspar de la Herrán (Hospital Universitario Donostia, San Sebastián, Spain); Pablo S Corona and Mayli Lung (Hospital Universitari Vall Hebron, Barcelona, Spain); Javier Garcés and Maite Ruiz Pérez de Pipaón (Hospital Universitario Virgen del Rocío, Sevilla, Spain); Juan Pablo Horcajada and Lluís Puig (Hospital del Mar, Barcelona, Spain); Carlos Rodríguez-Lucas and Cristina Rodríguez-Alonso (Hospital El Bierzo, Ponferrada, Spain); Helem H Vilchez and Antonio Ramírez (Hospital Universitari Son Espases, Palma, Spain); Jose María Bravo-Ferrer and Reinaldo Espíndola Roney (Hospital Universitario Virgen Macarena, Seville, Spain); Alex Soriano and Juan Carlos Martínez-Pastor (Hospital Clínic, Barcelona, Spain); Rosa Escudero and Patricia Ruiz Garbajosa (Hospital Universitario Ramón y Cajal, Madrid, Spain); Ana Granados and Ana María Martí-Garín (Hospital Parc Taulí, Sabadell, Spain); Isabel Mur and Alba Rivera (Hospital de la Santa Creu i Sant Pau, Barcelona, Spain); Antonio Ramos (Hospital Universitario Puerta de Hierro, Madrid, Spain); and Ferran Pérez-Villar and Mercè Garcia-González (Hospital Universitari Arnau de Vilanova, Lleida, Spain).

Conflicts of Interest: All authors declare no conflict of interest concerning this article. The funders had no role in the design of the study; in the collection, analyses, or interpretation of data; in the writing of the manuscript, or in the decision to publish the results.

References

1. Del Pozo, J.L.; Patel, R. Clinical practice. Infection associated with prosthetic joints. *N. Engl. J. Med.* **2009**, *361*, 787–794. [CrossRef] [PubMed]
2. Benito, N.; Franco, M.; Ribera, A.; Soriano, A.; Rodriguez-Pardo, D.; Sorli, L.; Fresco, G.; Fernandez-Sampedro, M.; Dolores Del Toro, M.; Guio, L.; et al. Time trends in the aetiology of prosthetic joint infections: A multicentre cohort study. *Clin. Microbiol. Infect.* **2016**, *22*, 732.e1–732.e8. [CrossRef] [PubMed]
3. Zimmerli, W.; Trampuz, A.; Ochsner, P.E. Prosthetic-joint infections. *N. Engl. J. Med.* **2004**, *351*, 1645–1654. [CrossRef] [PubMed]
4. Osmon, D.R.; Berbari, E.F.; Berendt, A.R.; Lew, D.; Zimmerli, W.; Steckelberg, J.M.; Rao, N.; Hanssen, A.; Wilson, W.R. Diagnosis and management of prosthetic joint infection: Clinical practice guidelines by the Infectious Diseases Society of America. *Clin. Infect. Dis.* **2013**, *56*, e1–e25. [CrossRef] [PubMed]
5. Aboltins, C.A.; Page, M.A.; Buising, K.L.; Jenney, A.W.; Daffy, J.R.; Choong, P.F.; Stanley, P.A. Treatment of staphylococcal prosthetic joint infections with debridement, prosthesis retention and oral rifampicin and fusidic acid. *Clin. Microbiol. Infect.* **2007**, *13*, 586–591. [CrossRef] [PubMed]

6. Brandt, C.M.; Sistrunk, W.W.; Duffy, M.C.; Hanssen, A.D.; Steckelberg, J.M.; Ilstrup, D.M.; Osmon, D.R. Staphylococcus aureus prosthetic joint infection treated with debridement and prosthesis retention. *Clin. Infect. Dis.* **1997**, *24*, 914–919. [CrossRef]
7. Byren, I.; Bejon, P.; Atkins, B.L.; Angus, B.; Masters, S.; McLardy-Smith, P.; Gundle, R.; Berendt, A. One hundred and twelve infected arthroplasties treated with 'DAIR' (debridement, antibiotics and implant retention): Antibiotic duration and outcome. *J. Antimicrob. Chemother.* **2009**, *63*, 1264–1271. [CrossRef]
8. Lora-Tamayo, J.; Murillo, O.; Iribarren, J.A.; Soriano, A.; Sanchez-Somolinos, M.; Baraia-Etxaburu, J.M.; Rico, A.; Palomino, J.; Rodriguez-Pardo, D.; Horcajada, J.P.; et al. A large multicenter study of methicillin-susceptible and methicillin-resistant Staphylococcus aureus prosthetic joint infections managed with implant retention. *Clin. Infect. Dis.* **2013**, *56*, 182–194. [CrossRef]
9. Marculescu, C.E.; Berbari, E.F.; Hanssen, A.D.; Steckelberg, J.M.; Harmsen, S.W.; Mandrekar, J.N.; Osmon, D.R. Outcome of prosthetic joint infections treated with debridement and retention of components. *Clin. Infect. Dis.* **2006**, *42*, 471–478. [CrossRef]
10. Brandt, C.M.; Duffy, M.C.; Berbari, E.F.; Hanssen, A.D.; Steckelberg, J.M.; Osmon, D.R. Staphylococcus aureus prosthetic joint infection treated with prosthesis removal and delayed reimplantation arthroplasty. *Mayo. Clin. Proc.* **1999**, *74*, 553–558. [CrossRef]
11. Senneville, E.; Joulie, D.; Legout, L.; Valette, M.; Dezeque, H.; Beltrand, E.; Rosele, B.; d'Escrivan, T.; Loiez, C.; Caillaux, M.; et al. Outcome and predictors of treatment failure in total hip/knee prosthetic joint infections due to Staphylococcus aureus. *Clin. Infect. Dis.* **2011**, *53*, 334–340. [CrossRef] [PubMed]
12. Rajgopal, A.; Panda, I.; Rao, A.; Dahiya, V.; Gupta, H. Does Prior Failed Debridement Compromise the Outcome of Subsequent Two-Stage Revision Done for Periprosthetic Joint Infection Following Total Knee Arthroplasty? *J. Arthroplast.* **2018**, *33*, 2588–2594. [CrossRef] [PubMed]
13. Sherrell, J.C.; Fehring, T.K.; Odum, S.; Hansen, E.; Zmistowski, B.; Dennos, A.; Kalore, N. The Chitranjan Ranawat Award: Fate of two-stage reimplantation after failed irrigation and debridement for periprosthetic knee infection. *Clin. Orthop. Relat. Res.* **2011**, *469*, 18–25. [CrossRef] [PubMed]
14. Zimmerli, W.; Widmer, A.F.; Blatter, M.; Frei, R.; Ochsner, P.E. Role of rifampin for treatment of orthopedic implant-related staphylococcal infections: A randomized controlled trial. Foreign-Body Infection (FBI) Study Group. *Jama* **1998**, *279*, 1537–1541. [CrossRef]
15. McPherson, E.J.; Woodson, C.; Holtom, P.; Roidis, N.; Shufelt, C.; Patzakis, M. Periprosthetic total hip infection: Outcomes using a staging system. *Clin. Orthop. Relat. Res.* **2002**, *403*, 8–15. [CrossRef]
16. Wouthuyzen-Bakker, M.; Sebillotte, M.; Lomas, J.; Taylor, A.; Palomares, E.B.; Murillo, O.; Parvizi, J.; Shohat, N.; Reinoso, J.C.; Sanchez, R.E.; et al. Clinical outcome and risk factors for failure in late acute prosthetic joint infections treated with debridement and implant retention. *J. Infect.* **2019**, *78*, 40–47. [CrossRef]
17. Tornero, E.; Morata, L.; Martinez-Pastor, J.C.; Bori, G.; Climent, C.; Garcia-Velez, D.M.; Garcia-Ramiro, S.; Bosch, J.; Mensa, J.; Soriano, A. KLIC-score for predicting early failure in prosthetic joint infections treated with debridement, implant retention and antibiotics. *Clin. Microbiol. Infect.* **2015**, *21*, 786.e9–786.e17. [CrossRef]
18. Bryan, A.J.; Abdel, M.P.; Sanders, T.L.; Fitzgerald, S.F.; Hanssen, A.D.; Berry, D.J. Irrigation and Debridement with Component Retention for Acute Infection After Hip Arthroplasty: Improved Results with Contemporary Management. *J. Bone Joint Surg. Am.* **2017**, *99*, 2011–2018. [CrossRef]
19. Wimmer, M.D.; Randau, T.M.; Friedrich, M.J.; Ploeger, M.M.; Schmolder, J.; Strauss, A.C.; Pennekamp, P.H.; Vavken, P.; Gravius, S. Outcome Predictors in Prosthetic Joint Infections–Validation of a risk stratification score for Prosthetic Joint Infections in 120 cases. *Acta Orthop. Belg.* **2016**, *82*, 143–148.
20. Amanatullah, D.; Dennis, D.; Oltra, E.G.; Marcelino Gomes, L.S.; Goodman, S.B.; Hamlin, B.; Hansen, E.; Hashemi-Nejad, A.; Holst, D.C.; Komnos, G.; et al. Hip and Knee Section, Diagnosis, Definitions: Proceedings of International Consensus on Orthopedic Infections. *J. Arthroplast.* **2019**, *34*, S329–S337. [CrossRef]
21. Gomez-Junyent, J.; Murillo, O.; Grau, I.; Benavent, E.; Ribera, A.; Cabo, X.; Tubau, F.; Ariza, J.; Pallares, R. Analysis of mortality in a cohort of 650 cases of bacteremic osteoarticular infections. *Semin. Arthritis Rheum.* **2018**, *48*, 327–333. [CrossRef] [PubMed]
22. Lora-Tamayo, J.; Euba, G.; Ribera, A.; Murillo, O.; Pedrero, S.; Garcia-Somoza, D.; Pujol, M.; Cabo, X.; Ariza, J. Infected hip hemiarthroplasties and total hip arthroplasties: Differential findings and prognosis. *J. Infect.* **2013**, *67*, 536–544. [CrossRef] [PubMed]
23. Kurtz, S.M.; Lau, E.C.; Son, M.S.; Chang, E.T.; Zimmerli, W.; Parvizi, J. Are We Winning or Losing the Battle With Periprosthetic Joint Infection: Trends in Periprosthetic Joint Infection and Mortality Risk for the Medicare Population. *J. Arthroplast.* **2018**, *33*, 3238–3245. [CrossRef] [PubMed]
24. Hart, W.J.; Jones, R.S. Two-stage revision of infected total knee replacements using articulating cement spacers and short-term antibiotic therapy. *J. Bone Joint Surg. Br.* **2006**, *88*, 1011–1015. [CrossRef] [PubMed]
25. Tibrewal, S.; Malagelada, F.; Jeyaseelan, L.; Posch, F.; Scott, G. Single-stage revision for the infected total knee replacement: Results from a single centre. *Bone Joint J.* **2014**, *96*, 759–764. [CrossRef]
26. Tsukayama, D.T.; Estrada, R.; Gustilo, R.B. Infection after total hip arthroplasty. A study of the treatment of one hundred and six infections. *J. Bone Joint Surg. Am.* **1996**, *78*, 512–523. [CrossRef]
27. Murray, P.R.; Jo Baron, E.; Jorgensen, J.H.; Landry, M.I.; Pfaller, M.A. *Manual of Clinical Microbiology*, 9th ed.; ASM Press: Washington, DC, USA, 2007.

28. Chotanaphuti, T.; Courtney, P.M.; Fram, B.; In den Kleef, N.J.; Kim, T.K.; Kuo, F.C.; Lustig, S.; Moojen, D.J.; Nijhof, M.; Oliashirazi, A.; et al. Hip and Knee Section, Treatment, Algorithm: Proceedings of International Consensus on Orthopedic Infections. *J. Arthroplast.* **2019**, *34*, S393–S397. [CrossRef]
29. Zimmerli, W.; Sendi, P. Orthopedic Implant-Associated Infections. In *Mandell, Douglas, and Bennett's Principles and Practice of Infectious Diseases*; Elsevier: Philadelphia, PA, USA, 2015; Volume I, pp. 1328–1340.
30. Tande, A.J.; Patel, R. Prosthetic joint infection. *Clin. Microbiol. Rev.* **2014**, *27*, 302–345. [CrossRef]

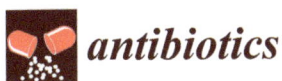

Article

Outcomes and Risk Factors in Prosthetic Joint Infections by multidrug-resistant Gram-negative Bacteria: A Retrospective Cohort Study

Raquel Bandeira da Silva [1] and Mauro José Salles [2,3,*]

[1] Department of Internal Medicine, Hospital São Francisco de Assis, Belo Horizonte 30360-290, Brazil; girassoisnojardim@gmail.com
[2] Division of Infectious Diseases, Santa Casa de São Paulo School of Medical Sciences, São Paulo 01221-020, Brazil
[3] Laboratório LEMC, Disciplina de Infectologia, Departamento de Medicina, Universidade Federal de São Paulo-Escola Paulista de Medicina (UNIFESP-EPM), São Paulo 04025-010, Brazil
* Correspondence: salles.infecto@gmail.com; Tel.: +55-11-985360055

Abstract: Gram-negative bacteria (GNB), including multidrug-resistant (MDR) pathogens, are gaining importance in the aetiology of prosthetic joint infection (PJI). This retrospective observational study identified independent risk factors (RFs) associated with MDR-GNB PJI and their influence on treatment outcomes. We assessed MDR bacteria causing hip and knee PJIs diagnosed at a Brazilian tertiary hospital from January 2014 to July 2018. RFs associated with MDR-GNB PJI were estimated by bivariate and multivariate analyses using prevalence ratios (PRs) with significance at $p < 0.05$. Kaplan–Meier analysis was performed to evaluate treatment outcomes. Overall, 98 PJI patients were analysed, including 56 with MDR-GNB and 42 with other bacteria. Independent RFs associated with MDR-GNB PJI were revision arthroplasty ($p = 0.002$), postoperative hematoma ($p < 0.001$), previous orthopaedic infection ($p = 0.002$) and early infection ($p = 0.001$). Extensively drug-resistant GNB ($p = 0.044$) and comorbidities ($p = 0.044$) were independently associated with MDR-GNB PJI treatment failure. In sum, MDR-GNB PJI was independently associated with previous orthopaedic surgery, postoperative local complications and pre-existing infections and was possibly related to selective pressure on bacterial skin colonisation by antibiotics prescribed for early PJI. Infections due to MDR-GNB and comorbidities were associated with higher treatment failure rates.

Keywords: surgical site infection; prosthetic joint infection; epidemiology; risk factors; multidrug-resistant Gram-negative bacteria; extensively drug-resistant; hematoma

1. Introduction

Joint replacement or arthroplasty aims to improve the mobility and quality of life of patients who experience painful symptoms or functional disability. However, prosthetic joint infection (PJI) is among the most feared complications that may result from such procedures, with an incidence of 1% to 2% among primary [1,2] and up to 4% among revision arthroplasties [3,4], respectively. Older patient age, revision arthroplasty, diabetes mellitus, rheumatoid arthritis, smoking, obesity and a high American Society of Anaesthesiologists (ASA) score are viewed as independent risk factors (RFs) for PJI [5–9].

Gram-positive cocci (GPC), such as *Staphylococcus aureus* and coagulase-negative staphylococci remain the primary etiological agents of PJI, with Gram-negative bacteria (GNB) identified less frequently [10]. Although few multicentre studies have described the microbiological epidemiology of PJI, the role played by GNB appears to be increasing. Rates of infections involving these organisms have ranged from 5% to 23% in previous investigations [4,7,10] but rates of greater than 40% have been reported for GNB-associated PJI in total knee arthroplasty (TKA) [11] and shoulder arthroplasty [6].

Due to the current scarcity of antibiotics able to control bone and biofilm infections, the emergence of MDR-GNB PJIs has become a growing concern in countries reporting high prevalence rates of MDR-GNB nosocomial infections, including postoperative infections [12,13]. Benito et al. [12] identified an increase in the prevalence of MDR-GNB arthroplasty infections from 5.3% between 2003 and 2004 to 8.1% between 2011 and 2012, with a corresponding increase in identified MDR-GNB strains, such as *Escherichia coli*, *Klebsiella pneumoniae*, *Pseudomonas aeruginosa* and *Morganella morganii*. In the same study, a worrying increase in the rates of quinolone-resistant MDR-GNB strains was identified; quinolones represent an important and effective class of antibiotics often used to treat PJIs. Fantoni et al. [13], in a multicentre study of GNB-associated PJI, identified higher rates of MDR strains (53.7%), including 13.5% that expressed resistance to carbapenems, which are considered the last-line antibiotics for GNB infections.

Although PJIs caused by GNB appear to be increasing in frequency, current literature describing the epidemiology of PJI caused by MDR-GNB remains scarce, and few studies to date have attempted to investigate the outcomes and RFs associated with MDR-GNB PJI. Herein we describe a cohort of patients presenting with MDR-GNB PJIs and identify the predisposing independent factors associated with PJI caused by MDR-GNB and their influence on treatment outcomes.

2. Materials and Methods

2.1. Study Design

This was a retrospective, single-centre cohort study involving the identification and analysis of information from patient records describing hip and knee PJIs caused by MDR-GNB between January 2014 and July 2018 at an orthopaedic referral hospital centre.

The primary study endpoint was the identification of independent predisposing factors associated with PJI caused by MDR-GNB. The secondary endpoint was the identification of independent variables influencing the treatment outcome of patients with MDR-GNB PJI. The study included individuals aged at least 18 years old who (a) met the criteria for arthroplasty infection as defined by the Musculoskeletal Infection Society (MSIS) [14] (Appendix A); (b) had at least one phenotypically indistinguishable aetiological agent that was identified in two or more samples of representative biological specimens; and (c) had at least one year of prospective follow-up data. Patients who underwent arthroplasty at an institution other than ours, had a follow-up period shorter than 12 months, did not meet the criteria for PJI as defined by the MSIS or had culture-negative results were excluded. Patients were selected from the infection database of the hospital infection control (IC) unit using surgical-site infection (SSI) notifications. Based on SSI notifications, patients' medical records and results of microbiological cultures were located in specific databases to determine whether each patient fulfilled the inclusion criteria. The study was reviewed and approved by the local ethics committee (approval no. 2,610,914) on 20 April 2018.

2.2. Definitions

The PJI onset date was defined according to the date of the first observation of typical infectious signs and symptoms. For the purposes of this study's analysis, only aetiological agents identified during the first debridement surgery were considered in cases subjected to multiple debridements. MDR-GNB was defined as the nonsusceptibility of the identified pathogen to at least one antimicrobial agent from three or more different antimicrobial classes (e.g., aminoglycosides, cephalosporins with an anti-*Pseudomonas* effect, carbapenems, fluoroquinolones, penicillin + β-lactamase inhibitors, monobactams and polymyxin). GNB that were extensively drug-resistant (XDR) to multiple antibiotics were defined as those lacking susceptibility to at least one antimicrobial agent from all but two classes of antimicrobials [15]. Early infections were defined as those with onset occurring less than three months after prosthesis placement. Long-term remission of PJI following treatment was defined as the absence of clinical, laboratory and radiological symptoms of infection at the last medical follow-up (with a minimum follow-up point of one year). Therapeutic failure was defined as infection recurrence at a previously controlled site; requirement for new surgery, a second course of antimicrobial therapy, chronic antibiotic suppression, excision arthroplasty or limb amputation, or death within the follow-up period [16,17].

2.3. Investigated Variables

To identify potential RFs associated with PJI caused by MDR-GNB as well as treatment outcomes for such infections, variables were obtained from patients' medical records and surgical description sheets were reviewed. The potential variables reviewed for association with MDR-GNB PJI were categorised into three distinct groups as follows: (a) variables related to the patient, (b) variables related to the surgical procedure and (c) variables related to the postoperative period. The patient-related variables included demographics, comorbidities, alcoholism, smoking habits, ASA Physical Status Classification score, previous use of antimicrobials in the last three months and previous orthopaedic infection. The variables related to the surgical procedure were arthroplasty joint location, total or partial arthroplasty, revision surgery and post-trauma or elective arthroplasty. The variables related to the postoperative period were a concomitant infection during the same hospitalisation, the presence of postoperative hematoma, the presence of sepsis at the time of infection diagnosis and early or late infection. Operative variables such as debridement and implant retention (DAIR) or any prosthesis exchange used for the treatment of PJI were assessed when RFs for MDR-GNB PJI were considered in the outcomes analysis.

2.4. Microbiological Analysis

The institutional microbiological protocol consisted of synovial fluid (aseptically inoculated into standard aerobic blood culture bottles) and tissue sample analyses. Tissues obtained from the surgical procedure were homogenised in 3 mL of brain–heart infusion broth for one minute and inoculated onto aerobic sheep blood agar, chocolate agar and anaerobic blood agar and into thioglycolate broth (BD Diagnostic Systems, Hunt Valley, MD, USA). The time limit for processing samples was six hours. Aerobic plates were incubated aerobically at 35 °C to 37 °C in 5% to 7% CO_2 for seven days, and anaerobic plates were anaerobically cultured at 37 °C for 14 days. Additionally, 0.5 mL of tissue homogenate was inoculated in thioglycolate broth for 14 days, and the turbid thioglycolate broth was subcultured on blood agar plates when cloudy. Colonies of microorganisms observed to be growing on the plates were identified, and their susceptibility to different antibiotics was tested according to standard microbiologic techniques [18]. The bacteria were identified by conventional biochemical and metabolic tests according to international standards and the definitions of the European Committee on Antimicrobial Susceptibility Testing (EUCAST) [18]. Sensitivity tests were performed using the disk-diffusion technique. If a minimum inhibitory concentration determination was necessary, automated or electronic test methods were used; the results are presented according to the EUCAST criteria that were valid at the time of testing [18].

2.5. Statistical Analysis

Qualitative variables for the overall study sample and the groups designated as infected by MDR-GNB and other bacteria, respectively, are described using mean and percentage values. Quantitative variables are described as using mean and standard deviation (SD), or median and interquartile range according to their observed distribution. Associations between qualitative variables were determined using the chi-squared test and Fisher's exact test, and comparisons of means between groups using interval-type variables were performed using the Student's t-test. Poisson regression was used to calculate prevalence ratios (PRs), using independent variables with significance levels below 25% ($p < 0.25$). Only those variables with a significance level below 5% ($p < 0.05$) were retained in the final model. To identify the variables related to treatment failure, Kaplan–Meier curves were constructed for each factor, and the log-rank test was used to compare the curves. Cox regression was used to identify predictor variables that influenced patient outcomes. All results were considered significant at a significance probability below 5% ($p < 0.05$). All data were analysed using the Statistical Package for the Social Sciences, version 23 (IBM Corporation, Armonk, NY, USA).

3. Results

3.1. Study Population

Overall, a total of 2672 arthroplasties were performed during the study period and a total of 115 PJI cases were assessed for inclusion in the study. Of these, 14 PJI cases that did not meet the MSIS criteria for infection and three PJI cases with negative cultures were excluded. Therefore, 98 PJI cases were analysed, including 56 (57.1%) and 42 (42.9%) caused by MDR-GNB and other microorganisms, respectively.

The demographic, clinical features, comorbidities, surgical procedures and postoperative characteristics of the study population are summarised in Table 1. The mean age in the study population was 67 years (SD: ± 13.2 years), and 58.2% of the patients were female. Perioperative risk assessment varied, with 21.4% of cases classified as ASA 1, 48% as ASA 2 and 30.6% as ASA 3 or 4, respectively. More than 70% of the patients had at least one comorbidity. Hip arthroplasty was the most frequent procedure (83.7%), while 39.8% of the patients underwent arthroplasty due to trauma.

Table 1. Demographics and clinical characteristics of the study population.

Characteristics	Number of Patients No. (%) Total = 98
Age (years) (mean ± S.D.)	67.3 ± 13.2
P50 (P25–P75)	69.5 (58.7–77)
Age group	
up to 50	10 (1.2)
51–60	23 (23.5)
61–70	20 (20.4)
71–80	31 (31.6)
over 80	14 (14.3)
Time between prosthesis and diagnosis (days) P50 (P25–P 75)	32 (20–242)
Variables related to the patient	
Comorbidities (yes)	71 (72.4)
SAH [a]	60 (61.2)
DM [b]	20 (20.4)
Malnutrition	8 (8.2)
Anemia	2 (2.0)
Neoplasm	1 (1.0)
Lung disease	5 (5.1)
Metabolic syndrome	18 (18.4)
Cardiovascular disease	5 (5.1)
Other comorbidities [c]	11 (11.3)
Previous use of an antimicrobial	37 (37.8)
Variables related to the surgical procedure	
Arthroplasty	
Total	75 (76.5)
Primary	56 (57.2)
Elective	59 (60.2)
Hip	82 (83.7)
DAIR [d]	69 (70.4)
Procedure duration greater than 2.5 h	5 (5.1)
Blood transfusion	16 (16.3)

Table 1. Cont.

Characteristics	Number of Patients No. (%) Total = 98
Variables related to the postoperative period	
Concomitant non-orthopedic infection	11 (11.2)
Previous ortopedic infection	19 (19.4)
Early infection	68 (69.4)
Sepsis	2 (2.0)

SAH [a]: Systemic arterial hypertension; DM [b]: Diabetes Mellitus; Other comorbidities [c]: rheumatoid arthritis, hypothyroidism, hyperthyroidism, depression. DAIR [d]: debridement and implant retention.

3.2. Microbial Identification

Overall, microbiological analysis yielded 104 microorganisms from 98 PJI patients. MDR-GNB was isolated from 30 patients (30.6%) and XDR-GNB from 26 (26.5%). The most prevalent pathogen was *Acinetobacter baumannii* (31.6%), followed by *S. aureus* among which 15.4% (16/104) were sensitive to methicillin (MSSA), and 4.8% (5/104) were methicillin-resistant (MRSA). Among patients with PJI caused by MDR or XDR-GNB, *A. baumannii* followed by *Enterobacter aerogenes*, *K. pneumoniae* and *E. coli* were the most commonly identified etiological agents. Microorganisms isolated from bone and soft tissue cultures of the 98 PJI patients included in this study are summarised in Table 2.

Table 2. Description of 104 microorganisms isolated from bone and soft tissue cultures of patients with PJI described in the study.

Microbial isolates in 56 episodes of MDR/XDR GNB [a] PJI [b]	60 (100)
Acinetobacter baumannii	31 (51.7)
Enterobacter aerogenes	8 (13.3)
Klebsiella pneumoniae	6 (10.0)
Escherichia coli	5 (8.3)
Proteus mirabilis	4 (6.7)
Pseudomonas aeruginosa	3 (5.0)
Others GNB-MDR	3 (5.0)
Microbial isolates in 42 episodes of others bacterias PJI [b]	44 (100)
MSSA [c]	16 (36.4)
Pseudomonas aeruginosa	6 (13.6)
MRSA [d]	5 (11.4)
Enterobacter aerogenes	4 (9.1)
Proteus mirabilis	3 (6.8)
Proteus vulgaris	2 (4.5)
Acinetobacter baumannii	2 (4.5)
Klebsiella pneumoniae	2 (4.5)
Morganella morganii	1 (2.3)
Enterobacter sakazakii	1 (2.3)
Enterobacter cloacae	1 (2.3)
Escherichia coli	1 (2.3)

MDR/XDR GNB [a]: Multidrug resistant/extensively drug-resistant, gram-negative bacteria; PJI [b]; prosthetic joint infection; MSSA [c]; Methicillin-sensitive *Staphylococcus aureus*, MRSA [d]; Methicillin-resistant *Staphylococcus aureus*.

3.3. Potential Predisposing Factors for PJI Caused by MDR-GNB and Clinical Outcomes

As compared with PJIs caused by other microorganisms, infections due to MDR- and XDR-GNB in the univariate analyses were significantly associated with male sex (70.7% vs. 29.3%; $p = 0.021$), revision arthroplasty (66.1% vs. 11.9%; $p = 0.000$), metabolic syndrome (10.7% vs. 28.6%; $p = 0.024$), alcoholism (21.4% vs. 4.8%; $p = 0.020$), nonelective arthroplasty (55.4% vs. 19.0%; $p = 0.000$), previous use of antibiotics in the last three months (55.4%

vs. 14.3%; $p = 0.000$), concomitant non-orthopaedic infection (19.6% vs. 4.8%; $p = 0.000$), previous orthopaedic infection (35.7% vs. 0%; $p = 0.000$), postoperative hematoma (51.8% vs. 2.4%; $p = 0.000$) and early infection (57.1% vs. 88.1%; $p = 0.001$). Age, ASA score, smoking and the surgical procedure lasting longer than 2.5 hours did not increase the risk for PJI caused by MDR- and XDR-GNB relative to the risk of PJI caused by other microorganisms (Table A1).

Variables identified as significant and clinically relevant in the univariate analysis were added to the multivariate model. In the multivariate model, the predisposing factors independently associated with PJI caused by MDR- and XDR-GNB were revision arthroplasty [PR: 1.7; 95% confidence interval (CI): 1.2–2.4; $p = 0.002$], previous orthopaedic infection (PR: 1.5; 95% CI: 1.1–2.1; $p = 0.002$), postoperative hematoma (PR: 2.6; 95% CI: 1.7–4.0; $p < 0.001$) and early infection (PR: 2.2; 95% CI: 1.4–3.5; $p = 0.001$) (Table 3).

Table 3. Predisposing factors independently associated with MDR-GNB [a] PJI [b] in the multivariate analysis.

Variables	Prevalence Ratio 95% CI	p-Value [c]
Revision arthroplasty	1.7 (1.2; 2.4)	0.002
Previous orthopedic infection	1.5 (1.1; 2.1)	0.020
Postoperative hematoma	2.6 (1.7; 4.0)	<0.001
Early infection	2.2 (1.4; 3.5)	0.001

MDR-GNB [a]: Multidrug resistant gram-negative bacteria; PJI [b]: prosthetic joint infection; p-values [c] < 0.05 were considered statistically significant.

No significant differences between groups were observed for the time between prosthesis placement and PJI diagnosis ($p = 0.066$) or the time between PJI diagnosis and treatment failure ($p = 0.063$) (Table A2). It is worth pointing out that the rate of PJI recurrence after treatment was lower among patients infected by MDR-/XDR-GNB than among those infected by other bacteria (4.1% and 6.1%, respectively). On the other hand, higher rates of death were observed in the MDR/XDR-GNB PJI group than in the 'other bacteria' PJI group (17.3% vs 5.1%; $p = 0.038$). Even though a comparison of the rate of treatment failure (recurrence/death) between groups (MDR- and XDR-GNB vs other microorganisms) showed no statistically significant difference ($p = 0.264$), a patient with PJI caused by XDR-GNB was 4.6 times more likely to progress to death than a patient with a PJI caused by other pathogens (odds ratio: 4.6; 95% CI: 1.4–15.7; $p = 0.010$). In contrast, progression to death was not more likely among patients with MDR-GNB PJIs than among those with PJIs caused by other microorganisms (odds ratio: 2.3; 95% IC: 0.6–7.9; $p = 0.200$). The risk of treatment failure was not significantly different between all GNB PJI cases and all GPC PJI cases ($p = 0.516$). Moreover, no significant differences in the outcome were observed when DAIR was performed versus the use of non-DAIR options (i.e., one-stage and two-stage exchange arthroplasty) ($p = 0.842$).

However, according to the multivariate model, infections caused by XDR-GNB (PR: 2.3; 95% CI: 1.0–5.2; $p = 0.044$) and the presence of comorbidities (PR: 2.9; 95% CI: 1.0–8.4; $p = 0.044$) were strong predictive RFs independently associated with therapeutic failure (Table A3). The higher rates of treatment failure associated with XDR-GNB PJI and patients with comorbidities is best illustrated in Figures 1 and 2.

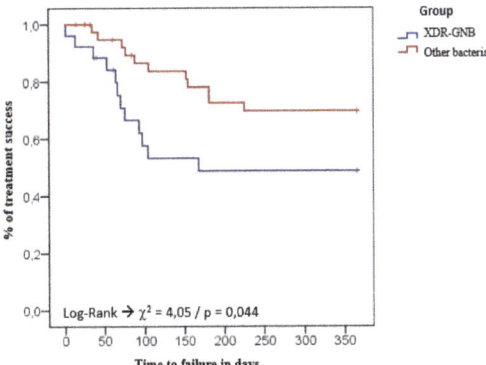

Figure 1. Kaplan–Meier survival curve for treatment failure (death/recurrence) considering PJIs caused by XDR-GNB and other bacteria.

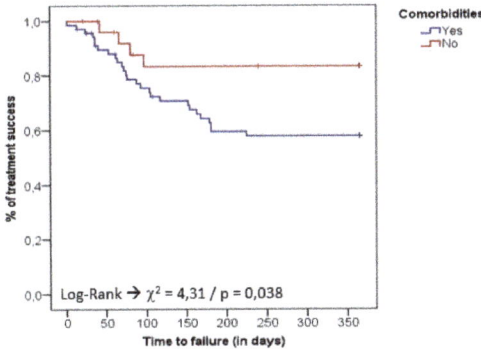

Figure 2. Kaplan–Meier survival curve for treatment failure (death/recurrence) among PJI patients with and without comorbidities.

4. Discussion

In this study, revision arthroplasty, previous orthopaedic infection and postoperative hematoma were independently associated with the risk of developing MDR-GNB PJI. These RFs are well-known to be associated with any deep periprosthetic infection; however, the relevance of any infection-associated findings may vary depending upon the epidemiological context of an orthopaedic referral centre. At our centre, located in a large city in a developing country, the likelihood of nosocomial SSI caused by MDR-GNB is high. Early PJI was an additional RF identified for MDR-GNB PJI. We argue that the high selective pressure imposed by empirical and broad-spectrum antibiotic therapy, which is often prescribed for early PJI, may have had a major role not only in the higher prevalence of GNB-PJI, but also impacting on the lower rates GPC infections (20.2%), including the lack of CNS that was not identified in this study cohort.

MDR-GNB were identified in more than half of the bacterial populations isolated in this cohort study. Many other authors have reported that the likelihood of GNB as the etiological agent of SSI is greater in Latin America than in more developed regions [19,20]. In a Latin American surveillance study that included several medical centres, 12,811 bacterial species were isolated from several types of nosocomial infections, including SSIs; 44.5% of cases were identified as GNB infections with high rates of MDR [20].

Importantly, *A. baumannii* accounted for 33.7% of all GNB isolated in our study. Despite the implementation of many IC measures at our institution, the IC team has been unable to eradicate *A. baumannii* from the hospital environment. It is likely that this species has become an endemic pathogen responsible for nosocomial infections, including SSIs. A high prevalence of *A. baumannii* has been reported in other Latin American countries as well [21]. Some authors have suggested that the tropical climates and higher temperatures in Latin America may result in increased numbers of *Acinetobacter* spp. colonising the human skin, increasing the risk of nosocomial infections [22,23]. Typically, patients who undergo arthroplasty receive immediate postoperative care in the intensive care unit, which has been characterised as an institutional environment associated with an overwhelmingly high rate of *A. baumannii* colonisation relative to in other hospital units. This factor may increase the risk of *A. baumannii*–associated PJI.

Although previous authors have reported an increased risk for PJI with revision surgery [24–26], an association between revision surgery and GNB-MDR PJI has not been reported before now. In our study, a preceding PJI episode was associated with a 1.5-fold increase in the chance that the new PJI would be caused by MDR-GNB. This represents new and important epidemiological information. The occurrence of a previous PJI implies the prolonged use of combined and broad-spectrum antibiotics, and a direct association between prolonged antibiotic use and greater rates of MDR-GNB infections has been reported previously [27,28]. In a study by Benito et al. [29] of 2524 episodes of PJI, negative-coagulase staphylococci was identified as the most commonly identified causative pathogen, but GNB were more frequently identified in cases of early infection. Additionally, MDR-GNB accounted for nearly one-quarter of early PJIs and were identified three times more frequently in early infections than in late infections. The study by Benito et al. [29], conducted in Spain, was the first cohort study to identify the role played by MDR-GNB in early PJI episodes. Our data corroborate the association.

The formation of hematoma or postoperative drainage for more than 2.5 days following arthroplasty has been identified previously as a predictor of wound infection for patients receiving hip and knee joint replacements [30]. In shoulder arthroplasty, an association between postoperative hematoma and subsequent PJI was documented by Cheung et al. [31] and Nagaya et al. [6]. Cheung et al. [31] identified various species of skin-associated microbiota in hematoma cultures, including *Cutibacterium acnes*, *Staphylococcus epidermidis* and other *Streptococcus* spp. The presence of postoperative hematoma in patients previously colonised with MDR-GNB may contribute to postarthroplasty infections, helping to explain our finding of postoperative hematoma as an independent risk factor for developing MDR-GNB PJI.

No significant differences in outcomes were observed when comparing infections caused by GNB and those caused by GPC. Uçkay and Bernard [32] reported similar success rates when treating PJIs caused by GPC or GNB. In contrast, several studies have linked GNB-associated PJI with high failure rates [16]. In our study, surgical options using DAIR had no impact on treatment outcomes, but XDR-PJI was independently associated with poor outcomes. In the study by Papadopoulos et al. [33], MDR- and XDR-GNB infections were associated with higher rates of therapeutic failure when DAIR was performed (52.2%) than when non-DAIR options were applied. Hiesh et al. [7] also reported worse outcomes when DAIR was the operative choice over non-DAIR options for GNB-associated PJI. Shohat et al. [17] reported higher failure rates for DAIR when treating PJIs caused by any MDR pathogens. However, in a study by Cobo et al. [34], the success rate of DAIR for early PJI was similar for GPC and GNB infections, with lower success rates reported for MRSA-affiliated PJI.

The impact of XDR-GNB on poor outcomes may be associated with the general lack of antibiotic options for eradicating these bacteria, especially biofilm-acting quinolones. In our study, all XDR samples were quinolone resistant. Additionally, comorbidities had an independent negative effect on outcomes, increasing the likelihood of poor outcomes 2.9-fold. Multiple comorbidities may impact PJI outcomes in several ways, such as an increased likelihood of adverse events associated with prolonged and combined antibiotic therapy. Chronic comorbidities, such as kidney and liver failure, have also been associated with reduced immune responses against bacteria, allowing for the development of bone and biofilm infections.

The present study had several limitations. This study was performed as an observational, retrospective study conducted at a single centre offering special orthopaedic care to a regional population located in a major city in a developing country. Consequently, the results may not apply to other hospitals. Furthermore, the patients enrolled in the cohort were heterogeneous. Matching MDR-GNB with other bacteria may have biased our analysis, although multivariate analyses were performed to adjust for this variability. Also, bacterial identification and susceptibility tests were performed using nonautomated methods, and no molecular and genotypic analyses were performed to identify clonal variants or similar patterns of resistance mechanisms. Besides, all potential SCN growing in a single tissue sample culture were considered contaminants and were excluded from the analysis, which may have biased our results. In addition, the type of surgical approach for hip arthroplasty was not assessed. However, this study identified a large number of MDR-GNB infections, with a high frequency of XDR strains.

5. Conclusions

We found that revision arthroplasty, previous orthopaedic infection, postoperative hematoma and early PJI were predisposing RFs for MDR-GNB PJI. Infections caused by XDR-GNB and comorbidities were both associated with poor outcomes. Despite the limitations of our cohort study, these results may reflect the epidemiology of certain developing regions with weak antibiotic stewardship programs. The increasing prevalence of antimicrobial resistance among PJIs poses a challenge for practitioners.

Author Contributions: Conceptualization, R.B.d.S. and M.J.S.; methodology, R.B.d.S. and M.J.S.; validation, M.J.S., formal analysis, M.J.S.; investigation R.B.d.S.; data curation, R.B.d.S.; writing—original draft preparation, R.B.d.S.; writing—review and editing, M.J.S.; visualization, M.J.S.; supervision, M.J.S.; project administration, R.B.d.S. All authors have read and agreed to the published version of the manuscript.

Funding: This research received no external funding.

Institutional Review Board Statement: "The study was conducted according to the guidelines of the Declaration of Helsinki and approved by Ethics Committee) of Fundação Hospitalar São Francisco de Assis (no. 2,610,914 on 20 April 2018).

Informed Consent Statement: Patient consent was waived due the research involves no more than minimal risk to the subject because is a retrospect observational study.

Data Availability Statement: Study data supporting our results were registered at an open access virtual platform for registration of studies on humans performed in Brazil. The Brazilian Registry of Clinical Trials (ReBEC) http://www.ensaiosclinicos.gov.br/rg/RBR-6ft5yb/ Register Number: RBR-6ft5yb.

Acknowledgments: We would like to thank the" Fundação Hospitalar São Francisco de Assis" for the support to conduct this study.

Conflicts of Interest: The authors declare no conflict of interest.

Appendix A

Presence of a major criteria
1. Sinus tract with evidence of communication of the joint or visualization of the prosthesis
or
2. Identification of the same phenotypically similar pathogen in two or more different periprosthetic tissue samples or in joint fluid

Presence of four or more minor criteria

1. Presence of purulent periprosthetic secretion
2. Identification of acute inflammatory reaction in histopathologic tests of periprosthetic tissue
3. A single culture with the identification of a microorganism
4. High leukocyte cellularity in the synovial fluid
5. High percentage of neutrophils in the synovial fluid
6. Increased serum levels of C-reactive protein (CRP) or erythrocyte sedimentation rate (ESR)

Appendix B

Table A1. Evaluation the influence of variables of interest on the outcome of PJI caused by MDR- GNB compared to other bacteria–univariate analysis.

Variables	PJI [a]		*p*-Value [c]
	MDR/XDR GNB [b] No. (%) N = 56	Other Bacteria No. (%) N = 42	
Demographic data			
Males	29 (70.7)	12 (29.3)	0.021 *
Females	27 (47.4)	30 (52.6)	
Age (years)		F	
Mean ± Standard deviation	68.2 ± 13.8	66.0 ± 1.4	0.415 ***
Age group			
up to 50	7 (70.0)	3 (30.0)	
51–60 years	13 (56.5)	10 (43.5)	
61–70 years	7 (35.0)	13 (65.0)	0.126 **
71–80 years	18 (58.1)	13 (41.9)	
above 80 years	11 (78.6)	3 (21.4)	
Variables related to the patient			
Presence of comorbidities	41 (73.2)	30 (71.4)	0.845 *
SAH [d]	33 (58.9)	27 (64.3)	0.590 *
DM [e]	12 (21.4)	8 (19.0)	0.772 *
Malnutrition	7 (12.5)	1 (2.4)	0.133 **
Anemia	2 (3.6)	0 (0)	0.505 **
Neoplasm	0 (0)	1 (2.4)	0.429 **
Lung disease	0 (0)	5 (9)	0.013 **
Metabolic syndrome	6 (10.7)	12 (28.6)	0.024 *
Cardiovascular disease	4 (7.1)	1 (2.4)	0.388 **
Other comorbidities [f]	4 (7.1)	7 (16.7)	0.197 **
Alcoholism	12 (21.4)	2 (4.8)	0.020 *
Smoking	9 (16.1)	4 (9.5)	0.344 *
ASA classification [g]			
1	8 (14.3)	13 (31.0)	
2	28 (50.0)	19 (45.2)	0.114 *
3 or 4	20 (35.7)	10 (23.8)	
Previous orthopedic infection	20 (35.7)	0 (0)	0.000 *
Previous use of antimicrobials (last three months)			
Yes	31 (55.4)	6 (14.3)	0.000 *
Quinolones	12 (21.4)	3 (7.1)	0.052 *
β-Lactam Antibiotics	20 (35.7)	4 (9.5)	0.003 *
Antimicrobial combination	10 (17.9)	1 (2.4)	0.000 **
Variables related to the surgical procedure			
Arthroplasty			
Total	41 (73.2)	34 (81.0)	0.371 *
Revision	66.1 (37)	11.9 (5)	0.000 *

Table A1. Cont.

Variables	PJI [a]		p-Value [c]
	MDR/XDR GNB [b] No. (%) N = 56	Other Bacteria No. (%) N = 42	
Non-elective	31 (55.4)	8 (19.0)	0.000 *
Hip	56 (100)	26 (61.9)	0.000 *
Duration of the procedure > 2.5 h	8 (14.3)	7 (16.7)	0.746 *
Blood transfusion	16 (28.6)	3 (7.1)	0.008 *
Variables related to the postoperative period			
Concomitant non-orthopedic infection	11 (19.6)	2 (4.8)	0.032 *
Previous orthopedic infection	20 (35.7)	0 (0)	0.000 *
Polymicrobial infection	4 (7.1)	4 (9.5)	0.721 **
Early infection	32 (57.1)	37 (88.1)	0.001 *
Postoperative hematoma	29 (51.8)	1 (2.4)	0.000 *
Sepsis associated with infection	2 (3.6)	0 (0)	0.505 **

PJI [a]: Prosthetic Joints Infections; MDR/XDR GNB [b]: Multidrug resistant/extensively drug-resistant, gram-negative bacteria; [c] p-values: <0.05 were considered statistically significant; SAH [d]: Systemic arterial hypertension; DM [e]: diabetes Mellitus; Other comorbidities [f]: rheumatoid arthritis, hypothyroidism, hyperthyroidism, depression; ASA [g]: American Anesthesiology Association. Significance probabilities refer to the Chi-squared test (*), Fisher's exact test (**), and Student's t-test (***).

Table A2. Comparative analysis between the two study groups regarding the time elapsed between prosthesis and diagnosis and time to therapeutic failure.

Variable	PJI by MDR-GNB	Descriptive Measures			p *
		Min-Max	Median (P_{25}–P_{75})	Mean ± SD	
Time elapsed between prosthesis and diagnosis (days)	Yes	7.0–5.040.0	37.0 (20.3–472.5)	453.1 ± 934.7	0.066
	No	7.0–1.825.0	30.0 (20.0–39.3)	95.4 ± 285.4	
Time to failure (days)	Yes	1.0–179.0	68.0 (37.0–102.3)	77.1 ± 50.1	0.063
	No	34.0–225.0	105.0 (72.0–181.0)	119.1 ± 62.9	

* Significance probability refers to the Mann-Whitney test.

Table A3. Evaluation of the influence of variables of interest on the time to therapeutic failure–univariate and multivariate analysis.

Variables	Univariate Analysis	Prevalence Ratio 95% CI	p-Value [a]
PJI [b] by GNB [c]	0.087	-	-
PJI by MDR-GNB [d]		1.0 (0.4; 2.5)	0.991
PJI by XDR-GNB [e]		2.3 (1.0; 5.2)	0.044
DAIR [f] surgical strategy	0.842	-	-
Presence of comorbidities	0.038	2.9 (1.0; 8.4)	0.044

p-values [a] < 0.05 were considered statistically significant. PJI [b]: Prosthetic Joints Infections; GNB [c]: Gram-negative bacteria; MDR-GNB [d]: multidrug-resistant, gram-negative bacteria; XDR-GNB [e]: extensively-resistant, gram-negative bacteria; DAIR [f]: debridement and implant retention. Significance probabilities in the univariate analysis refer to Log-Rank test. Significance probabilities in the multivariate analysis refer to Cox regression.

References

1. Kozak, L.J.; DeFrances, C.J.; Hall, M.J. National Hospital Discharge Survey: 2004 Annual Summary with Detailed Diagnosis and Procedure Data. *Vital. Health Stat.* **2006**, *13*, 1–209.
2. Corvec, S.; Portillo, M.E.; Pasticci, B.M.; Borens, O.; Trampuz, A. Epidemiology and New Developments in the Diagnosis of Prosthetic Joint Infection. *Int. J. Artif. Organs* **2012**, *35*, 923–934. [CrossRef] [PubMed]
3. Ong, K.L.; Kurtz, S.M.; Lau, E.; Bozic, K.J.; Berry, D.J.; Parvizi, J. Prosthetic Joint Infection Risk After Total Hip Arthroplasty in the Medicare Population. *J. Arthroplast.* **2009**, *24* (Suppl. 6), 105–109. [CrossRef]

4. Martínez-Pastor, J.C.; Muñoz-Mahamud, E.; Vilchez, F.; García-Ramiro, S.; Bori, G.; Sierra, J.; Martínez, J.A.; Font, L.; Mensa, J.; Soriano, A. Outcome of Acute Prosthetic Joint Infections Due to Gram-Negative Bacilli Treated with Open Debridement and Retention of the Prosthesis. *Antimicrob. Agents Chemother.* **2009**, *53*, 4772–4777. [CrossRef]
5. Tande, A.J.; Patel, R. Prosthetic Joint Infection. *Clin. Microbiol. Rev.* **2014**, *27*, 302–345. [CrossRef]
6. Nagaya, L.H.; Salles, M.J.C.; Takikawa, L.S.C.; Fregoneze, M.; Doneux, P.; Da Silva, L.A.; Sella, G.D.V.; Miyazaki, A.N.; Checchia, S.L. Infections after shoulder arthroplasty are correlated with higher anesthetic risk score: A case-control study in Brazil. *Braz. J. Infect. Dis.* **2017**, *21*, 613–619. [CrossRef] [PubMed]
7. Hsieh, P.; Lee, M.S.; Hsu, K.; Chang, Y.; Shih, H.; Ueng, S.W. Gram-Negative Prosthetic Joint Infections: Risk Factors and Outcome of Treatment. *Clin. Infect. Dis.* **2009**, *49*, 1036–1043. [CrossRef]
8. Namba, R.S.; Inacio, M.C.; Paxton, E.W. Risk Factors Associated with Deep Surgical Site Infections After Primary Total Knee Arthroplasty: An Analysis of 56,216 Knees. *J. Bone Jt. Surg. Am. Vol.* **2013**, *95*, 775–782. [CrossRef]
9. Malinzak, R.A.; Ritter, M.A.; Berend, M.E.; Meding, J.B.; Olberding, E.M.; Davis, K.E. Morbidly Obese, Diabetic, Younger, and Unilateral Joint Arthroplasty Patients Have Elevated Total Joint Arthroplasty Infection Rates. *J. Arthroplast.* **2009**, *24* (Suppl. 6), 84–88. [CrossRef]
10. Zimmerli, W.; Trampuz, A.; Ochsner, P.E. Prosthetic-Joint Infections. *N. Engl. J. Med.* **2004**, *351*, 1645–1654. [CrossRef]
11. Pradella, J.G.D.P.; Bovo, M.; Salles, M.J.C.; Klautau, G.B.; De Camargo, O.A.P.; Cury, R.D.P.L. Infected primary knee arthroplasty: Risk factors for surgical treatment failure. *Rev. Bras. Ortop.* **2013**, *48*, 432–437. [CrossRef]
12. Benito, N.; Franco, M.; Ribera, A.; Soriano, A.; Rodriguez-Pardo, D.; Sorlí, L.; Fresco, G.; Fernández-Sampedro, M.; Del Toro, M.D.; Guío, L.; et al. Time trends in the aetiology of prosthetic joint infections: A multicentre cohort study. *Clin. Microbiol. Infect.* **2016**, *22*, 732.e1–732.e8. [CrossRef] [PubMed]
13. Fantoni, M.; Borrè, S.; Rostagno, R.; Riccio, G.; Carrega, G.; Giovannenze, F.; Taccari, F. Epidemiological and clinical features of prosthetic joint infections caused by gram-negative bacteria. *Eur. Rev. Med. Pharmacol. Sci.* **2019**, *23*, 187–194.
14. Parvizi, J.; Zmistowski, B.; Berbari, E.F.; Bauer, T.W.; Springer, B.D.; Della Valle, C.J.; Garvin, K.L.; Mont, M.A.; Wongworawat, M.D.; Zalavras, C.G. New Definition for Periprosthetic Joint Infection: From the Workgroup of the Musculoskeletal Infection Society. *Clin. Orthop. Relat. Res.* **2011**, *469*, 2992–2994. [CrossRef] [PubMed]
15. Magiorakos, A.-P.; Srinivasan, A.; Carey, R.B.; Carmeli, Y.; Falagas, M.E.; Giske, C.G.; Harbarth, S.; Hindler, J.F.; Kahlmeter, G.; Olsson-Liljequist, B.; et al. Multidrug-resistant, extensively drug-resistant and pandrug-resistant bacteria: An international expert proposal for interim standard definitions for acquired resistance. *Clin. Microbiol. Infect.* **2012**, *18*, 268–281. [CrossRef] [PubMed]
16. Kandel, C.E.; Jenkinson, R.; Daneman, N.; Backstein, D.; Hansen, B.E.; Muller, M.P.; Katz, K.C.; Widdifield, J.; Bogoch, E.; Ward, S.; et al. Predictors of Treatment Failure for Hip and Knee Prosthetic Joint Infections in the Setting of 1- and 2-Stage Exchange Arthroplasty: A Multicenter Retrospective Cohort. *Open Forum Infect. Dis.* **2019**, *6*, ofz452. [CrossRef]
17. Shohat, N.; Goswami, K.; Tan, T.L.; Fillingham, Y.; Parvizi, J. Increased Failure after Irrigation and Debridement for Acute Hematogenous Periprosthetic Joint Infection. *J. Bone Jt. Surg. Am. Vol.* **2019**, *101*, 696–703. [CrossRef]
18. Leclercq, R.; Cantón, R.; Brown, D.; Giske, C.; Heisig, P.; MacGowan, A.; Mouton, J.; Nordmann, P.; Rodloff, A.; Rossolini, G.; et al. EUCAST expert rules in antimicrobial susceptibility testing. *Clin. Microbiol. Infect.* **2013**, *19*, 141–160. [CrossRef]
19. Villegas, M.V.; Blanco, M.G.; Sifuentes-Osornio, J.; Rossi, F. Increasing prevalence of extended-spectrum-betalactamase among Gram-negative bacilli in Latin America: 2008 update from the Study for Monitoring Antimicrobial Resistance Trends (SMART). *Braz. J. Infect. Dis.* **2011**, *15*, 34–39. [CrossRef]
20. Gales, A.C.; Castanheira, M.; Jones, R.N.; Sader, H.S. Antimicrobial resistance among Gram-negative bacilli isolated from Latin America: Results from SENTRY Antimicrobial Surveillance Program (Latin America, 2008–2010). *Diagn. Microbiol. Infect. Dis.* **2012**, *73*, 354–360. [CrossRef]
21. Vega, S.; Dowzicky, M.J. Antimicrobial susceptibility among Gram-positive and Gram-negative organisms collected from the Latin American region between 2004 and 2015 as part of the Tigecycline Evaluation and Surveillance Trial. *Ann. Clin. Microbiol. Antimicrob.* **2017**, *16*, 1–16. [CrossRef]
22. Kim, Y.A.; Kim, J.J.; Won, D.J.; Lee, K. Seasonal and Temperature-Associated Increase in Community-Onset Acinetobacter baumannii Complex Colonization or Infection. *Ann. Lab. Med.* **2018**, *38*, 266–270. [CrossRef] [PubMed]
23. Perencevich, E.N.; McGregor, J.C.; Shardell, M.; Furuno, J.P.; Harris, A.D.; Morris, J.G.; Fisman, D.N.; Johnson, J.A. Summer Peaks in the Incidences of Gram-Negative Bacterial Infection Among Hospitalized Patients. *Infect. Control. Hosp. Epidemiol.* **2008**, *29*, 1124–1131. [CrossRef] [PubMed]
24. Jacobs, A.M.E.; Bénard, M.; Meis, J.F.; Van Hellemondt, G.; Goosen, J.H.M. The unsuspected prosthetic joint infection. *Bone Jt. J.* **2017**, *99-B*, 1482–1489. [CrossRef] [PubMed]
25. Hoell, S.; Moeller, A.; Gosheger, G.; Hardes, J.; Dieckmann, R.; Schulz, D. Two-stage revision arthroplasty for periprosthetic joint infections: What is the value of cultures and white cell count in synovial fluid and CRP in serum before second stage reimplantation? *Arch. Orthop. Trauma Surg.* **2016**, *136*, 447–452. [CrossRef] [PubMed]
26. Kunutsor, S.K.; Whitehouse, M.R.; Blom, A.W.; Beswick, A.D.; Team, I. Patient-Related Risk Factors for Periprosthetic Joint Infection after Total Joint Arthroplasty: A Systematic Review and Meta-Analysis. *PLoS ONE* **2016**, *11*, e0150866. [CrossRef]
27. Liu, P.; Li, X.; Luo, M.; Xu, X.; Su, K.; Chen, S.; Qing, Y.; Li, Y.; Qiu, J. Risk Factors for Carbapenem-Resistant Klebsiella pneumoniaeInfection: A Meta-Analysis. *Microb. Drug Resist.* **2018**, *24*, 190–198. [CrossRef] [PubMed]

28. Raman, G.; Avendano, E.E.; Chan, J.; Merchant, S.; Puzniak, L. Risk factors for hospitalized patients with resistant or multidrug-resistant Pseudomonas aeruginosa infections: A systematic review and meta-analysis. *Antimicrob. Resist. Infect. Control.* **2018**, *7*, 79. [CrossRef]
29. Benito, N.; Mur, I.; Ribera, A.; Soriano, A.; Rodríguez-Pardo, D.; Sorlí, L.; Cobo, J.; Fernández-Sampedro, M.; Del Toro, M.D.; Guío, L.; et al. The Different Microbial Etiology of Prosthetic Joint Infections according to Route of Acquisition and Time after Prosthesis Implantation, Including the Role of Multidrug-Resistant Organisms. *J. Clin. Med.* **2019**, *8*, 673. [CrossRef]
30. Saleh, K.; Olson, M.; Resig, S.; Bershadsky, B.; Kuskowski, M.; Gioe, T.; Robinson, H.; Schmidt, R.; McElfresh, E. Predictors of wound infection in hip and knee joint replacement: Results from a 20 year surveillance program. *J. Orthop. Res.* **2002**, *20*, 506–515. [CrossRef]
31. Cheung, E.V.; Sperling, J.W.; Cofield, R.H. Infection Associated With Hematoma Formation After Shoulder Arthroplasty. *Clin. Orthop. Relat. Res.* **2008**, *466*, 1363–1367. [CrossRef] [PubMed]
32. Uçkay, I.; Bernard, L. Gram-Negative versus Gram-Positive Prosthetic Joint Infections. *Clin. Infect. Dis.* **2010**, *50*, 795. [CrossRef] [PubMed]
33. Papadopoulos, A.; Ribera, A.; Mavrogenis, A.F.; Rodriguez-Pardo, L.; Bonnet, E.; Josésalles, M.; Del Toro, M.D.; Nguyen, S.; Blanco-García, A.; Skaliczki, G.; et al. Corrigendum to "Multidrug-resistant and extensively drug-resistant Gram-negative prosthetic joint infections: Role of surgery and impact of colistin administration". *Int. J. Antimicrob. Agents* **2019**, *53*, 538–539. [CrossRef] [PubMed]
34. Cobo, J.; Miguel, L.G.S.; Euba, G.; Rodríguez, D.; García-Lechuz, J.; Riera, M.; Falgueras, L.; Palomino, J.; Benito, N.; Del Toro, M.; et al. Early prosthetic joint infection: Outcomes with debridement and implant retention followed by antibiotic therapy. *Clin. Microbiol. Infect.* **2011**, *17*, 1632–1637. [CrossRef]

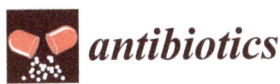

Article

Prosthetic Shoulder Joint Infection by *Cutibacterium acnes*: Does Rifampin Improve Prognosis? A Retrospective, Multicenter, Observational Study

Helem H. Vilchez [1,*], Rosa Escudero-Sanchez [2], Marta Fernandez-Sampedro [3], Oscar Murillo [4], Álvaro Auñón [5], Dolors Rodríguez-Pardo [6], Alfredo Jover-Sáenz [7], Mª Dolores del Toro [8], Alicia Rico [9], Luis Falgueras [10], Julia Praena-Segovia [11], Laura Guío [12], José A. Iribarren [13], Jaime Lora-Tamayo [14], Natividad Benito [15], Laura Morata [16], Antonio Ramirez [17], Melchor Riera [1], Study Group on Osteoarticular Infections (GEIO) [†] and the Spanish Network for Research in Infectious Pathology (REIPI) [†]

[1] Infectious Diseases Unit, Internal Medicine Department, Hospital Universitari Son Espases, Fundació Institut d'Investigació Sanitària Illes Balears (IdISBa), 07120 Palma de Mallorca, Spain; melchor.riera@ssib.es
[2] Infectious Diseases Department, Hospital Universitario Ramón y Cajal, 28034 Madrid, Spain; rosa.escudero0@gmail.com
[3] Infectious Diseases Unit, Department of Medicine, Hospital Universitario Marqués de Valdecilla-IDIVAL, 39008 Cantabria, Spain; martafersam@yahoo.es
[4] Infectious Diseases Department, Hospital Universitari de Bellvitge, 08907 Barcelona, Spain; omurillo@bellvitgehospital.cat
[5] Bone and Joint Infection Unit, Department of Orthopaedic Surgery, IIS-Fundación Jiménez Díaz, 28040 Madrid, Spain; alvaro.aunon@gmail.com
[6] Infectious Diseases Department, Hospital Universitari Vall d'Hebron, Universitat Autònoma de Barcelona, 08035 Barcelona, Spain; mariadrp7@gmail.com
[7] Unit of Nosocomial Infection, Hospital Universitari Arnau de Vilanova, 25198 Lleida, Spain; ajover.lleida.ics@gencat.cat
[8] Clinical Unit of Infectious Diseases, Microbiology and Preventive Medicine, Hospital Universitario Virgen Macarena CSIC, Instituto de Biomedicina de Sevilla (IBiS), Universidad de Sevilla, 41009 Sevilla, Spain; mdeltoro@us.es
[9] Infectious Diseases Unit and Clinical Microbiology, Hospital Universitario La Paz, 28046 Madrid, Spain; alicia.rico@salud.madrid.org
[10] Infectious Diseases Department, Corporació Sanitària Parc Taulí, 08208 Barcelona, Spain; lfalgueras@tauli.cat
[11] Clinical Unit of Infectious Diseases, Microbiology and Preventive Medicine, University Hospital Virgen del Rocio, 41013 Sevilla, Spain; juliapraena@gmail.com
[12] Infectious Diseases Department, Hospital Universitario Cruces, 48903 Vizcaya, Spain; LAURA.GUIOCARRION@osakidetza.eus
[13] Infectious Diseases Department, Hospital Universitario Donostia, Instituto BioDonostia, 20014 San Sebastián, Spain; JOSEANTONIO.IRIBARRENLOYARTE@osakidetza.eus
[14] Infectious Diseases Unit, Internal Medicine Department, Hospital Universitario 12 de Octubre, Instituto de Investigación Hospital 12 de Octubre "i + 12", 28041 Madrid, Spain; sirsilverdelea@yahoo.com
[15] Infectious Diseases Unit, Hospital de la Santa Creu i Sant Pau-Institut d'Investigació Biomèdica Sant Pau, Departament de Medicine, Universitat Autònoma de Barcelona, 08041 Barcelona, Spain; nbenito@santpau.cat
[16] Department of Infectious Diseases, Hospital Clínic of Barcelona, IDIBAPS, University of Barcelona, 08036 Barcelona, Spain; LMORATA@clinic.cat
[17] Microbiologic Department, Hospital Universitari Son Espases, 07120 Palma de Mallorca, Spain; antonio.ramirez@ssib.es
* Correspondence: helemh.vilchez@ssib.es; Tel.: +34-653419331
† Membership of the GEIO and REIPI are provided in the Acknowledgments.

Abstract: This retrospective, multicenter observational study aimed to describe the outcomes of surgical and medical treatment of *C. acnes*-related prosthetic joint infection (PJI) and the potential benefit of rifampin-based therapies. Patients with *C. acnes*-related PJI who were diagnosed and treated between January 2003 and December 2016 were included. We analyzed 44 patients with *C. acnes*-related PJI (median age, 67.5 years (IQR, 57.3–75.8)); 75% were men. The majority (61.4%) had late chronic infection according to the Tsukayama classification. All patients received surgical treatment, and most antibiotic regimens (43.2%) included β-lactam. Thirty-four patients (87.17%) were cured; five showed relapse. The final outcome (cure vs. relapse) showed a nonsignificant trend toward higher failure frequency among patients with previous prosthesis (OR: 6.89; 95% CI: 0.80–58.90) or prior surgery and infection (OR: 10.67; 95% IC: 1.08–105.28) in the same joint. Patients treated with clindamycin alone had a higher recurrence rate (40.0% vs. 8.8%). Rifampin treatment did not decrease recurrence in patients treated with β-lactams. Prior prosthesis, surgery, or infection in the same joint might be related to recurrence, and rifampin-based combinations do not seem to improve prognosis. Debridement and implant retention appear a safe option for surgical treatment of early PJI.

Keywords: *Cutibacterium acnes*; prosthetic joint infection; surgical and medical treatment

1. Introduction

Cutibacterium (formerly known as *Propionibacterium*) *acnes* is an anaerobic Gram-positive bacillus and a skin commensal organism with a predilection for pilosebaceous follicles, and it was formerly considered a contaminant. Moreover, *C. acnes* has been identified as a cause of biomaterial-related infections (BRIs) involving arthroplasty, cerebrospinal fluid (CSF) shunts, and spinal instrumentation, among others [1–3]. In recent years, with improved diagnosis methodology, including prolonged incubation protocols, *C. acnes* has become the microorganism most frequently related to infections involving shoulder prostheses. This infection type has become an emerging problem, but the relevant data are still limited [1,4,5].

Cutibacterium infections are usually characterized by a paucity of classical infections or inflammation symptoms, and they are often characterized by the absence of elevated inflammatory markers [1,6].

The role of *C. acnes* in prosthetic joint infections (PJIs) might be underestimated for the following reasons: (1) it is a common contaminant of the skin; (2) it needs a special transport medium; (3) it has delayed growth (up to 14 days); (4) the cultures need to be rechecked or discarded within 3 to 5 days of incubation. The advent of matrix-assisted laser desorption ionization time-of-flight mass spectrometry (MALDI-TOF MS) for the routine diagnosis of bacterial infections in clinical laboratories has increased the speed and ease of anaerobic bacteria identification [4,7,8].

Cutibacterium appears to have a greater predilection for infections involving the shoulder joint compared to other anatomical regions. The risk factors for *C. acnes*-related orthopedic infection include a history of joint surgery prior to the index surgery and male sex [9,10].

C. acnes is usually susceptible to a wide range of common antibiotics but there are no clinical trials or extensive observational studies that allow us to know the best antibiotic regimen or surgical procedure in these patients. The Infectious Diseases Society of America (IDSA) guidelines recommend penicillin or ceftriaxone as first-line treatment for *C. acnes*-related PJIs, with clindamycin or vancomycin as alternatives, and minocycline or doxycycline for suppressive therapy [11]. However, there have also been reports of increased antimicrobial resistance in biofilm-associated *C. acnes* isolates in vitro. In vitro and animal models of *C. acnes* biofilms suggest the efficacy of rifampin against *C. acnes*-related foreign-body infections [12,13], but adjunctive rifampin therapy is not included in the IDSA recommendations for *C. acnes*-related PJI management.

Despite its antimicrobial susceptibility, *C. acnes* is sometimes remarkably difficult to eradicate; therefore, medical management of PJIs without surgical intervention has been considered to result in poorer clinical outcomes [2].

The aim of this study was to describe the epidemiological, clinical, and biological characteristics, as well as the outcomes of surgical and medical treatment, of *C. acnes*-related PJI and the potential benefit of rifampin-based therapeutic combinations.

2. Results

Forty-six cases of *C. acnes*-related PJI were identified, of which two patients were excluded because both had co-infections with a microorganism other than CNS. Finally, we included 44 patients with *C. acnes*-related PJI. The median patient age was 67.5 years (IQR, 57.3–75.8); 75% of the patients were men. The number of cases included, according to year, is shown in Figure 1.

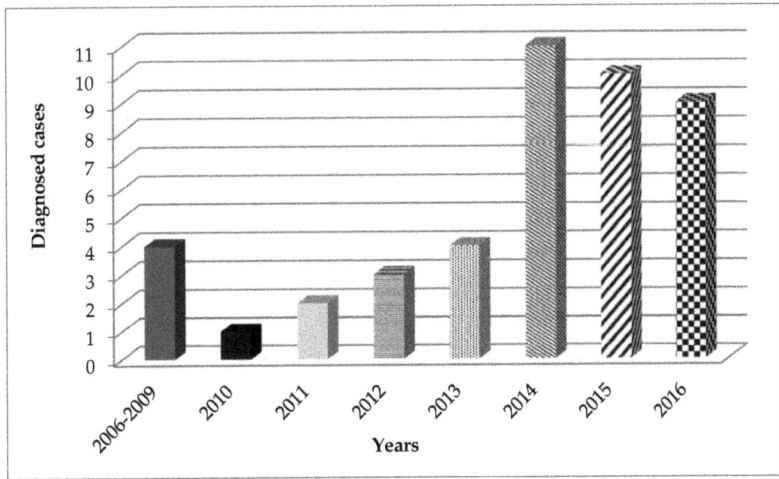

Figure 1. Cases frequency by year.

2.1. Patient Baseline and Clinical Characteristics

Demographic data, comorbidities, risk factors predisposing to PJI, signs and symptoms, and laboratory data at presentation are shown in Table 1. Most cases were classified as late chronic infection (type 2) or positive intraoperative culture (type 4), with 25% being acute prosthetic infections according to the Tsukayama classification. However, according to the Zimmerli classification, the most frequent type of infection was early infection (52.3%), while delayed and late infections were present in 47.7% of cases.

Table 1. Demographic, clinical, and laboratory characteristics of shoulder PJI due to *C. acnes*.

Variable	No (%) [a]
Age, years [b]	67.5 (IQR, 57.3–75.8)
Male	33 (75)
Charlson Index [b]	3.0 (IQR, 0.0–4.0)
Comorbidities	
Diabetes mellitus	13 (29.5)
Oncologic diseases	8 (18.2)
Renal insufficiency	3 (6.8)
Immunosuppressive treatment	2 (4.5)
Others	14 (31.8)
Time to diagnosis, days [b]	78.0 (IQR, 10.0–431.0)
Previous prosthesis	5 (11.4)
Previous surgery	5 (11.4)
Previous infections	5 (11.4)
Prosthesis infection	
Right shoulder	24 (54.5)
Left shoulder	20 (45.5)

Table 1. Cont.

Variable	No (%) [a]
Clinical characteristics	
Fever	8 (18.2)
Joint pain	33 (75)
Swelling	23 (52.3)
Fistula	7 (15.9)
Purulent wound drainage	12 (27.3)
Laboratory parameters [b]	
WBC count, cells/mm^3	8245.0 (IRQ, 6427.5–10,367.5)
CRP, mg/dL	14.0 (IQR, 6.0–32.3)
ESR, mm/h	46.0 (IQR, 22.0–71.0)
Type of shoulder PJI	
• **Tsukayama classification**	
Early postoperative infection	11 (25.0)
Late chronic infection	27 (61.4)
Positive intraoperative infection	6 (13.6)
• **Zimmerli classification**	
Early infection	23 (52.3)
Delayed or low-grade infection	14 (31.8)
Late infection	7 (15.9)

Abbreviations: CRP, C-reactive protein; ESR, erythrocyte sedimentation rate; WBC, white blood cell. [a] Data are the number (%) of cases. [b] Median (IQR, interquartile ranges).

2.2. Microbiological Characteristics and Antimicrobial Susceptibility Patterns

With regard to microbiological data, diagnosis was performed preoperatively and/or intraoperatively in all patients. In 17 (38.6%) of the 44 patients, C. acnes was found in the joint fluid aspiration. In 42 (95.5%) of 44 patients, C. acnes was found in intraoperative samples. There were 15 patients with C. acnes isolation in both samples (joint and intraoperative).

Three or more positive cultures were obtained in 32 patients (72.7%), two cultures were obtained in seven patients (15.9%), and only one culture was obtained in five patients (11.4%), where the infection was demonstrated by histopathologic inflammation and positive sonicate fluid from the prosthetic material culture. All tested isolates were susceptible to β-lactams (penicillin), vancomycin, and rifampin (Table 2).

Table 2. Samples and microbiological characteristics of shoulder PJI due to C. acnes.

Variable	Patients No. (%) [a]
Samples taken for culture	
Joint aspirate fluid	17 (38.6)
Intraoperative sample	42 (95.5)
Joint fluid + intraoperative samples	15 (34.1)
Microorganisms isolated	
Only P. acnes	35 (79.5)
Co-infection with S. epidermidis	9 (20.5)
Microbial susceptibility [b]	
Penicillin	39 (100)
Vancomycin	27 (100)
Clindamycin	38 (97.4)
Tetracycline	13 (100)
Rifampin	23 (100)

Abbreviations: CLSI, Clinical and Laboratory Standards Institute; EUCAST, European Committee on Antimicrobial susceptibility testing. [a] Data are the number (%) of cases; susceptibilities determined as per CLSI/EUCAST breakpoints. [b] All antibiotics were not tested in all strains isolated.

2.3. Surgical and Medical Therapy

All patients received surgical treatment: two-stage procedure (38.6%), debridement and implant retention (DAIR) (36.4%), one-stage procedure (18.2%), arthrodesis (2.3%), and resection arthroplasty (4.5%). When we compared the surgical treatment received with the type of infection according to the Tsukayama classification, there was an expected association between performing DAIR and early postoperative infection (Table 3).

Table 3. Comparison between the types of treatment with type of infection of shoulder PJI due to *C. acnes*.

Treatment	Type of Infection No. (%) [a]			Total (n = 44)	p
	Type 4 [b] (n = 6)	Type 2 [b] (n = 27)	Type 1 [b] (n = 11)		
Antibiotic					
Amoxicillin	3 (50.0)	13 (48.1)	3 (27.3)	19 (43.2)	0.558
Clindamycin	3 (50.0)	8 (29.6)	3 (27.3)	14 (31.8)	0.650
Rifampin	2 (33.3)	11 (40.7)	6 (54.5)	19 (43.2)	0.677
Surgical					
Debridement and retention	0	6 (22.2)	10 (90.9)	16 (36.4)	0.000
2-stage procedure	1 (16.7)	15 (55.6)	1 (9.1)	17 (38.6)	0.013
1-stage procedure	4 (66.7)	4 (14.8)	0 (0)	8 (18.2)	0.006
Arthrodesis	0	1 (3.7)	0 (0)	1 (2.3)	1
Resection arthroplasty	1 (16.7)	1 (3.7)	0 (0)	2 (4.5)	0.315

[a] Data are the number (%) of cases. [b] Tsukayama classification: early postoperative infection (Type 1), late chronic infection (Type 2), and positive intraoperative cultures (Type 4).

The majority (43.2%) of antibiotic regimens used β-lactam (amoxicillin), while clindamycin was used in 31.8% and other antibiotics (linezolid, quinolones, doxycycline, and glycopeptides—vancomycin and teicoplanin) were used in 22.7%. Rifampin was administered concurrently with at least one of the aforementioned antibiotics in 19 patients (43%), with two cases of rifampin treatment being discontinued due to adverse reactions. When we compared the type of antibiotic treatment with the type of infection, we observed no significant differences (Table 3). The median duration of antibiotic therapy was 56 days (IQR, 44–84 days).

2.4. Treatment Outcomes

Among the 44 patients included, 39 were evaluable for treatment outcome. At the last follow-up, five patients were lost, 34 patients were considered cured, and five had microbiologically confirmed recurrence. Three patients died due to noninfectious causes (acute pulmonary edema, advanced renal neoplasm, and cardiorespiratory arrest); these patients were followed up for more than 12 months with favorable infection outcomes.

We compared patients with a favorable outcome to those who failed treatment (Table 4). All patients in the failure group were male, but there was no significant difference in the clinical presentation, treatment received, or type of infection. A nonsignificant trend toward a higher frequency of failure was observed among patients with previous prosthesis (odds ratio (OR): 6.89; 95% confidence interval (CI): 0.80–58.90; $p = 0.078$) and previous surgery and infection in the same joint (OR: 10.67; 95% IC: 1.08–105.28; $p = 0.043$). In addition, we observed a higher frequency of recurrence in diabetic patients (OR: 4.87; 95% IC: 0.69–34.50; $p = 0.113$) and those who were treated only with clindamycin (OR: 6.89; 95% IC: 0.80–58.90; $p = 0.078$) than those who only received amoxicillin (OR: 0.357; 95% CI: 0.04–3.55; $p = 0.379$) or rifampin-based combinations (OR: 0.844; 95% CI: 0.12–5.72; $p = 0.862$).

Table 4. Comparison of final outcomes.

Variable	Outcome		p
	Cured (N = 34)	Recurrence (N = 5)	
Age, years (Median)	68 (IQR, 57.8–76.3)	69 (IQ, 42.5–73.5)	0.378
Gender, No. (%)			
Male	24 (70.6)	5 (100)	0.302
Female	10 (29.4)	0 (0)	
Charlson Index (Median)	2.95 (IQR, 0–4.03)	2.0 (IQR, 0–4.50)	0.729
Comorbidities, No. (%)			
Diabetes	8 (23.5)	3 (60)	0.125
Renal insufficiency	2 (5.9)	1 (20)	0.345
Oncologic disease	7 (20.6)		0.563
Immunosuppressive therapy	2 (5.9)		1
Previous prosthesis, No. (%)	3 (8.8)	2 (40)	0.114
Previous surgery, No. (%)	2 (5.9)	2 (40)	0.072
Previous infections, No. (%)	2 (5.9)	2 (40)	0.072
Prosthesis infection, No. (%)			
Right shoulder	18 (53)	3 (60)	1
Left shoulder	16 (47)	2 (40)	
Time to diagnosis, days (Median)	67 (IQR, 9–199)	70 (IQR, 7–1537)	0.823
Type of infection No. (%)			
• Tsukayama classification			1
Early postoperative infection	10 (29.4)	1 (20.0)	
Late chronic infection	20 (58.8)	3 (60.0)	
Positive intraoperative cultures	4 (11.8)	1 (20.0)	
• Zimmerli classification			0.823
Early infection	19 (55.9)	3 (60)	
Delayed or low-grade infection	11 (32.4)	1 (20)	
Late infection	4 (11.8)	1 (20)	
Surgical treatment, No. (%)			
Prosthesis retention	13 (38.2)	2 (40)	1
1-stage procedure	5 (14.7)	1 (20)	1
2-stage procedure	13 (38.2)	2 (40)	1
Arthrodesis	1 (2.9)	0	1
Resection arthroplasty	2 (5.9)	0	1
Antimicrobial treatment, No. (%)			
Amoxicillin	14 (41.2)	1 (20)	0.631
Clindamycin	3 (8.8)	2 (40)	0.114
Other	2 (5.9)	0	1
Amoxicillin plus rifampin	3 (8.8)	1 (20)	0.436
Clindamycin plus rifampin	5 (14.7)	1 (20)	1
Other plus rifampin	7 (20.6)	0	0.563

Regarding surgical treatment, 15/39 patients (38.5%) underwent DAIR, with 13 having favorable outcomes (Figure 2). When analyzed according to both classifications, for patients classified by the Tsukayama guidelines, 9/13 cured patients (69.23%) had type 1 infections and 4/13 (30.77%) had type 2, with one case of recurrence for type 1 and another recurrence for type 2. According to the Zimmerli classification, 12/13 of the cured patients (92.30%) had early infections and 1/13 (7.7%) had a delayed infection, with both recurrences being classified as early infections. Of the 24 patients treated with prosthesis removal, only three had recurrence (12.5%) (Table 4).

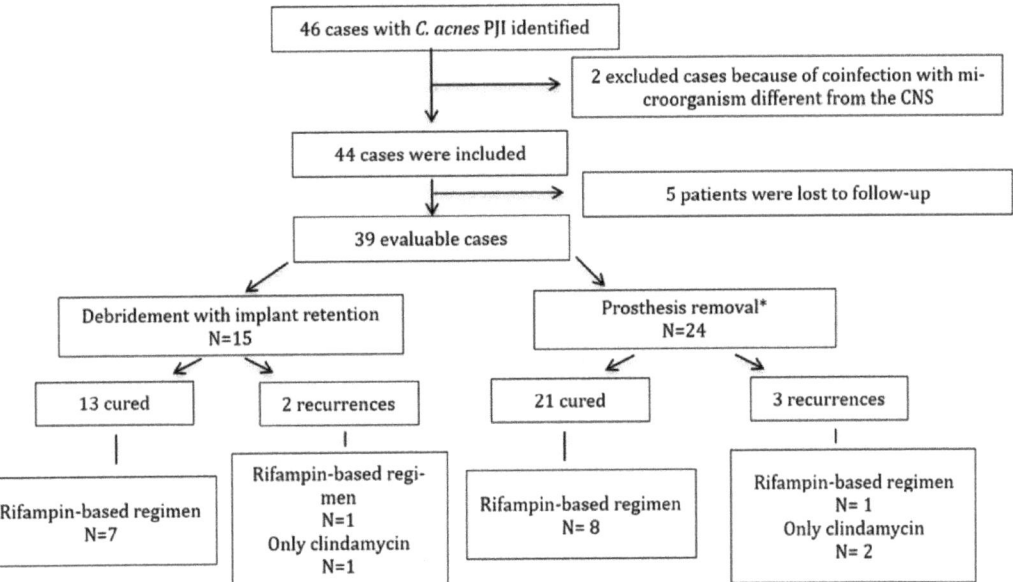

Figure 2. Flowchart of failure rates according to the medical and surgical approaches used. * Fifteen patients were treated with a two-stage procedure, six were treated with a one-stage procedure, one was treated with arthrodesis, and two were treated with resection arthroplasty.

Among the 39 evaluable patients, 17 were treated with rifampin. There were no differences in the outcome of patients treated with rifampin-based combinations. There were five patients with positive intraoperative cultures, with one being treated with rifampin therapy and cured, while the others (4/5) did not receive rifampin and recurrences were observed. Of the 15 patients treated with DAIR, eight (53.3%) received rifampin-based regimens, while seven did not, and one recurrence was observed in each group, but this was not significant (Figure 2). We analyzed 11 patients who received clindamycin treatment (six associated with rifampin) and there were three instances of recurrence (all isolates were susceptible to clindamycin).

The epidemiological, clinical, and treatment data of the five patients who showed recurrence are presented in Table 5.

Table 5. Individual clinical characteristics and treatment of the five recurrence cases.

Patient	Age, Years [a]	Sex	Comorbid Factors	Clinical Signs and Symptoms	Delay in Diagnosis, Days	Type of Infection		Treatment		
						Tsukayama [b]	Zimmerli	Type of Surgery	Antibiotic Regimen	Duration, Days
1	69	Male		Fever	407	Type 2	Delayed infection	1-stage procedure	Amoxicillin	57
2	74	Male	DM, CKD	Joint pain, joint swelling	70	Type 2	Early infection	DAIR	Amoxicillin plus Rifampin	138
3	52	Male	DM	Joint pain, joint swelling, fistula	2667	Type 2	Late infection	2-stage procedure	Clindamycin plus Rifampin	112
4	73	Male	DM		0	Type 4	Early infection	2-stage procedure	Clindamycin	60
5	33	Male		Joint pain, joint swelling, fistula, purulent wound drainage	14	Type 1	Early infection	DAIR	Clindamycin	175

Abbreviations: DM, diabetes mellitus; CKD, Chronic kidney disease. [a] Mean age (SD), 60.2 (SD 17.6) years. [b] Tsukayama classification: early postoperative infection (Type 1), late chronic infection (Type 2), and positive intraoperative cultures (Type 4).

3. Discussion

In this retrospective multicenter study, we described 44 patients with shoulder PJI due to *C. acnes* over a period of 14 years. The diagnosis of this infection is difficult due to the absence of classical clinical evidence, as well as the challenges associated with culturing the microorganism. In this 14 year series, we observed an increase in the number of diagnosed cases of this infection, which is probably due to the extended incubation time that has been demonstrated in other studies for maximizing the recovery of *C. acnes* from PJI specimens [1,7,14–17].

Previous studies have argued that the shoulder has a propensity for infection with *C. acnes* because it is the anaerobic dominant bacteria from healthy skin, particularly in moist areas (axilla), where a higher *C. acnes* bacterial burden is observed in men compared to women [17–19]. Moreover, previous series have reported that male gender is a risk factor for the development of this infection [1,9,20]. These previous findings would explain our results in which a male predominance of PJI was observed.

The most frequent types of infection in this study, according to the Tsukayama classification, were late chronic or positive intraoperative cultures, which is similar to that reported in other studies [1,21,22]; this is due to the paucity of classical symptoms and the absence of elevated inflammatory markers that delay diagnosis. However, when we classified the infection type according to the Zimmerli classification, early infection was the most frequent.

In our study, the most frequent symptom was joint pain. This is consistent with other studies in which pain and functional limitations without either fever or constitutional symptoms were the most frequent clinical presentations [6,7,23].

Previous surgery in the same joint has been linked to an increased risk of *C. acnes*-related PJI because repeated manipulation of the joint causes changes in the anatomical structure; this increases the duration of surgery, which is a major risk factor for shoulder PJI from this microorganism [20,24,25]. We observed that previous prosthesis, infection, or surgery in the same joint might be related with recurrence, but we could not demonstrate a significant association, possibly due to small sample size.

In our study, all isolates tested were susceptible to penicillin, vancomycin, and rifampin, with approximately 2.5% being resistant to clindamycin. These observed susceptibility patterns were similar to those of other studies [1,7,22], which suggested that the broad antimicrobial susceptibility of *C. acnes* appeared to be maintained.

Previous clinical studies and case reports provide little information regarding the optimal treatment for *C. acnes*-related PJI. In our study, all patients received antibiotic and surgical treatment. As expected, we observed significant differences between surgery type (DAIR, two-stage surgery, and one-stage surgery), as well as the type of prosthetic infection. Regarding surgical treatment, prosthesis retention and the two-stage procedure were the most frequent surgical procedures performed, unlike previous articles, which suggests that prosthesis exchange should be the treatment of choice in most cases [2,5,26]. We observed that, in the cases of early infection according to the Zimmerli classification, DAIR treatment may be a safe option.

In terms of antimicrobial treatment, the outcomes with or without adjunctive rifampin therapy were similar to other studies [1,22]. This finding is striking, particularly in cases treated with debridement and implant retention, because this antibiotic has antibiofilm activity and its effectiveness for the eradication of *C. acnes* has been demonstrated both in vitro and in vivo in an animal model of foreign-body infection [12]. However, another explanation could be that the presence of a high inoculum in the biofilms forms in a foreign body (i.e., a prosthetic joint). In this state, the microorganism produces mutations that can lead to some degree of resistance, which is observed as a reduced susceptibility to rifampin; this phenomenon was reported in a study by Furustrand et al. [27], where it was demonstrated in vitro.

On the other hand, we observed a nonsignificant trend toward a higher frequency of failure among 11 patients who received clindamycin (cured 72.7% vs. recurrence 27.3%). The IDSA guidelines recommend clindamycin as an alternative treatment to β-lactams, because the majority of tested isolates were susceptible; for this reason, the use of clindamycin has been evaluated in previous studies [1–3]. However, future clinical trials will be needed to compare antibiotic therapy between β-lactams and clindamycin in *C. acnes*-related PJI.

The strength of this multicenter study is that only patients with a proven diagnosis of *C. acnes*-related PJI were included. Currently, most studies include all types of bone infection due to this microorganism, which makes it difficult to determine the best management and evolution of this entity.

This study did have some limitations. This was a retrospective observational study that did not have predefined therapeutic procedures, and this could have induced bias. Moreover, the follow-up time was limited to a 1 year period. However, in PJIs caused by microorganisms as paucisymptomatic as *C. acnes*, in which DAIR has been performed, a longer follow-up time might be necessary.

4. Methods

4.1. Study Design, Patients, and Settings

This multicenter, retrospective observational study was conducted at 16 hospitals belonging to the Prosthetic Joint Infection Group of the Spanish Network for Research in Infectious Diseases between January 2003 and December 2016.

Patients aged 18 years and older with shoulder PJIs that were caused by *C. acnes* and diagnosed between January 2003 and December 2016 were included, regardless of the age of the implant at the time of the initial symptoms. Polymicrobial infections with coagulase-negative staphylococci (CNS) were also included.

4.2. Data Collection

Cases were identified by searching the databases of previously recorded consecutive PJIs or the general archives at each participating hospital.

Medical chart abstraction was performed using a standardized case report form to retrieve demographic, clinical, and laboratory data. Demographic data included age and sex. Laboratory data included erythrocyte sedimentation rate (ESR), C-reactive protein (CRP), and white blood cell (WBC) counts. Clinical data consisted of comorbidities, immunosuppressive therapy, Charlson index, previous exposure to antibiotics (7 days), hospitalization in the previous 90 days (of at least 2 days), and receipt of hemodialysis. We also collected the following information regarding arthroplasty: date of implantation, site, primary or revision arthroplasty, previous infections in the same joint (date and microorganism), cemented versus uncemented arthroplasty, use of antibiotics in bone cement, and date of diagnosis. The time from index surgery to diagnosis was recorded as the time from the last surgical procedure performed pre diagnosis to the first positive *C. acnes* culture, with classification of the PJI, type and number of cultured samples, and their results also being recorded.

Information regarding surgical treatment, exchange of removable pieces of the prosthesis (in at least one debridement surgery), and the type and duration of antimicrobials used was also collected, as well as patient outcomes and the date of the last follow-up visit.

4.3. Definitions

A PJI was defined on the basis of previously detailed criteria [1,11]. The *C. acnes* etiology was confirmed if ≥2 specimens were positive for *C. acnes*, or if one culture specimen was positive for *C. acnes*, with no other organism detected on culture and concurrent evidence of joint purulence, histopathological inflammation, or a sinus tract communicating with the prosthesis. PJI was assigned according to the Tsukayama and Zimmerli classifications [28–30].

4.4. Follow-Up and Treatment Success

Antimicrobial therapeutic regimens and treatment outcomes were assessed through the last recorded clinical visit. Decisions on therapeutic regimens were based on the clinical judgment of the infectious disease and surgical specialist providers. The type, delivery method, and duration of antimicrobial therapy were recorded.

After being discharged, patients were followed-up according to the protocol of each participating center. The follow-up period was calculated from surgery due to infection: debridement, one-stage exchange, two-stage exchange, or other procedures (arthrodesis/resection arthroplasty). Among patients in remission, only those with at least 1 year of follow-up were included in the outcome analysis.

Cure was defined as the absence of signs and symptoms of infection at the conclusion of a minimum 1 year follow-up period after antibiotic therapy, which did not result in unplanned additional surgical debridement for putative persistent infection. Treatment failure was established on the basis of the following criteria: (1) persistence of symptoms and clinical signs of infection during treatment that led to a change in the surgical strategy (except for new surgical debridement during the first month after an initial debridement); (2) the recurrence of symptoms and clinical signs of infection once the surgical strategy was completed, with isolation of the same microorganism; (3) the need for suppressive antibiotic treatment against *C. acnes*; (4) infection-related death. Any case of reinfection by microorganisms other than *C. acnes* detected during the follow-up period was not considered a failure.

4.5. Microbiological Methods

Culture specimens were collected and processed at each participating institution, following the Spanish guidelines for the microbiological diagnosis of bone and joint infections [31,32]. Identification testing of isolates was performed in the clinical microbiology laboratory at each center using standard microbiological techniques. The susceptibilities of *C. acnes* isolates were tested against standard antimicrobial agents. Isolates were classified as susceptible according to the minimum inhibitory concentration (MIC) breakpoints set by the Clinical and Laboratory Standards Institute (CLSI) or the European Committee on Antimicrobial Susceptibility Testing (EUCAST).

4.6. Statistical Analysis

The descriptive analysis for defining the patient's characteristics was done by frequencies and percentages for categorical variables and measures of central tendency and dispersion for numerical variables. The non-normally distributed continuous variables were expressed by median and interquartile range (IQR). For evaluating the differences between favorable outcome and failed treatment, the Mann–Whitney *U* test was used to compare continuous variables and the chi-squared and Fisher exact tests were used for comparing categorical variables. Moreover, univariate logistic regression was used for evaluating the recurrence risk. A p-value <0.05 was considered statistically significant. Statistical analyses were performed using SPSS software version 26 (IBM Inc., Armonk, NY, USA).

5. Conclusions

Physicians should be aware of the increase in the frequency of shoulder PJIs caused by *C. acnes* because there are few clinical symptoms and an absence of elevated inflammatory markers. On the other hand, patients with type 1 infections according to the Tsukayama classification or early infection by the Zimmerli classification could be treated with DAIR. According to our data, rifampin therapy does not seem to improve outcomes, and clindamycin seems to be associated with a worse prognosis. Randomized studies with a greater number of patients are necessary to establish the optimal antimicrobial treatment.

Author Contributions: Conceptualization and methodology, H.H.V. and M.R.; formal analysis, H.H.V., M.R., and J.L.-T.; investigation, H.H.V.; resources, H.H.V., R.E.-S., M.F.-S., O.M., Á.A., D.R.-P., A.J.-S., M.D.d.T., A.R. (Alicia Rico), L.F., J.P.-S., L.G., J.A.I., J.L.-T., N.B., L.M., A.R. (Antonio Ramirez), M.R., and Antonio Ramirez data curation, H.H.V.; writing—original draft preparation, H.H.V.; writing—review and editing, R.E.-S., M.F.-S., O.M., Á.A., D.R.-P., A.J.-S., M.D.d.T., A.R. (Alicia Rico), L.F., J.P.-S., L.G., J.A.I., J.L.-T., N.B., L.M., A.R. (Antonio Ramirez), and M.R.; visualization, H.H.V., M.R. and J.L.-T.; supervision, M.R. and J.L.-T.; project administration, H.H.V. and M.R. All authors have read and agreed to the published version of the manuscript.

Funding: This work received no specific funding from the public, private, or not-for-profit sectors.

Institutional Review Board Statement: The study was conducted according to the guidelines of the Declaration of Helsinki, and approved by the Ethics Committee for Clinical Research of the Balearic Islands, Spain (IB3404/17PI).

Informed Consent Statement: Patient consent was waived due to this is a retrospective and observational study, the information is collected from the medical archives of each hospital and there is neither intervention in the patient's treatment nor in the epidemiological and clinical information.

Data Availability Statement: The data presented in this study are available on request from the corresponding author. The data are not publicly available due to ethical concerns.

Acknowledgments: We acknowledge Aina Millán Pons for the statistical analysis and Antonio Vanrell for the creation of the database. We also thank Jonathan McFarland for improving the English language and to all doctors belonging to the 16 hospitals of the Prosthetic Joint Infection Group of the Spanish Network for Research in Infectious Diseases that participated in this study. GEIO Study Collaborators: Javier Cobo [1], Luis Estelles [2], Julia Laporte [3], Javier Ariza [3], Bernadette G. Pfang [4], Jaime Esteban [4], Carles Pilgrau [5], Mayli Lung [6], Pablo S. Corona [7], Ferrán Perez-Villar [8], Mercé Gracía-Gonzalez [9], Oriol Gasch [10], Maite Ruiz [11], Javier Garcés [12], Mikel Mancheño-Losa [13], Isabel Mur[14], Pere Coll [15], Xavier Crusi [16], Alex Soriano [17] [1] Infectious Diseases Department, Hospital Universitario Ramón y Cajal, Madrid, España. [2] Infectious Diseases Unit, Department of Medicine, Hospital Universitario Marqués de Valdecilla-IDIVAL, Cantabria, Spain. [3] Infectious Diseases Department, Hospital Universitari de Bellvitge, Barcelona, Spain. [4] Department of Internal Medicine. Bone and Joint Infection Unit. IIS-Fundación Jiménez Díaz. Madrid, Spain. [5] Infectious Diseases Department. Hospital Universitari Vall d'Hebron, Universitat Autònoma de Barcelona, Barcelona, Spain. [6] Microbiology Department. Hospital Universitari Vall d'Hebron, Universitat Autònoma de Barcelona, Barcelona, Spain. [7] Reconstructive and Septic surgery Division. Department of Orthopedic Surgery. Hospital Universitari Vall d'Hebron, Universitat Autònoma de Barcelona, Barcelona, Spain. [8] Orthopedic Surgery and Traumatology Departmet, Hospital Universitari Arnau de Vilanova. Lleida, Spain. [9] Microbiology Department, Hospital Universitari Arnau de Vilanova. Lleida, Spain. [10] Infectious Diseases Department, Corporació Sanitària Parc Taulí, Barcelona, Spain. [11] Microbiology Department, University Hospital Virgen del Rocio, Sevilla, Spain. [12] Orthopedic Surgery and Traumatology Department, University Hospital Virgen del Rocio, Sevilla, Spain. [13] Infectious Diseases Unit, Internal Medicine Department, Hospital Universitario 12 de Octubre, Instituto de Investigación Hospital 12 de Octubre "i + 12", Madrid, Spain. [14] Infectious Diseases Unit. Hospital de la Santa Creu i Sant Pau-Institut d'Investigació Biomèdica Sant Pau; Departament of Medicine, Universitat Autònoma de Barcelona, Barcelona, Spain. [15] Department of clinical Microbiology. Hospital de la Santa Creu i Sant Pau-Institut d'Investigació Biomèdica Sant Pau; Departament of Medicine, Universitat Autònoma de Barcelona, Barcelona, Spain. [16] Department of Orthopedic and Traumatology. Hospital de la Santa Creu i Sant Pau-Institut d'Investigació Biomèdica Sant Pau; Departament of Medicine, Universitat Autònoma de Barcelona, Barcelona, Spain. [17] Department of Infectious diseases, Hospital Clínic of Barcelona, IDIBAPS, University of Barcelona, Barcelona, Spain.

Conflicts of Interest: The authors declare no conflict of interest.

References

1. Piggott, D.A.; Higgins, Y.M.; Melia, M.T.; Ellis, B.; Carroll, K.C.; McFarland, E.G.; Auwaerter, P.G. Characteristics and Treatment Outcomes of Propionibacterium acnes Prosthetic Shoulder Infections in Adults. *Open Forum Infect. Dis.* **2015**, *3*, ofv191. [CrossRef]
2. Lutz, M.F.; Berthelot, P.; Fresard, A.; Cazorla, C.; Carricajo, A.; Vautrin, A.C.; Fessy, M.-H.; Lucht, F. Arthroplastic and osteo-synthetic infections due to Propionibacterium acnes: A retrospective study of 52 cases, 1995–2002. *Eur. J. Clin. Microbiol. Infect. Dis.* **2005**, *24*, 739–744. [CrossRef]
3. Levy, P.Y.; Fenollar, F.; Stein, A.; Borrione, F.; Cohen, E.; Lebail, B.; Raoult, D. Propionibacterium acnes post-operative shoulder arthritis: An emerging clinical entity. *Clin. Infect. Dis.* **2008**, *46*, 1884–1886. [CrossRef]
4. Walter, G.; Vernier, M.; Pinelli, P.O.; Million, M.; Coulange, M.; Seng, P.; Stein, A. Bone and joint infections due to anaerobic bacteria: An analysis of 61 cases and review of the literature. *Eur. J. Clin. Microbiol. Infect. Dis.* **2014**, *33*, 1355–1364. [CrossRef] [PubMed]
5. Achermann, Y.; Sahin, F.; Schwyzer, H.; Kolling, C.; Wüst, J.; Vogt, M. Characteristics and outcome of 16 periprosthetic shoulder joint infections. *Infection* **2012**, *41*, 613–620. [CrossRef] [PubMed]
6. Cooper, M.E.; Trivedi, N.N.; Sivasundaram, L.; Karns, M.R.; Voos, J.E.; Gillespie, R.J. Diagnosis and man-agement of periprosthetic joint infection after shoulder arthroplasty. *JBJS Rev.* **2019**, *7*, e3. [CrossRef]
7. Wang, B.; Toye, B.; Desjardins, M.; Lapner, P.; Lee, C. A 7-year retrospective review from 2005 to 2011 of Propionibacterium acnes shoulder infections in Ottawa, Ontario, Canada. *Diagn. Microbiol. Infect. Dis.* **2013**, *75*, 195–199. [CrossRef] [PubMed]
8. Nodzo, S.R.; Boyle, K.K.; Bhimani, S.; Duquin, T.R.; Miller, A.O.; Westrich, G.H. Propionibacterium acnes Host Inflammatory Response During Periprosthetic Infection Is Joint Specific. *HSS J.* **2017**, *13*, 159–164. [CrossRef] [PubMed]
9. Kanafani, Z.A.; Pien, B.C.; Varkey, J.; Basmania, C.; Kaye, K.S.; Sexton, D.J. Postoperative Joint Infections Due to Propionibacterium Species: A Case-Control Study. *Clin. Infect. Dis.* **2009**, *49*, 1083–1085. [CrossRef] [PubMed]
10. Matsen, F.A.; Whitson, A.; Neradilek, M.B.; Pottinger, P.S.; Bertelsen, A.; Hsu, J.E. Factors predictive of Cutibacterium peripros-thetic shoulder infections: A retrospective study of 342 prosthetic revisions. *J. Shoulder Elb. Surg.* **2020**, *29*, 1177–1187. [CrossRef]
11. Osmon, D.R.; Berbari, E.F.; Berendt, A.R.; Lew, D.; Zimmerli, W.; Steckelberg, J.M.; Rao, N.; Hanssen, A.; Wilson, W.R. Diagnosis and management of prosthetic joint infection: Clinical practice guidelines by the infectious diseases Society of America. *Clin. Infect. Dis.* **2013**, *56*, e1–e25. [CrossRef] [PubMed]
12. Tafin, U.F.; Corvec, S.; Betrisey, B.; Zimmerli, W.; Trampuz, A. Role of rifampin against Propionibacte-rium acnes biofilm in vitro and in an experimental foreign-body infection model. *Antimicrob. Agents Chemother.* **2012**, *56*, 1885–1891. [CrossRef] [PubMed]
13. Sendi, P.; Zimmerli, W. Antimicrobial treatment concepts for orthopaedic device-related infection. *Clin. Microbiol. Infect.* **2012**, *18*, 1176–1184. [CrossRef] [PubMed]
14. Butler-Wu, S.M.; Burns, E.M.; Pottinger, P.S.; Magaret, A.S.; Rakeman, J.L.; Matsen, F.A.; Cookson, B.T. Optimization of Periprosthetic Culture for Diagnosis of Propionibacterium acnes Prosthetic Joint Infection. *J. Clin. Microbiol.* **2011**, *49*, 2490–2495. [CrossRef]
15. Frangiamore, S.J.; Saleh, A.; Grosso, M.J.; Alolabi, B.; Bauer, T.W.; Iannotti, J.P.; Ricchetti, E.T. Early versus late cul-ture growth of Propionibacterium acnes in revision shoulder arthroplasty. *J. Bone Jt. Surg. Am. Vol.* **2015**, *97*, 1149–1158. [CrossRef] [PubMed]
16. Hsu, J.E.; Somerson, J.S.; Vo, K.V.; Matsen, F.A. What is a "periprosthetic shoulder infection"? A systematic review of two decades of publications. *Int. Orthop.* **2017**, *41*, 813–822. [CrossRef] [PubMed]
17. Dodson, C.C.; Craig, E.V.; Cordasco, F.A.; Dines, D.M.; Dines, J.S.; DiCarlo, E.; Brause, B.D.; Warren, R.F. Propionibacterium ac-nes infection after shoulder arthroplasty: A diagnostic challenge. *J. Shoulder Elb. Surg.* **2010**, *19*, 303–307. [CrossRef] [PubMed]
18. Patel, A.; Calfee, R.P.; Plante, M.; Fischer, S.A.; Green, A. Propionibacterium acnes colonization of the human shoulder. *J. Shoulder Elb. Surg.* **2009**, *18*, 897–902. [CrossRef]
19. Zeller, V.; Ghorbani, A.; Strady, C.; Leonard, P.; Mamoudy, P.; Desplaces, N. Propionibacterium acnes: An agent of prosthetic joint infection and colonization. *J. Infect.* **2007**, *55*, 119–124. [CrossRef]
20. Egglestone, A.; Ingoe, H.; Rees, J.; Thomas, M.; Jeavons, R.; Rangan, A. Scoping review: Diagnosis and management of periprosthetic joint infection in shoulder arthroplasty. *Shoulder Elb.* **2019**, *11*, 167–181. [CrossRef]
21. Levy, O.; Iyer, S.; Atoun, E.; Peter, N.; Hous, N.; Cash, D.; Musa, F.; Narvani, A. Propionibacterium acnes: An underestimated etiology in the pathogenesis of osteoarthritis? *J. Shoulder Elb. Surg.* **2013**, *22*, 505–511. [CrossRef]
22. Garrigues, G.E.; Zmistowski, B.; Cooper, A.M.; Green, A.; Abboud, J.; Beasley, J.; Belay, E.S.; Benito, N.; Cil, A.; Clark, B.; et al. Proceedings from the 2018 International Consensus Meeting on Orthopedic Infections: Management of periprosthetic shoulder infection. *J. Shoulder Elb. Surg.* **2019**, *28*, S67–S99. [CrossRef]
23. Sperling, J.W.; Kozak, T.K.; Hanssen, A.D.; Cofield, R.H. Infection after Shoulder Arthroplasty. *Clin. Orthop. Relat. Res.* **2001**, *382*, 206–216. [CrossRef]

24. Fink, B.; Sevelda, F. Periprosthetic Joint Infection of Shoulder Arthroplasties: Diagnostic and Treatment Options. *BioMed Res. Int.* **2017**, *2017*, 1–10. [CrossRef]
25. Simha, S.; Shields, E.J.; Wiater, J.M. Periprosthetic Infections of the Shoulder. *JBJS Rev.* **2018**, *6*, e6. [CrossRef] [PubMed]
26. Paxton, E.S.; Green, A.; Krueger, V.S. Periprosthetic Infections of the Shoulder: Diagnosis and Management. *J. Am. Acad. Orthop. Surg.* **2019**, *27*, E935–E944. [CrossRef] [PubMed]
27. Furustrand Tafin, U.; Trampuz, A.; Corvec, S. In vitro emergence of rifampicin resistance in Propionibacterium acnes and molecular characterization of mutations in the rpoB gene. *J. Antimicrob. Chemother.* **2013**, *68*, 523–528. [CrossRef]
28. Tsukayama, D.T.; Estrada, R.; Gustilo, R.B. Infection after Total Hip Arthroplasty A Study of the Treatment of One Hundred and Six Infections. Available online: http://journals.lww.com/jbjsjournal (accessed on 7 March 2021).
29. Zimmerli, W.; Trampuz, A.; Ochsner, P.E. Prosthetic-Joint Infections. *N. Engl. J. Med.* **2004**, *351*, 1645. Available online: www.nejm.org (accessed on 21 March 2021). [CrossRef] [PubMed]
30. Trampuz, A.; Zimmerli, W. Prosthetic joint infections: Update in diagnosis and treatment. *Swiss Med. Wkly.* **2005**, *135*, 243–251.
31. Jaime, E.; Mercedes, M.; Antonia, M.M.; Mar, S.-S. Diagnostico microbiológico de las infecciones osteoarticulares. Procedimientos en Microbiol Clínica Recomendaciones de la Sociedad Española Enfermedades Infecciosas y Microbiol Clínica. 2009, p. 1. Available online: http://www.seimc.org/documentos/protocolos/microbiologia (accessed on 21 March 2021).
32. Marín, M.; Esteban, J.; Meseguer, M.A.; Sánchez-Somolinos, M. Diagnóstico microbiolgico de las infecciones osteoarticulares. *Enferm. Infecc. Microbiol. Clin.* **2010**, *28*, 534–540. [CrossRef]

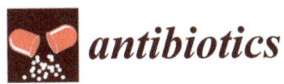

Perspective

Candida Periprosthetic Joint Infection: Is It Curable?

Laura Escolà-Vergé [1,2,3,*], Dolors Rodríguez-Pardo [1,2,3], Pablo S. Corona [2,3,4] and Carles Pigrau [1,2,3]

1. Infectious Diseases Department, Hospital Universitari Vall d'Hebron, Universitat Autònoma de Barcelona, Passeig Vall d'Hebron 119-129, 08035 Barcelona, Spain; dolorodriguez@vhebron.net (D.R.-P.); cpigraus@gmail.com (C.P.)
2. Spanish Network for Research in Infectious Diseases (REIPI RD16/0016/0003), Instituto de Salud Carlos III, 28029 Madrid, Spain; pcorona@vhebron.net
3. Study Group on Osteoarticular Infections of the Spanish Society of Clinical Microbiology and Infectious Diseases (GEIO-SEIMC), 28003 Madrid, Spain
4. Septic and Reconstructive Surgery Unit (UCSO), Orthopaedic Surgery Department, Vall d'Hebron University Hospital, Passeig Vall d'Hebron 119-129, 08035 Barcelona, Spain
* Correspondence: lauraescola@gmail.com; Tel.: +34-932-746-090; Fax: +34-934-894-091

Abstract: Candida periprosthetic joint infection (CPJI) is a rare and very difficult to treat infection, and high-quality evidence regarding the best management is scarce. *Candida* spp. adhere to medical devices and grow forming biofilms, which contribute to the persistence and relapse of this infection. Typically, CPJI presents as a chronic infection in a patient with multiple previous surgeries and long courses of antibiotic therapy. In a retrospective series of cases, the surgical approach with higher rates of success consists of a two-stage exchange surgery, but the best antifungal treatment and duration of antifungal treatment are still unclear, and the efficacy of using an antifungal agent-loaded cement spacer is still controversial. Until more evidence is available, focusing on prevention and identifying patients at risk of CPJI seems more than reasonable.

Keywords: *Candida* spp.; periprosthetic joint infection; fungus; biofilm; antifungal-loaded cement spacer; two-stage exchange surgery

1. Introduction

Periprosthetic joint infection (PJI), which occurs in approximately 1–2% of all procedures, is one of the most feared complications after arthroplasty due to its associated comorbidities and the possible need for implant removal [1]. Candida periprosthetic joint infection (CPJI) represents a rare etiology among all PJIs; sometimes it is very difficult to diagnose, and it is especially difficult to treat when the prosthetic material cannot be removed [2]. In addition, we have no clear guidelines regarding the best antifungal management in these cases [3–7], and evidence is based on small retrospective series.

2. Epidemiology

There have been a few recent studies analyzing the prevalence of these infections, and most of them are retrospective in nature [8–11]. A Spanish retrospective multicenter study that analyzed the etiology of PJIs from 2003 to 2012 found that a fungal etiology represented 1.3% of all culture-positive PJIs (n = 2288), and *Candida* spp. were responsible for 90% of all fungal infections [9]. A smaller retrospective multicenter study performed in Australia from 2006 to 2008 found that CPJI accounted for 0.7% (1/152) of all culture-positive infections [10], and another study that compared the etiology of PJIs between two referral centers in Europe and in the United States between 2000 and 2011 found that fungal PJIs were responsible for 2.3% of 772 cases and 0.3% of 898 cases, respectively [11].

The species of *Candida* depends on the local epidemiology of the geographical area. In two multicenter studies in Spain [2,9] and one in the United States [12], *C. albicans* was the most frequently isolated fungus (55–65%), followed by *C. parapsilosis* (13–33%).

Other species, such as *C. glabrata* and *C. tropicalis*, were more anecdotic (3–7% and 2–4%, respectively). Smaller series have found similar results [13,14], and in a recent review of the literature, *C. albicans* (47.3%) was the most frequent strain isolated, followed by *C. parapsilosis* (22.3%) [15], but epidemiology may still vary among regions.

3. Pathogenesis and Risk Factors

Colonization by *Candida* spp. is regarded as the first step for subsequent infection [16], and *Candida* spp. are common commensals of the human skin and gut microbiota in healthy individuals [17–19]. Invasive disease, which encompasses both candidemia and deep-seated infections, usually results from an abnormal or increased number of fungi combined with alterations in the cutaneous and mucosal barriers due to weakening of host immunity [16,17], which permits the transition from *Candida* sp. commensalism to opportunism. Three possible routes of CPJI development have been described: (1) the hematogenous route from an infected catheter or a urinary or intraabdominal source; (2) direct inoculation during prosthesis implantation, revision surgery, or even after arthrocentesis, especially in colonized patients; and (3) extension into synovial fluid from contiguous infected tissues.

Candida spp. have specific properties allowing them to adhere to surfaces and form biofilms, especially on prosthetic devices, which permits the development of persister cells, facilitating antifungal resistance, and explains treatment failure when the implant is not removed. In vitro experiments have shown that *C. albicans* biofilm formation begins with the adherence of yeast to a substrate and thereafter yeast cells proliferate across the surface and produce filamentous forms, including hyphae and pseudohyphae. As the biofilm matures, an extracellular matrix accumulates, facilitating antifungal resistance, notably to azoles and polyenes, through different mechanisms [20], which may explain the high failure rates in CPJI when the implant is not removed. Finally, non-adherent yeast cells are released from the biofilm into the surrounding medium (the dispersal step). *C. albicans*, the most frequent causative agent of CPJI, has been reported to form larger and more complex biofilms than other *Candida* species [21].

All parts of the immune system are involved in the response to this infection. For example, deficiencies in the T-helper 17 lymphocyte cell line impair the mucosal immune response to *Candida* spp. and facilitate Candida infections. Neutrophil dysfunction or leukopenia also predisposes patients to suffer invasive candidiasis, and complement or immunoglobulin deficiency or alteration is associated with complicated disease as well [17]. The regulatory pathways and mechanisms that govern Candida biofilm development are very complex [20]; gene expression of *C. albicans* is regulated by both a continuous host–pathogen interplay and by distinct genetic mechanisms [19], but this is not the scope of this review.

However, there are other factors that are not only easier to identify than alterations in host immunity but also probably more prevalent in patients with CPJIs and may play a major role in the pathogenesis of invasive candidiasis. The most reported factors are as follows [17]: (1) the long-term or repeated use of broad-spectrum antibiotics, especially in the previous 3 months, which depletes commensal gut bacteria, enabling *Candida* sp. overgrowth. Many antibiotics are known to promote fungal growth and pathogenicity because they disrupt the microbiota and eliminate anaerobic bacteria in the gut which could have otherwise inhibited the fungi, and studies show that the introduction of small amounts of *C. albicans* to mice after antibiotic treatment caused significant changes in the gut microbiota, which may persist in the long term [22]. (2) Breach of the cutaneous and gastrointestinal barriers by chemotherapy, surgery, gastrointestinal perforation, or instrumentation, such as central venous catheters, which may facilitate *Candida* sp. translocation into the bloodstream. (3) Immunosuppression secondary to malignant diseases, immunodeficiencies, or immunosuppressive therapy. Other risk factors reported in patients with CPJIs have been older age [18], diabetes, rheumatoid arthritis, malnutrition, and tuberculosis, which probably also reflect alterations in host immunity [2,12–14,23]. Other series have also identified that multiple previous surgeries at the site of the CPJI are also a risk factor [2,13,23,24]. A recent retrospective case–control study that compared fungal PJIs with bacterial PJIs found that recent antibiotic consumption (OR: 3.4; 95% CI: 1.2–9.3) and prolonged wound drainage (OR: 7.3; 95% CI: 2.02–26.95) were significantly associated with CPJI [13]. In our experience, patients treated with long courses of linezolid for multidrug-resistant chronic bacterial PJIs tend to present mucocutaneous candidiasis, and their colonization may persist for an unknown duration, which could also be another risk factor for hip CPJI.

Although it has not been deeply studied, considering the pathogenesis of the disease, previous *Candida* spp. colonization in the urine or *Candida* intertrigo may also be risk factors in patients undergoing hip arthroplasty [2,13]. In a multicenter retrospective study of patients with CPJIs, we found 14% of patients with *Candida* intertrigo and 9% of patients with a previous urinary tract infection (three with positive blood cultures) caused by the same *Candida* spp. before the diagnosis of CPJI [2].

4. Clinical Manifestations and Diagnosis

CPJIs are usually chronic infections characterized by pain, swelling, and sinus tracts. Implant loosening may be observed on radiography in nearly 50% of cases, as previously reported in some studies [2,25]. In fact, the median duration from the index surgery and the diagnosis of CPJI averaged 17–25 months [12,13]. Blood tests could show no leukocytosis, and the C-reactive protein (CRP) level and erythrocyte sedimentation rate are usually normal or mildly elevated [2,12]. The same recently published study comparing patients with CPJIs with those with bacterial PJIs showed that patients with CPJIs had lower median CRP values (2.95 mg/dL vs. 5.99 mg/dL) and lower synovial fluid leukocyte levels (13,953 cells/mm^3 vs. 33,198 cell/mm^3) [13].

The criteria to diagnose CPJI are not well established, and the same criteria used in diagnosing bacterial PJIs may not be reliable in some cases. The Infectious Diseases Society of America (IDSA) guidelines [3], a previous International Consensus on PJIs [6], and a recent European Bone and Joint Infection Society (EBJIS) consensus [26] consider two or more intraoperative cultures or the combination of preoperative aspiration and intraoperative cultures yielding the same organism definitive evidence of a PJI [3]. However, when reviewing published series of CPJI cases, the microbiological criteria changed from one study to another. Some authors consider that one positive preoperative aspiration culture and/or a positive intraoperative culture is sufficient [9], while others require two positive cultures [2,13] or one positive culture with additional criteria for PJIs [2,24]. In our opinion, when *Candida* spp. are found in only one intraoperative culture, the case should be evaluated carefully, and treating the Candida etiology should be considered, especially in patients with other risk factors for CPJI such as previous antibiotic therapy or multiple previous surgeries (Figure 1). In fact, even if another microorganism is isolated in two or more cultures, polymicrobial infection is not infrequent, particularly in the hip location, being found in 16% to 26% of cases, depending on the series [2,12], and this should not be a criterion for discarding the value of one positive culture for *Candida* spp.

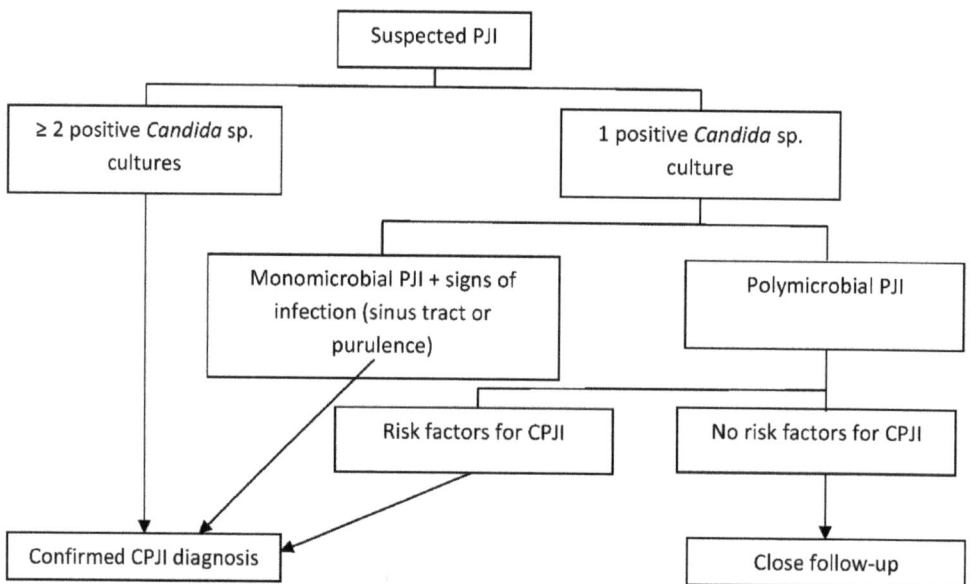

Figure 1. Diagnosis of Candida periprosthetic joint infection.

5. Medical and Surgical Treatment

International guidelines on candidiasis and PJIs [5,7] recommend, with limited evidence, the combination of prosthesis removal and reimplantation in two stages. They recommend a prolonged period of antifungal therapy for at least 12 weeks after resection arthroplasty and at least 6 weeks after prosthesis implantation, without specifying the best antifungal option [5]. They state that the use of antifungal agent-loaded cement spacers is controversial.

The fact that *Candida* spp. grow and form biofilms on medical devices makes these microorganisms highly resistant to antifungal agents and the host immune system [27–30]. Therefore, the best surgical approach is to remove the prosthetic material to avoid the problem of antifungals penetrating and acting within the biofilm. In this sense, a two-stage exchange arthroplasty strategy is probably the best option when feasible to eradicate the infection and to preserve joint function [15], with variable success rates from 14% to almost 100% depending on the series and on the definition of success [2,12,14,23–25,31–35]. In patients with reduced mobility, particularly old patients with multiple previous surgeries in the same location, a resection arthroplasty may be the best alternative. There is less evidence of success with a one-stage exchange arthroplasty strategy, which has been reported in only a few cases [15,36,37]. In a recent review of the literature of 76 episodes of CPJI, one-stage exchange arthroplasty was performed only in three patients with a favorable outcome [15], but in another series of 11 CPJI episodes, it was performed in four with success in two [14]. However, due to the publication bias, the small amount of experience and the difficulty of curing this type of infection, with a high rate of relapses, in our opinion, this procedure should be used only in very selected cases. Irrigation and debridement with prosthesis retention usually fails to cure the infection (cure rates from 0% to 20%), especially in cases of chronic infection [2,12,23,32,35]. Table 1 summarizes the type of treatment, the duration of follow-up and the outcome of the larger case series (number of patients ≥ 10) of CPJI.

Table 1. Treatment, follow-up, and outcome of the largest series (number of patients ≥ 10) of Candida periprosthetic joint infection.

Study (Year)	Number of Patients (n)	Surgical Treatment (n)	Antifungal Treatment (n)	Antifungal-Loaded Cement Spacers (n)	Follow-Up	Outcome (n)
Saconi et al. (2020) [14]	11	Resection arthroplasty 6	Fluconazol 6	No	Range 5.6–74 months	Remission 5 Lost to follow-up 1
		One-stage exchange 4	Fluconazol 2 Itraconazol 1 Micafungin 1	No	Range 2.1–84 months	Remission 2 Failure 1 Lost to follow-up 1
		Two-stage exchange 1	Voriconazol, itraconazol 1	No	48 months	Remission 1
Escola-Vergé et al. (2018) [2]	35	Prosthesis removal 20	Azoles 13 Antibiofilm-containing regimen * 6 No antifungal 1	Amphotericin B 3	24 months	Remission 13 Failure 7
		Debridement with prosthesis retention 15	Azoles 10 Antibiofilm-containing regimen * 5	No	24 months	Remission 4 Failure 11
Brown et al. (2018) [24]	25	Two-stage exchange 11		Amphotericin B 10		Remission 5 Failure 6
		Debridement with prosthesis retention 5		No		Failure 5
		Resection arthroplasty 5	Fluconazol 25	No	Not reported	Remission 2 Failure 3
		Prosthesis retention and suppressive therapy 3		No		Remission 3
		One-stage exchange 1		No		Remission 1
Gao et al. (2018) [35]	14	Two-stage exchange 14	Fluconazol 11 Caspofungin, fluconazol 1 Vorinconazol 1 Amphotericin B, caspofungin, fluconazol, voriconazol 1	Amphotericin B 3 Voriconazol 2 Fluconazol 2	Mean 65.1 months Range 25–129 months	Remission 10 Failure 4
Ueng et al. (2013) [31]	16	Two-stage exchange 9	Fluconazol 9	Amphotericin B 5	Mean 41 months Range 28–90 months	Remission 8 Failure 1
		Resection arthroplasty 7	Fluconazol 7	Amphotericin B 1		Remission 4 Failure 3

Table 1. *Cont.*

Study (Year)	Number of Patients (n)	Surgical Treatment (n)	Antifungal Treatment (n)	Antifungal-Loaded Cement Spacers (n)	Follow-Up	Outcome (n)
Hwang et al. (2012) [32]	28	Two-stage exchange 24	Amphotericin B 21 Amphotericin B, fluconazol 3	No	Mean 4.3 years Range 2.6–6.1 years	Remission 22 Failure 2
		Debridement with prosthesis retention 4	Fluconazol 4	No		Failure 4
García-Oltra et al. (2011) [23]	10	Two-stage exchange 7	Fluconazol 5 Anidulafungin, fluconazol 1 Caspofungin, fluconazol 1	No	Mean 31 months Range 2–67 months	Failure 7
		Debridement with prosthesis retention 3	Fluconazol 3	No		Failure 3
Azzam et al. (2009) [12]	31	Two-stage exchange 19	Fluconazol 23 Caspofungin, fluconazol 3 Amphotericin B 5	Amphotericin B 5	Mean 45 months Range from 24 months to 11 years	Remission 9 Failure 10
		Resection arthroplasty 10 (5 with previous debridement failure)				Remission 6 Failure 4
		Debridement with prosthesis retention 7		No		Failure 7

* Antibiofilm-containing regimen: amphotericin B or an echinocandin.

Fluconazole is active against most CPJI isolates, and it shows good penetration into synovial fluid and less toxicity than amphotericin B, but its activity against *Candida* sp. biofilms is limited. However, the antifungals that have demonstrated better activity against biofilms are echinocandins and liposomal formulations of amphotericin B [27–29,38]. In the absence of clear recommendations for systemic antifungal treatment, the most frequently used antifungals have been fluconazole followed by amphotericin B in older series and [15] by echinocandins in recent series [2], with different outcomes, especially in relation to the type of surgical approach (Table 1). However, due to the rarity of this infection, there will probably not be randomized clinical trials regarding the best antifungal treatment. In our retrospective multicenter study, we found better results when amphotericin B or echinocandins rather than fluconazole were combined with implant removal [2], with remission rates higher than 80% vs. 62%, similar to values reported in previous studies [32,39]. Therefore, we would recommend the use of an antifungal with antibiofilm activity, amphotericin B or an echinocandin, after resection arthroplasty and after prosthesis implantation, following our proposed diagram of treatment in Figure 2.

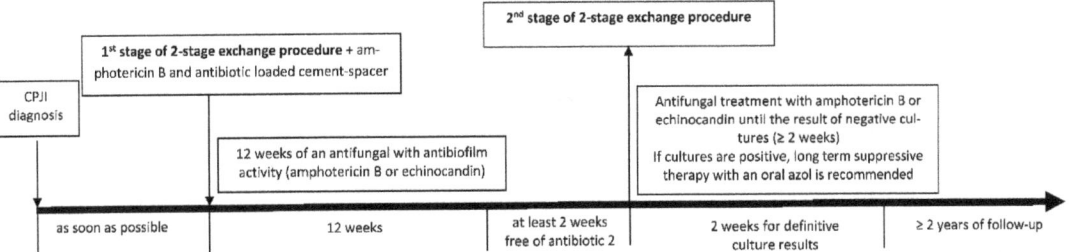

Figure 2. Our proposal for optimal treatment of Candida periprosthetic joint infection.

On the other hand, few studies have evaluated the efficacy of using an antifungal agent-loaded cement spacer in staged exchange arthroplasty for CPJI, so the indication to use it remains controversial. Moreover, there is no consensus on which antifungal agent should be used and at what dose to achieve the optimal balance between cement stability and drug elution. There have been some cases in which amphotericin B deoxycholate or an azole (mainly fluconazole or voriconazole) was mixed with the cement in the spacer [2,15,35,40–42], with different outcomes. In our clinical practice, amphotericin B (200 mg of amphotericin B deoxycholate for every 40 g of bone cement) is often used because of its broad antifungal spectrum and antibiofilm activity, its heat stability, and its availability in powder form. However, amphotericin B has been proven to behave differently than water-soluble antibacterial agents [43,44], and it is not clear whether the local dose is sufficiently high to elute from cement spacers [27,39,42–44] or whether it is toxic to osteoblasts [45]. An in vitro study found that the elution of 800 mg of liposomal amphotericin B was higher than that of the same dose of deoxycholate amphotericin B when mixed with acrylic bone cement, although it was associated with a loss of compressive strength [46]. In addition, some authors and ourselves have concerns about using only antifungal agents in cement spacers, and we prefer to combine amphotericin B with vancomycin plus gentamycin to avoid bacterial superinfections [15]. Until more evidence is available, we believe that using antifungal agent-loaded cement spacers (preferably with amphotericin B and combined with antibacterial agents) in staged exchange arthroplasty seems reasonable to avoid relapses secondary to fungi that may remain adhered to the bone and cement spacer.

Another unsolved issue is the duration of antifungal treatment. Although short antifungal courses (6 weeks) were successful in a small series when using a staged exchange procedure [33], the median duration of antifungal treatment in larger studies was 3 months [2,12,25,34], consistent with IDSA guideline recommendations [5]. In our opinion, at least 3 months of antifungal treatment are necessary, especially with a drug with antibiofilm activity (an echinocandin or amphotericin B) and combined with implant removal whenever possible, preferably in the form of a two-stage exchange procedure to maintain joint functionality (Figure 2). In patients with high surgical risk for whom prostheses cannot be removed, suppressive therapy with azoles may be an alternative treatment to maintain joint functionality [2].

6. Prognosis and Prevention

The prognosis of patients with CPJIs varies depending on the medical and surgical approach. Often, aggressive surgical treatment is dismissed due to the patient's comorbidities, and resection arthroplasty or amputation is performed, resulting in poor patient functionality, but at least curing the infection. On the other hand, even if performing the best strategy (a two-stage exchange), some patients may persist with the infection or relapse. A recent study found that the main risk factors for two-stage exchange failure are hemodialysis, obesity, multiple previous procedures, diabetes, corticosteroid therapy, hypoalbuminemia, immunosuppression, rheumatological diseases, coagulation disorders, and infection due to multidrug-resistant bacteria or fungal species [47]. Therefore, if some of these risk factors coexist in a patient with CPJI, a resection arthroplasty, agreed with the patient, may be the best alternative to cure the infection even if it implies loosing functionality. Unfortunately, we have no score of risk that helps us in making the best decision. In addition, due to the formation of biofilms by Candida spp., CPJIs, when treated, may take several months or even years to relapse. Patient follow-up varies among some studies, and this makes it difficult to establish when CPJI can be considered cured. In our personal experience, due to the chronic nature of CPJI, follow-up periods shorter than 2 years may not be able to detect some relapses.

As histories of previous antibiotic therapy or surgery are not modifiable, we believe that searching for and treating Candida intertrigo in patients with risk factors for CPJI would be a reasonable, cost-effective measure [2,13]. Therefore, although there is no strong evidence to support this hypothesis, we believe that patients with previous Candida infection or clinical Candida colonization may benefit from the addition of fluconazole to standard prophylaxis before hip arthroplasty. Another more debatable measure would be including fluconazole in surgical prophylaxis for patients with an advanced age, diabetes, a long course of antibiotic therapy in the previous months (especially if it was with linezolid) and multiple previous orthopedic surgeries. As these factors may be difficult to evaluate retrospectively, prospective multicenter studies are needed.

Given the poor prognosis of this type of infection, until more evidence is available regarding the best antifungal treatment, the duration of treatment, and the efficacy of using antifungal agent-loaded cement spacers, focusing on CPJI prevention remains essential.

Author Contributions: L.E.-V. and C.P. contributed to the conception, methodology, writing of the original draft, and writing of the review and editing with the assistance of a medical writer. D.R.-P. and P.S.C. contributed to the review and editing of the manuscript. All authors have read and agreed to the published version of the manuscript.

Funding: This research did not receive any specific grant from funding agencies in the public, commercial, or not-for-profit sectors.

Conflicts of Interest: The authors declare no conflict of interest.

Abbreviations

PJI	periprosthetic joint infection
CPJI	Candida periprosthetic joint infection

References

1. Tande, A.J.; Patel, R. Prosthetic Joint Infection. *Clin. Microbiol. Rev.* **2014**, *27*, 302–345. [CrossRef] [PubMed]
2. Escolà-Vergé, L.; Rodríguez-Pardo, D.; Lora-Tamayo, J.; Morata, L.; Murillo, O.; Vilchez, H.; Sorli, L.; Carrión, L.G.; Barbero, J.M.; Palomino-Nicás, J.; et al. Candida Periprosthetic Joint Infection: A Rare and Difficult-to-Treat Infection. *J. Infect.* **2018**, *77*, 151–157. [CrossRef]
3. Osmon, D.R.; Berbari, E.F.; Berendt, A.R.; Lew, D.; Zimmerli, W.; Steckelberg, J.M.; Rao, N.; Hanssen, A.; Wilson, W.R. Diagnosis and Management of Prosthetic Joint Infection: Clinical Practice Guidelines by the Infectious Diseases Society of America. *Clin. Infect. Dis.* **2013**, *56*, e1–e25. [CrossRef] [PubMed]
4. Ariza, J.; Cobo, J.; Baraia-Etxaburu, J.; Benito, N.; Bori, G.; Cabo, J.; Corona, P.; Esteban, J.; Horcajada, J.P.; Lora-Tamayo, J.; et al. Executive Summary of Management of Prosthetic Joint Infections. Clinical Practice Guidelines by the Spanish Society of Infectious Diseases and Clinical Microbiology (SEIMC). *Enferm. Infect. Microbiol. Clin.* **2017**, *35*, 189–195. [CrossRef]
5. Pappas, P.G.; Kauffman, C.A.; Andes, D.R.; Clancy, C.J.; Marr, K.A.; Ostrosky-Zeichner, L.; Reboli, A.C.; Schuster, M.G.; Vazquez, J.A.; Walsh, T.J.; et al. Clinical Practice Guideline for the Management of Candidiasis: 2016 Update by the Infectious Diseases Society of America. *Clin. Infect. Dis.* **2015**, civ933. [CrossRef]
6. Parvizi, J.; Gehrke, T.; Chen, A.F. Proceedings of the International Consensus on Periprosthetic Joint Infection. *Bone Jt. J.* **2013**, *95*, 1450–1452. [CrossRef]
7. Belden, K.; Cao, L.; Chen, J.; Deng, T.; Fu, J.; Guan, H.; Jia, C.; Kong, X.; Kuo, F.-C.; Li, R.; et al. Hip and Knee Section, Fungal Periprosthetic Joint Infection, Diagnosis and Treatment: Proceedings of International Consensus on Orthopedic Infections. *J. Arthroplast.* **2019**, *34*, S387–S391. [CrossRef]
8. Benito, N.; Mur, I.; Ribera, A.; Soriano, A.; Rodríguez-Pardo, D.; Sorlí, L.; Cobo, J.; Fernández-Sampedro, M.; del Toro, M.; Guío, L.; et al. The Different Microbial Etiology of Prosthetic Joint Infections According to Route of Acquisition and Time after Prosthesis Implantation, Including the Role of Multidrug-Resistant Organisms. *J. Clin. Med.* **2019**, *8*, 673. [CrossRef]
9. Benito, N.; Franco, M.; Ribera, A.; Soriano, A.; Rodriguez-Pardo, D.; Sorlí, L.; Fresco, G.; Fernández-Sampedro, M.; Dolores Del Toro, M.; Guío, L.; et al. Time Trends in the Aetiology of Prosthetic Joint Infections: A Multicentre Cohort Study. *Clin. Microbiol. Infect.* **2016**, *22*, 732.e1–732.e8. [CrossRef]
10. Peel, T.N.; Cheng, A.C.; Buising, K.L.; Choong, P.F.M. Microbiological Aetiology, Epidemiology, and Clinical Profile of Prosthetic Joint Infections: Are Current Antibiotic Prophylaxis Guidelines Effective? *Antimicrob. Agents Chemother.* **2012**, *56*, 2386–2391. [CrossRef] [PubMed]
11. Aggarwal, V.K.; Bakhshi, H.; Ecker, N.U.; Parvizi, J.; Gehrke, T.; Kendoff, D. Organism Profile in Periprosthetic Joint Infection: Pathogens Differ at Two Arthroplasty Infection Referral Centers in Europe and in the United States. *J. Knee Surg.* **2014**, *27*, 399–406. [CrossRef]
12. Azzam, K.; Parvizi, J.; Jungkind, D.; Hanssen, A.; Fehring, T.; Springer, B.; Bozic, K.; Della Valle, C.; Pulido, L.; Barrack, R. Microbiological, Clinical, and Surgical Features of Fungal Prosthetic Joint Infections: A Multi-Institutional Experience. *J. Bone Jt. Surg. Am. Vol.* **2009**, *91*, 142–149. [CrossRef] [PubMed]
13. Riaz, T.; Tande, A.J.; Steed, L.L.; Demos, H.A.; Salgado, C.D.; Osmon, D.R.; Marculescu, C.E. Risk Factors for Fungal Prosthetic Joint Infection. *J. Bone Jt. Infect.* **2020**, *5*, 76–81. [CrossRef] [PubMed]
14. Saconi, E.S.; de Carvalho, V.C. Prosthetic Joint Infection Due to Candida Species. *Medicine* **2020**, *99*, e19735. [CrossRef] [PubMed]
15. Cobo, F.; Rodríguez-Granger, J.; Sampedro, A.; Aliaga-Martínez, L.; Navarro-Marí, J.M. Candida Prosthetic Joint Infection. A Review of Treatment Methods. *J. Bone Jt. Infect.* **2017**, *2*, 114–121. [CrossRef]
16. Pappas, P.G.; Lionakis, M.S.; Arendrup, M.C.; Ostrosky-Zeichner, L.; Kullberg, B.J. Invasive Candidiasis. *Nat. Rev. Dis. Primers* **2018**, *4*, 18026. [CrossRef] [PubMed]
17. McCarty, T.P.; Pappas, P.G. Invasive Candidiasis. *Infect. Dis. Clin. N. Am.* **2016**, *30*, 103–124. [CrossRef] [PubMed]
18. Kullberg, B.J.; Arendrup, M.C. Invasive Candidiasis. *N. Engl. J. Med.* **2015**, *373*, 1445–1456. [CrossRef]
19. Hube, B. From Commensal to Pathogen: Stage- and Tissue-Specific Gene Expression of *Candida albicans*. *Curr. Opin. Microbiol.* **2004**, *7*, 336–341. [CrossRef]
20. Finkel, J.S.; Mitchell, A.P. Genetic Control of *Candida albicans* Biofilm Development. *Nat. Rev. Microbiol.* **2011**, *9*, 109–118. [CrossRef]
21. Kuhn, D.M. Comparison of Biofilms Formed by Candidaalbicans and Candidaparapsilosis on Bioprosthetic Surfaces. *Infect. Immun.* **2002**, *70*, 878–888. [CrossRef] [PubMed]
22. Sam, Q.; Chang, M.; Chai, L. The Fungal Mycobiome and Its Interaction with Gut Bacteria in the Host. *Int. J. Mol. Sci.* **2017**, *18*, 330. [CrossRef] [PubMed]
23. García-Oltra, E.; García-Ramiro, S.; Martínez, J.C.; Tibau, R.; Bori, G.; Bosch, J.; Mensa, J.; Soriano, A. Prosthetic joint infection by *Candida* spp. *Rev. Esp. Quimioter.* **2011**, *24*, 37–41. [PubMed]
24. Brown, T.S.; Petis, S.M.; Osmon, D.R.; Mabry, T.M.; Berry, D.J.; Hanssen, A.D.; Abdel, M.P. Periprosthetic Joint Infection With Fungal Pathogens. *J. Arthroplast.* **2018**, *33*, 2605–2612. [CrossRef]
25. Kuiper, J.W.; van den Bekerom, M.P.; van der Stappen, J.; Nolte, P.A.; Colen, S. 2-Stage Revision Recommended for Treatment of Fungal Hip and Knee Prosthetic Joint Infections: An Analysis of 164 Patients, 156 from the Literature and 8 Own Cases. *Acta Orthop.* **2013**, *84*, 517–523. [CrossRef]

26. McNally, M.; Sousa, R.; Wouthuyzen-Bakker, M.; Chen, A.F.; Soriano, A.; Vogely, H.C.; Clauss, M.; Higuera, C.A.; Trebše, R. The EBJIS Definition of Periprosthetic Joint Infection: A Practical Guide for Clinicians. *Bone Jt. J.* **2021**, *103*, 18–25. [CrossRef]
27. Kuhn, D.M.; George, T.; Chandra, J.; Mukherjee, P.K.; Ghannoum, M.A. Antifungal Susceptibility of Candida Biofilms: Unique Efficacy of Amphotericin B Lipid Formulations and Echinocandins. *Antimicrob. Agents Chemother.* **2002**, *46*, 1773–1780. [CrossRef]
28. Nett, J.E. Future Directions for Anti-Biofilm Therapeutics Targeting *Candida*. *Expert Rev. Anti Infect. Ther.* **2014**, *12*, 375–382. [CrossRef]
29. Iñigo, M.; Pemán, J.; Del Pozo, J.L. Antifungal Activity against Candida Biofilms. *Int. J. Artif. Organs* **2012**, *35*, 780–791. [CrossRef]
30. Mukherjee, P.K.; Chandra, J. Candida Biofilms: Development, Architecture, and Resistance. *Microbiol. Spectrum.* **2015**, *3*. [CrossRef]
31. Ueng, S.W.N.; Lee, C.-Y.; Hu, C.; Hsieh, P.-H.; Chang, Y. What Is the Success of Treatment of Hip and Knee Candidal Periprosthetic Joint Infection? *Clin. Orthop. Relat. Res.* **2013**, *471*, 3002–3009. [CrossRef]
32. Hwang, B.H.; Yoon, J.Y.; Nam, C.H.; Jung, K.A.; Lee, S.C.; Han, C.D.; Moon, S.H. Fungal Peri-Prosthetic Joint Infection after Primary Total Knee Replacement. *J. Bone Jt. Surg. Br.* **2012**, *94*, 656–659. [CrossRef] [PubMed]
33. Anagnostakos, K.; Kelm, J.; Schmitt, E.; Jung, J. Fungal Periprosthetic Hip and Knee Joint Infections. *J. Arthroplast.* **2012**, *27*, 293–298. [CrossRef] [PubMed]
34. Phelan, D.M.; Osmon, D.R.; Keating, M.R.; Hanssen, A.D. Delayed Reimplantation Arthroplasty for Candidal Prosthetic Joint Infection: A Report of 4 Cases and Review of the Literature. *Clin. Infect. Dis.* **2002**, *34*, 930–938. [CrossRef] [PubMed]
35. Gao, Z.; Li, X.; Du, Y.; Peng, Y.; Wu, W.; Zhou, Y. Success Rate of Fungal Peri-Prosthetic Joint Infection Treated by 2-Stage Revision and Potential Risk Factors of Treatment Failure: A Retrospective Study. *Med. Sci. Monit.* **2018**, *24*, 5549–5557. [CrossRef] [PubMed]
36. Selmon, G.P.F.; Slater, R.N.S.; Shepperd, J.N.; Wright, E.P. Successful 1-Stage Exchange Total Knee Arthroplasty for Fungal Infection. *J. Arthroplast.* **1998**, *13*, 114–115. [CrossRef]
37. Klatte, T.O.; Kendoff, D.; Kamath, A.F.; Jonen, V.; Rueger, J.M.; Frommelt, L.; Gebauer, M.; Gehrke, T. Single-Stage Revision for Fungal Peri-Prosthetic Joint Infection: A Single-Centre Experience. *Bone Jt. J.* **2014**, *96-B*, 492–496. [CrossRef]
38. Katragkou, A.; Chatzimoschou, A.; Simitsopoulou, M.; Dalakiouridou, M.; Diza-Mataftsi, E.; Tsantali, C.; Roilides, E. Differential Activities of Newer Antifungal Agents against Candida Albicans and Candida Parapsilosis Biofilms. *Antimicrob. Agents Chemother.* **2008**, *52*, 357–360. [CrossRef]
39. Schoof, B.; Jakobs, O.; Schmidl, S.; Klatte, T.O.; Frommelt, L.; Gehrke, T.; Gebauer, M. Fungal Periprosthetic Joint Infection of the Hip: A Systematic Review. *Orthop. Rev.* **2015**, *7*. [CrossRef]
40. Bruce, A.S.W.; Kerry, R.M.; Norman, P.; Stockley, I. Fluconazole-Impregnated Beads in the Management of Fungal Infection of Prosthetic Joints. *J. Bone Jt. Surg. Br. Vol.* **2001**, *83*, 183–184. [CrossRef]
41. Deelstra, J.J.; Neut, D.; Jutte, P.C. Successful Treatment of Candida Albicans–Infected Total Hip Prosthesis with Staged Procedure Using an Antifungal-Loaded Cement Spacer. *J. Arthroplast.* **2013**, *28*, 374.e5–374.e8. [CrossRef] [PubMed]
42. Marra, F.; Robbins, G.M.; Masri, B.A.; Duncan, C.; Wasan, K.M.; Kwong, E.H.; Jewesson, P.J. Amphotericin B-Loaded Bone Cement to Treat Osteomyelitis Caused by *Candida albicans*. *Can. J. Surg.* **2001**, *44*, 383.
43. Goss, B.; Lutton, C.; Weinrauch, P.; Jabur, M.; Gillett, G.; Crawford, R. Elution and Mechanical Properties of Antifungal Bone Cement. *J. Arthroplast.* **2007**, *22*, 902–908. [CrossRef]
44. Kweon, C.; McLaren, A.C.; Leon, C.; McLemore, R. Amphotericin B Delivery From Bone Cement Increases With Porosity but Strength Decreases. *Clin. Orthop. Relat. Res.* **2011**, *469*, 3002–3007. [CrossRef] [PubMed]
45. Harmsen, S.; McLaren, A.C.; Pauken, C.; McLemore, R. Amphotericin B Is Cytotoxic at Locally Delivered Concentrations. *Clin. Orthop. Relat. Res.* **2011**, *469*, 3016–3021. [CrossRef] [PubMed]
46. Cunningham, B.; McLaren, A.C.; Pauken, C.; McLemore, R. Liposomal Formulation Increases Local Delivery of Amphotericin from Bone Cement: A Pilot Study. *Clin. Orthop. Relat. Res.* **2012**, *470*, 2671–2676. [CrossRef]
47. Fagotti, L.; Tatka, J.; Salles, M.J.C.; Queiroz, M.C. Risk Factors and Treatment Options for Failure of a Two-Stage Exchange. *Curr. Rev. Musculoskelet. Med.* **2018**, *11*, 420–427. [CrossRef] [PubMed]

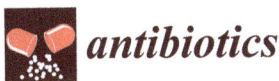

Article

A New Antifungal-Loaded Sol-Gel Can Prevent *Candida albicans* Prosthetic Joint Infection

Hugo Garlito-Díaz [1,2], Jaime Esteban [3,*], Aranzazu Mediero [4], Rafael Alfredo Carias-Cálix [5], Beatriz Toirac [6], Francisca Mulero [7], Víctor Faus-Rodrigo [8], Antonia Jiménez-Morales [6,9], Emilio Calvo [1,2] and John Jairo Aguilera-Correa [3,*]

1. Department of Orthopaedic Surgery, Infanta Elena University Hospital, 28342 Valdemoro, Spain; hugo.garlito@quironsalud.es (H.G.-D.); ecalvo@fjd.es (E.C.)
2. Department of Orthopaedic Surgery, Fundación Jiménez Diaz University Hospital, 28040 Madrid, Spain
3. Department of Clinical Microbiology, IIS-Fundación Jiménez Diaz, UAM, 28040 Madrid, Spain
4. Bone and Joint Research Unit, IIS-Fundación Jiménez Diaz, UAM, 28040 Madrid, Spain; aranzazu.mediero@quironsalud.es
5. Pathology Department, Fundación Jiménez Diaz University Hospital, UAM, 28040 Madrid, Spain; Rafael.carias@quironsalud.es
6. Materials Science and Engineering Department, University Carlos III of Madrid, 28040 Madrid, Spain; btoirac@ing.uc3m.es (B.T.); toni@ing.uc3m.es (A.J.-M.)
7. Molecular Imaging Unit, Spanish National Cancer Research Centre (CNIO), 28040 Madrid, Spain; fmulero@cnio.es
8. Experimental Surgery and Animal Research Service, IIS-Fundación Jiménez Diaz, UAM, 28040 Madrid, Spain; victor.faus@quironsalud.es
9. Álvaro Alonso Barba Technological Institute of Chemistry and Materials, Carlos III University of Madrid, 28040 Madrid, Spain
* Correspondence: jesteban@fjd.es (J.E.); john.aguilera@fjd.es (J.J.A.-C.); Tel.: +34-91-550-4900 (J.E.)

Abstract: Fungal PJI is one of the most feared complications after arthroplasty. Although a rare finding, its high associated morbidity and mortality makes it an important object of study. The most frequent species causing fungal PJI is *C. albicans*. New technology to treat this type of PJI involves organic–inorganic sol-gels loaded with antifungals, as proposed in this study, in which anidulafungin is associated with organophosphates. This study aimed to evaluate the efficacy of an anidulafungin-loaded organic–inorganic sol-gel in preventing prosthetic joint infection (PJI), caused by *Candida albicans* using an in vivo murine model that evaluates many different variables. Fifty percent (3/6) of mice in the *C. albicans*-infected, non-coated, chemical-polished (CP)-implant group had positive culture and 100% of the animals in the *C. albicans*-infected, anidulafungin-loaded, sol-gel coated (CP + A)-implant group had a negative culture (0/6) ($p = 0.023$). Taking the microbiology and pathology results into account, 54.5% (6/11) of *C. albicans*-infected CP-implant mice were diagnosed with a PJI, whilst only 9.1% (1/11) of *C. albicans*-infected CP + A-implant mice were PJI-positive ($p = 0.011$). No differences were observed between the bone mineral content and bone mineral density of noninfected CP and noninfected CP + A ($p = 0.835$, and $p = 0.181$, respectively). No histological or histochemical differences were found in the tissue area occupied by the implant among CP and CP + A. Only 2 of the 6 behavioural variables evaluated exhibited changes during the study: limping and piloerection. In conclusion, the anidulafungin-loaded sol-gel coating showed an excellent antifungal response in vivo and can prevent PJI due to *C. albicans* in this experimental model.

Keywords: sol-gel; anidulafungin; prosthetic joint infection; *Candida albicans*

1. Introduction

Osteoarthritis is one of the most common musculoskeletal diseases worldwide, and is the most well-known cause of disability among elderly people [1]. The social and economic burden of osteoarthritis-related loss of work is also high [2]. Joint replacement is a treatment approach that improves quality of life in many individuals worldwide. Although already used routinely, prosthesis implantation is likely to continue to rise in the coming years [3,4]. The primary cause of device failure is prosthetic joint infection (PJI), a disease involving joint prosthesis and nearby tissue. Advances in the study of the transmission, diagnosis, and treatment of PJI over the last 25 years have led to an improvement in outcomes following this difficult complication. PJI occurs rarely (1–2% of all cases), although its effects are often devastating due to the high associated morbidity and substantial costs [2,5,6]. Additionally, the economic burden of PJI is expected to rise in the coming years with increasing life expectancy and the resulting increase in the number of patients undergoing arthroplasty replacements [7].

The most frequently isolated pathogens from PJI are Gram-positive bacteria, especially *Staphylococcus* species, and Gram-negative microorganisms. Nevertheless, other microorganisms, such as fungi, can also cause PJI, particularly *Candida* species [8–13]. *C. albicans* is the most frequent pathogen isolated, followed by *C. parapsilosis* [10]. Most fungal PJIs present with an insidious, chronic clinical course and are associated with risk factors such as advanced age, previous infection with *Candida*, prior antimicrobial use, multiple surgeries on the joint, immunosuppression, and diabetes [10,14–16]. Despite being a rare infection (<1%), up to a quarter of cases can progress to candidemia, which carries an associated mortality of up to 40% [17]. This type of PJI poses a challenge for clinicians and requires a multidisciplinary approach, including systemic antibiotics, local therapies, and surgery [18–20]. The systemic and prophylactic treatment of PJIs may be ineffective, as antimicrobials are incapable of reaching the prosthesis–tissue interface due to the continued presence of necrotic and/or avascular tissue after surgery [21].

To address this problem, local antibiotic therapy was proposed as an alternative and/or adjuvant to systemic prophylaxis or treatment, preventing systemic toxicity and favouring drug release directly within the implant site [22]. Organic–inorganic sol-gels loaded with antifungals were used in this approach. Recently, the incorporation of organophosphate [tris(trimethylsilyl) phosphite] in this sol-gel, made of two silanes (3-methacryloxypropyl trimethoxysilane and 2-tetramethyl orthosilicate), has been shown to enhance the adhesion of sol-gel on metallic surfaces and increase cell proliferation [23]. Recently, some studies have reported the excellent biosafety and bactericidal capacity of these materials, showing that they completely inhibit the formation of biofilm by *S. epidermidis* in venous catheters without deleterious procoagulant effects in the animal model [24]. Furthermore, new studies show that sol-gel coatings loaded with fluconazole can prevent and locally treat yeast PJI, specifically those caused by the *Candida* species [25].

This study aimed to evaluate the efficacy of an anidulafungin-loaded, organic–inorganic sol-gel in preventing PJI caused by *C. albicans* using an in vivo murine model.

2. Results
2.1. Animal Monitoring

The median weight of the mice over time by group is shown in Figure 1a,b. Only the group of mice infected with *C. albicans* (Cal 35) after the insertion of an anidulafungin-loaded, coated, chemically polished (CP + A) implant showed a significant increase in weight of 44.23 mg per day ($p = 0.0189$). The weight of the remaining groups showed no change over time ($p > 0.05$).

Only two of the six behavioural variables evaluated exhibited changes during the study: limping and piloerection. In the groups with uncoated CP implants, limping decreased significantly over time in both noninfected and Cal35-infected groups ($p = 0.025$, and $p = 0.026$, respectively). The slope of the limping was higher in the Cal35-infected group than in the noninfected one: -0.6694% per day versus -0.5198% per day, respectively (Figure 1c). In both groups of mice with a CP + A implant, limping stayed constant over time ($p > 0.05$) (Figure 1d).

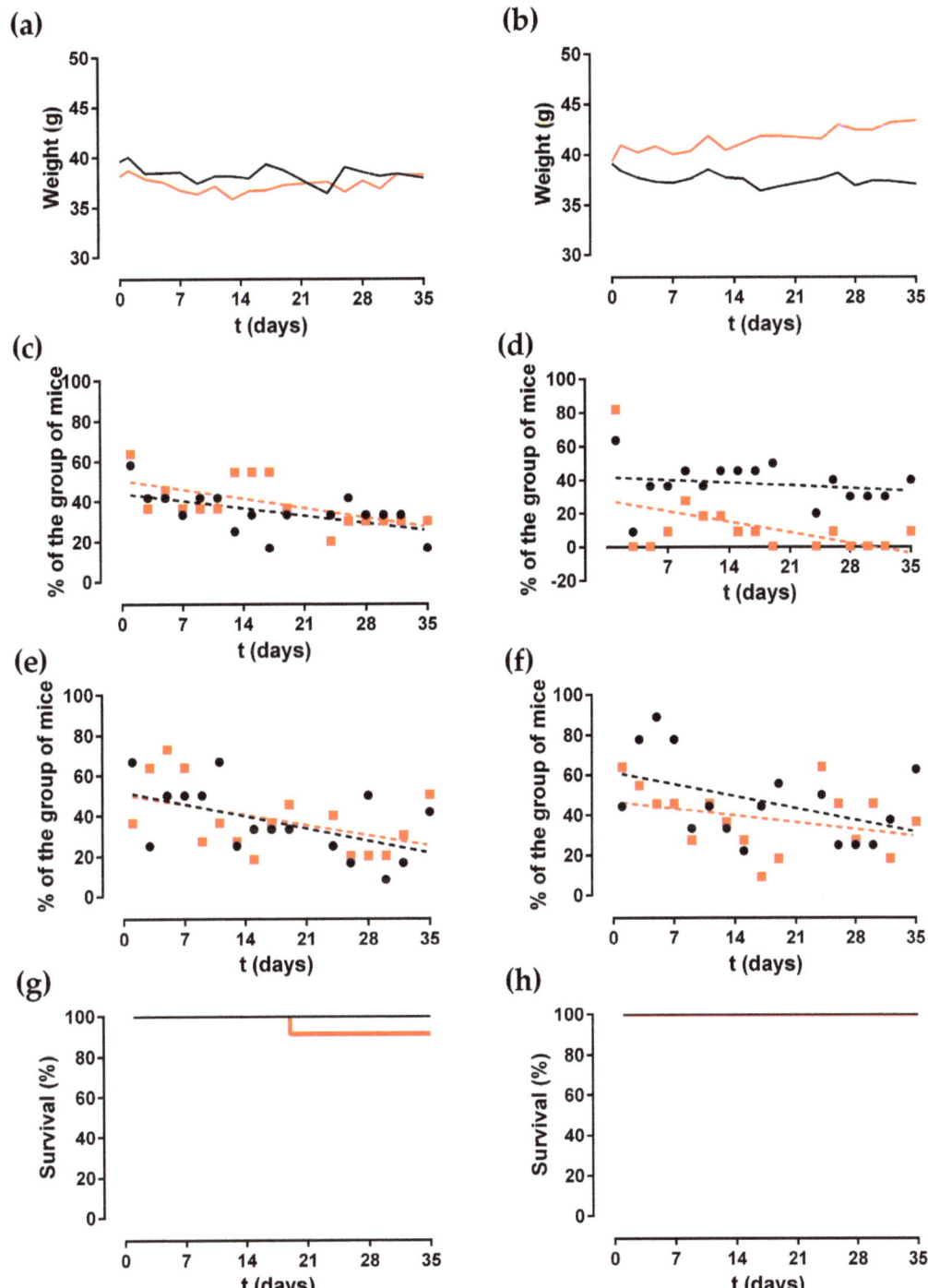

Figure 1. Median weight (**a,b**), limping (**c,d**), piloerection (**e,f**), and survival (**g,h**) in different noninfected groups (black) and in the Cal 35-infected group (red) with insertion of CP (left column) and CP + A implant (right column) over time.

In the groups of animals with CP implants, only the noninfected group showed a significant decrease in piloerection over time ($p = 0.031$), with a slope of -0.8635% per day (Figure 1e). In the mice with an inserted CP + A-implant, piloerection stayed constant over time in both groups (Figure 1f).

Survival was significantly lower in the Cal35-infected group with CP implants than in the noninfected group as of day 19 ($p = 0.002$) (Figure 1g). Only one mouse (9.1%) in the Cal35-infected group with CP implants died of candidemia (Figure 2). Only one mouse in the Cal35-infected group with CP + A implants died because of a Cytomegalovirus infection (Figure 3); for this reason, this mouse was withdrawn from the survival analysis. Taking this into account, no survival differences were detected between CP + A-implants group and Cal35-infected mice with the CP + A-implants group (Figure 1h).

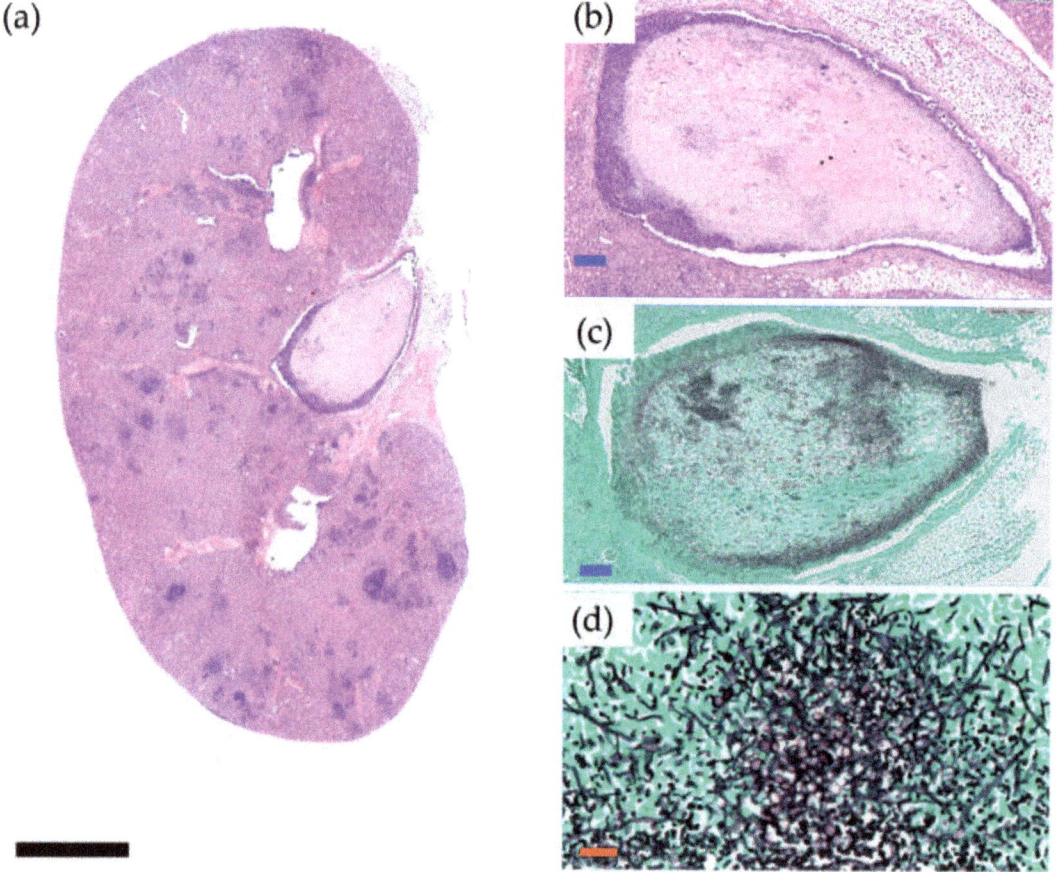

Figure 2. Histological section of the kidney of a mouse belonging to the Cal35-infected CP-implant group that died of candidemia (**a**) and histological sections at higher magnifications in haematoxylin and eosin staining (**b**) and Groccot's stain (**c**,**d**). Black, blue, and red bars represent 2 mm, 50 μm, and 20 μm, respectively.

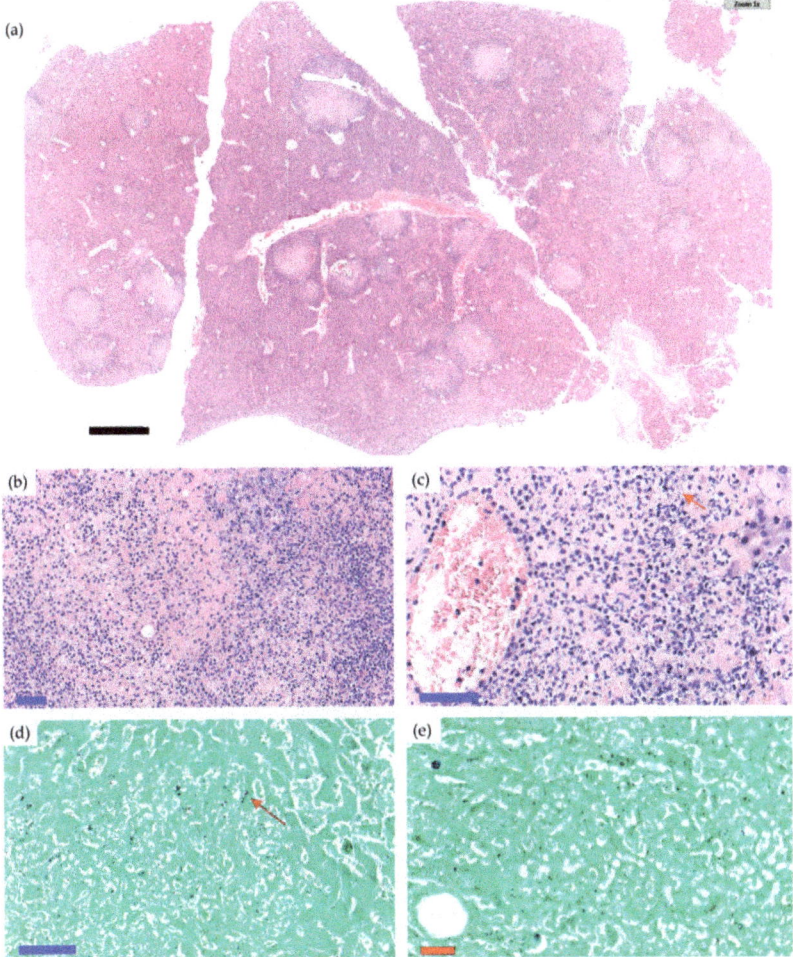

Figure 3. Histological section of the liver of a mouse of the CP Cal35 group that died of CMV infection (**a**) and histological sections with a greater increase in H&E (**b**,**c**) and Groccot's silver stain (**d**,**e**). Black, blue, and red bars represent 2 mm, 50 µm, and 20 µm, respectively. The liver of the animal showed parenchyma with foci of necrosis and a polymorphonuclear-type inflammatory infiltration accompanied by occasional Grocott-positive intracellular inclusions inside some hepatocytes, which was compatible with a cytomegalovirus infection. An acute necrotising inflammatory reaction was detected around the central veins.

2.2. Microbiological and Pathological Results

The femur culture of the noninfected groups was negative for all of mice. Three of the 11 stamps from Cal35-infected CP-implant mice revealed the presence of yeast in the synovial fluid on Gram staining (Figure 4). All of the stamps from the Cal35-infected mice with CP + A-implants were negative. Each Cal-35-infected group composed of 11 mice was divided into two subgroups: six animals were used for microbiological studies and five for pathological studies.

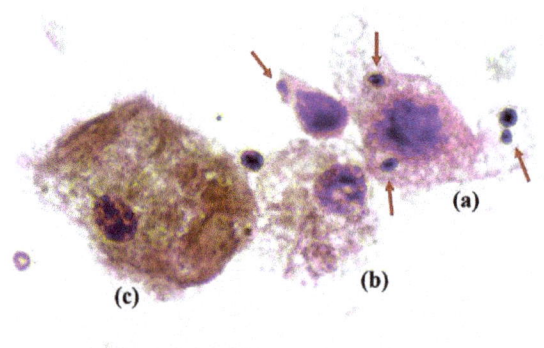

Figure 4. Cytological image of a Gram stain showing a macrophage (a,b) phagocytizing multiple yeasts (red arrows), and a myocyte (c).

Fifty percent (3/6; 95%CI: 0.099–0.900) of mice in the Cal 35-infected group of mice with CP implants had positive culture, whilst 100% of the Cal 35-infected animals with CP + A-implants had a negative culture (0/6) ($p = 0.023$). No statistically significant difference was observed in the quantity of yeast per gram of femur between the 2 Cal35-infected groups ($p = 0.091$) (Figure 5). The mouse that died in the Cal35-infected group with CP implants had granulomas in both kidneys and a concentration of 4.02 $\log_{10}$ (colony-forming units per femur, CFU/femur) on the outside of the operated femur, 5.51 $\log_{10}(CFU/g)$ in the operated femur, 5.47 $\log_{10}(CFU/g)$ in the kidney, and 25.5 CFU/cm^2 of the implant surface. The renal parenchyma showed extensive Grocott-positive fungal involvement accompanied by intense acute polymorphonuclear-type inflammation, which presented a patchy distribution pattern affecting both the renal cortex and medulla and the pyelocaliceal system (Figure 2).

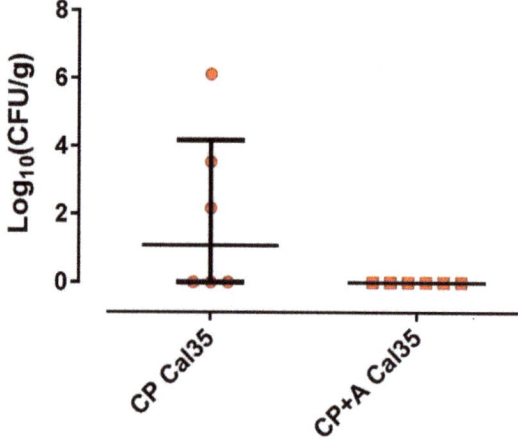

Figure 5. Quantity of yeast per gram of femur from each group of mice.

In the Cal35-infected group with CP implants, acute osteomyelitis was observed in four of the five femurs (Figure 6a); no chronic osteomyelitis was diagnosed, and the presence of yeast was also detected in four of the five femurs on Grocott's silver staining (Figure 6b). In the Cal35-infected group with CP + A-implants, acute osteomyelitis was observed in two of the five femurs (Figure 6c,d), chronic osteomyelitis was diagnosed in two of the five femurs, and presence of yeast was detected in only one of the five femurs following Grocott´s silver staining; the latter also showed the presence of acute osteomyelitis. Only one mouse (9.1%) in the noninfected group of animals with a CP + A-implant died (Figure 3). The deceased mouse from this group showed signs of having had diarrhoea, enteritis, and hepatomegaly. Furthermore, when the operated femur, both kidneys, and a piece of the liver were sent for microbiological study, no growth in aerobic or facultative anaerobic bacteria or fungi was detected.

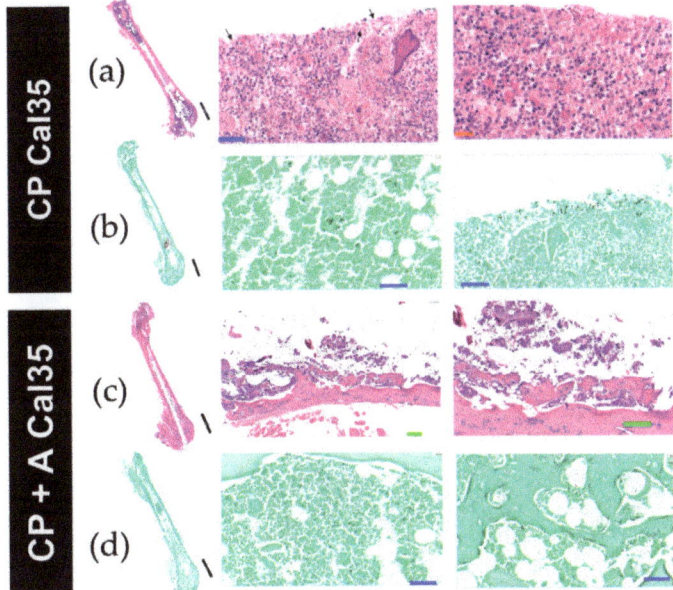

Figure 6. Histological images with H&E stain (**a,c**) and Grocott's stain (**b,d**) of Cal-35–infected mice with implant without CP coating (**a,b**) and mice infected with implant and anidulafungin coating CP + A (**c,d**). The black, green, blue, and red bars represent 2 mm, 200 μm, 50 μm, and 20 μm, respectively.

Taking both the microbiology results and pathology results into account, 54.5% of the Cal35-infected mice with CP implants were diagnosed with a PJI, whilst only 9.1% of the Cal35-infected mice with CP + A-implants were PJI-positive. Therefore, the PJI positivity was significantly higher in the Cal35-infected CP-implant group than in the Cal-35 CP + A-implant group ($p = 0.011$).

The presence of round or ovoid structures accompanied by signs of germination was noteworthy, as was as the presence of other septate structures corresponding to pseudo-hyphae and hyphae, visible with Grocott's stain. No other infectious agents were observed in the samples studied.

2.3. Microcomputed Tomography and Bone Histology

No differences were observed between the bone mineral content (BMC) and bone mineral density (BMD) of the groups of mice with CP- and CP + A-implants ($p = 0.835$, and $p = 0.181$, respectively). The BMD results were perfectly comparable as there were no differences in BMC between the compared groups (Figure 7).

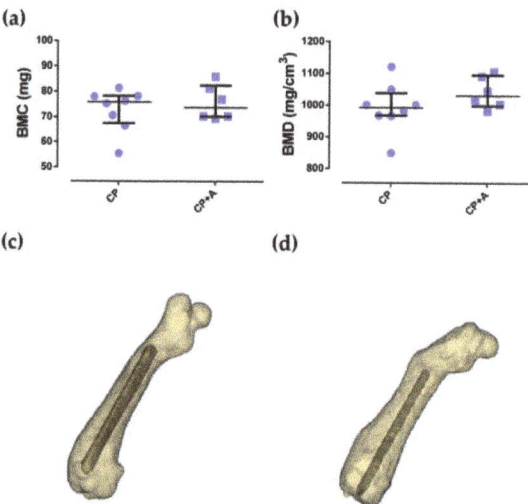

Figure 7. Bone mineral content (BMC) (**a**) and bone mineral density (BMD) (**b**) and their three-dimensional reconstructions of a representative sample of the CP group (**c**) and CP + A group (**d**).

Hematoxilin-eosin staining showed no differences in tissue in the area occupied by the implant among the mice with CP- and CP + A-implants. When bone markers were analysed in the defect area, no changes were observed among the different animals, in alkaline phosphatase (ALP) staining, Cathepsin K or cluster of differentiation 68 (CD68) (Figure 8).

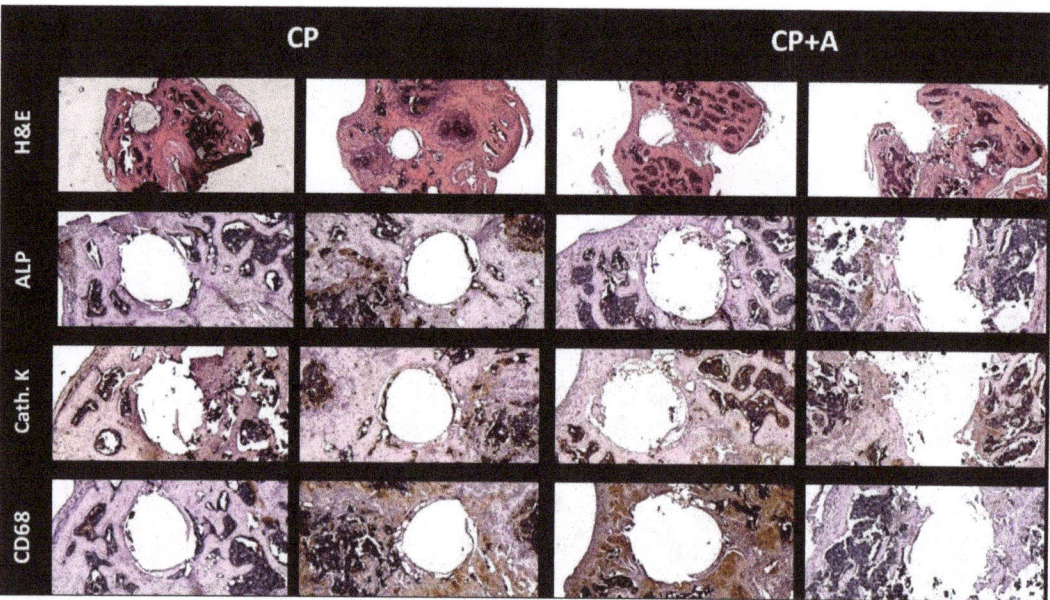

Figure 8. Immunohistochemistry for markers of different bone cells. Long bones were processed and immunohistology staining was carried out. Representative images stained for haematoxylin-eosin (H&E), tartrate-resistant acid phosphatase (TRAP) staining, cathepsin K (cath. K), alkaline phosphatase (ALP), and macrophages (cluster of differentiation 68, CD68). H&E images were taken at 4× magnification. All immunostaining images were taken at 10× magnification.

The viable medullary zones are of a habitual trilinear aspect and were arranged in the peripheral ends of the bone (epiphysis).

3. Discussion

In this study, we demonstrate the in vivo efficacy of anidulafungin-loaded sol-gel to prevent PJI caused by *C. albicans* using a murine model. We describe a novel approach to sol-gel technology applied to Ti materials using anidulafungin to locally prevent the development of yeast biofilms.

The most frequent clinical manifestations of PJI are pain, joint swelling or effusion, erythema or warmth around the joint, fever, drainage, and the presence of a sinus tract connecting to the prosthesis [2]. In our in vivo model, joint pain was evaluated by monitoring mice weight, limping, and piloerection. Weight remained constant over time in all groups, except the Cal35-infected CP + A-implant group, where the mice increased in weight over time. This discrepancy in weight is uncertain, but it could be attributed to the effect of dexamethasone, which has been shown to both increase [26] and reduce mouse weight [27,28]. Moreover, it is known that enrofloxacin does not impede weight gain [29]. Infection seems to decrease limping more significantly, as can be seen in the CP-implant groups. *C. albicans*-caused infections were characterised by a chronic, indolent, and relapsing course [10–12]. This indolent course may be the result of the release of neutrophil extracellular traps (NETs) triggered by farnesol, a crucial quorum-sensing molecule of *C. albicans* [13]. The accumulation of NETs can reduce inflammation through the degeneration of cytokines and chemokines [14]. This could explain why *C. albicans*-infected CP-implant mice stopped limping before the noninfected CP-implant animals. In the CP + A-implant groups, limping decreased faster in *C. albicans*-infected mice compared to noninfected mice. This finding is uncertain but could be attributed to the indolent course provoked by the presence of *C. albicans* on the implant, although these yeasts are not viable. Piloerection did not show a clear difference between noninfected and Cal35-infected mice in non-coated or coated implants over time, contrasting with other bacterial PJI in vivo models [30]. The survival of our animal model varied according to the group. One of 11 mice from the Cal35-infected CP-implant group died as a result of renal "fungus balls" caused by *C. albicans* infection [18,19]. These balls are most likely the result of haematogenous seeding from septic arthritis of the knee joint [20]. This highlights the high mortality associated with candidemia derived from *Candida* bone and joint diseases [21,22,31]. However, these results must be interpreted cautiously, particularly when there is a difference of only one individual. Likewise, one of the 11 mice from the noninfected CP + A-implant group perished due to an acute hepato-digestive infection caused by mouse cytomegalovirus. This virus can be latent in different organs (e.g., liver) in immunocompetent mice, and cause acute infection in immunodeficient ones [32]. Furthermore, this virus can be detected as Grocott-positive intranuclear inclusions in pathological samples [33].

The microbiological and histological results obtained in this study revealed the difficulty of inducing this type of infection despite having used two of the most important pharmacological risk factors, i.e., immunosuppression [34] and broad-spectrum antibiotic therapy [35]. This fact could underline the importance of other risk factors, such as systemic disease, diabetes mellitus, revision arthroplasty, type of prosthesis (monoblock or modular), and type of fixation (uncemented, cemented, hybrid, or with plain or antibiotic-loaded cement) [27–29,31,34]. The most important finding of this work is that anidulafungin-loaded sol-gel coating, when applied to orthopaedic implants, can prevent Candida PJI in an in vivo model. Interestingly, some kind of osteomyelitis was detected in three mice, though no presence of yeast was observed. This finding may be due to both the presence of dead yeast killed by anidulafungin and the inhibition of yeast phagocytosis that dexamethasone therapy exerts on phagocytes [36], thereby explaining the inflammation in absence of yeast proliferation. Our results are consistent with other previously published in vitro studies [25]. Moreover, anidulafungin-loaded coating had a non-harmful effect on bone mineralisation according to the microcomputed tomographic images, and no changes in bone markers were found among groups, thus supporting the results obtained in previous research, based on sol-gel processes [30]. Hence, the fixation of an anidulafungin-loaded sol-gel coated implant is likely to be at least as effective as an uncoated implant.

In recent years, several types of coating have been presented for clinical use: natural, peptide, ceramic, and synthetic coatings [37,38]. Most were designed for osteointegration and antibacterial purposes [30,39–42]. To our knowledge, few studies have developed these coatings to be loaded with antifungals associated with sol-gel technology, as proposed in this work [25]. As fungal PJI prediction is difficult, the use of anidulafungin-loaded sol-gel may be recommended in those patients who have risk factors for developing fungal PJI [35]. This would reduce the personal and healthcare costs associated with this type of infection and its relapses following delayed reimplantation arthroplasty after a follow-up of more than 50 months [43].

However, this study is not exempt from limitations. Firstly, the form of implant infection may have reduced yeast viability on anidulafungin-loaded sol-gel before implantation. No alternative form of infection was possible according to the results obtained in pilot studies (data not shown). Secondly, the results would be more robust with an equal number of samples allocated for microbiological and pathological analyses, although our number of specimens is nearly double that of similar, recently published studies [30]. This unexpected limitation stems from the low infectivity shown by *C. albicans* (approximately 50%), as evidenced in this study. Thirdly, this type of technology can carry other antifungals, e.g., fluconazole [22], which provides it with an antifungal ability against both *C. albicans* and some non-*C. albicans* species, and which should be evaluated using in vivo models for preventive use in some special cases. Fourthly, the death caused by cytomegalovirus suggests that this animal model should be replicated in an Animal Biosafety Level-2 facility, where moderately immunosuppressed animals are less exposed to environmental pathogens.

4. Materials and Methods

4.1. Sol-Gel Synthesis and Coating of Titanium Implants

The Ti-6Al-4V implants were made from 0.6-mm thick Kirschner wires provided by Depuy Synthes (Johnson & Johnson, New Brunswick, NJ, USA). Each wire was cut into implants measuring 1 cm in length. Subsequently, these were chemically polished (CP), as previously described [44], to achieve a surface finish more closely resembling that used in routine clinical practice.

Hybrid organic–inorganic sol-gel coatings composed of a mixture of organopolysyloxanes, including methacryloxypropyltrimethoxy silane (MAPTMS, 98%, Acros Organics, Thermo Fisher Scientific, Waltham, MA, USA) and tetramethyl orthosilane (TMOS, 98%, Acros Organics, Thermo Fisher Scientific, Waltham, MA, USA) and biofunctionalised with tris(trimethylsilyl)phosphite (92%, Sigma-Aldrich, St. Louis, MO, USA) were prepared following a previously published methodology [23]. The coating was loaded with 0.99 mg/mL of anidulafungin (Pfizer, New York, NY, USA) by adding the drug to the aqueous phase during its preparation [22]. Finally, the Ti-6Al-4V implants for the in vivo model were coated by dipping them in anidulafungin and allowing them to dry for at least 1 h at 60 °C (CP + A).

4.2. Animal Surgical Model and Monitoring

We used one clinical strain isolated in the clinical microbiology department of Fundación Jiménez Díaz University Hospital: a strain of *C. albicans* from an 81-year-old woman with infection of a hip prosthesis (Cal35). The antifungal susceptibility profile of Cal35 was obtained by the Vitek 2 AST-YS08 yeast susceptibility test (bioMérieux, Marcy l'Etoile, France). Cal35 was susceptible to all antifungals tested, i.e., amphotericin B (≤ 0.25 µg/mL), caspofungin (≤ 0.25 µg/mL), flucytosine (≤ 1 µg/mL), fluconazole (2 µg/mL), micafungin (≤ 0.06 µg/mL), and voriconazole (≤ 0.12 µg/mL). Surgical intervention of the in vivo model was based on a modified model previously described by Aguilera-Correa et al. [30]. The intervention consisted of placing the implant into the right femur of RjOrl:SWISS

(CD1) mice (Janvier Labs, France) through the knee using an aseptic surgical technique (Figures 9 and 10). Two main modifications were made. Firstly, all mice were premedicated with 4 mg/L of dexamethasone [45] (B.Braun, Melsungen, Germany) and 0.1 mg/L of enrofloxacin (ganadexil 5%, Industrial Veterinaria, S.A.—Invesa, Spain) [46] in sterile drinking water one week before surgery and for the entire duration of the study. Secondly, the implant infection procedure consisted of incubating 1 mL of a 2.00 McFarland standard of Cal-35 strain in saline (B.Braun, Melsungen, Germany) with each implant in a 12-well plate at 37 °C and 5% CO_2 for 120 min. After incubation, each implant was rinsed two times in saline. This form of implant infection aims to adhere the yeast to the surface of the implant, due to the impossibility of injecting planktonic yeasts into the femur. In pilot studies conducted prior to this, in vivo model animals infected by planktonic yeasts in the femur before implantation of the prosthesis died from *Candida* infections associated with the liver, kidneys, or lungs (data not shown).

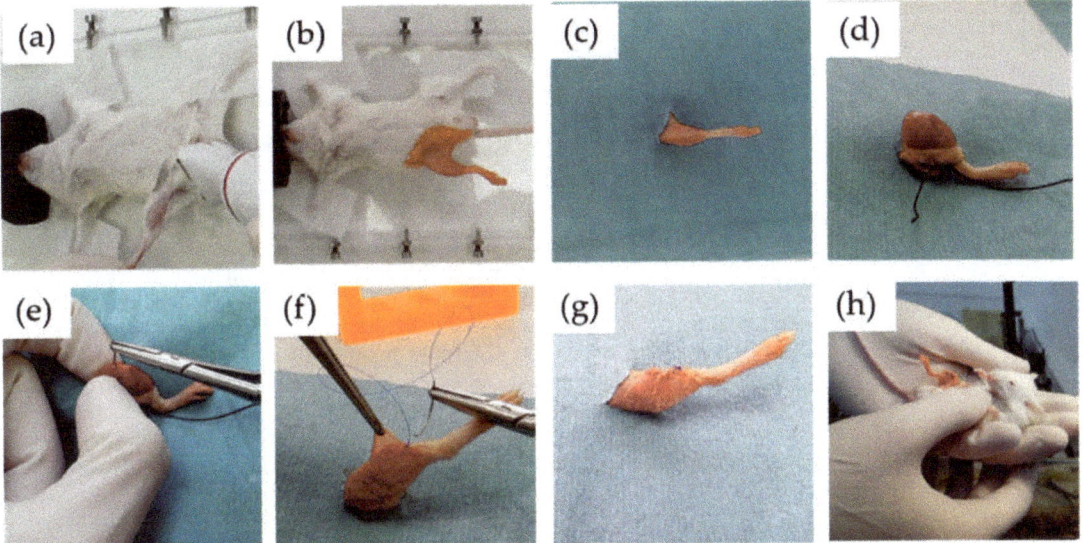

Figure 9. Surgical procedure: inhaled anaesthesia and shaving of the limb (**a**), antiseptic washing and isolation of the surgical field (**b,c**), skin dissection and exposure of the bony entry point (**d**), retrograde introduction of the biomaterial into the femur of the mouse (**e**), suture and cleaning of the surgical wound (**f,g**), awakening and care of the animal (**h**).

Sixteen-week-old male mice with femoral implants were randomly distributed into four groups: one group with a CP implant without infection (CP group, $n = 11$), a group with a CP implant with infection induced by Cal35 (CP Cal35 group, $n = 11$), the third with a CP implant coated with anidulafungin-loaded sol-gel without infection (CP + A group, $n = 11$), and the fourth with a CP implant coated with anidulafungin-loaded sol-gel with infection induced by Cal35 (CP + A Cal35 group, $n = 11$). The sample size was estimated by Wilcoxon Mann–Whitney test and an a priori type of power analysis, considering $d = 1.5$, $\alpha = 0.05$, $(1-\beta) = 0.95$, allocation ratio = 1 by using G*Power 3.1.9.7 software [47]. The d parameter is based on the assumption that the anidulafungin-loaded coating is able to reduce the yeast concentration by at least 80% per gram of bone when compared to the uncoated implant group. The statistical power of the sample was 0.9522. All the animals were included in the study and there were no exclusions.

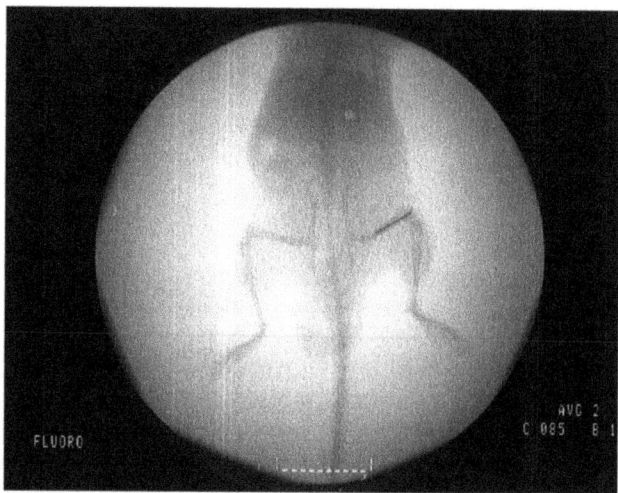

Figure 10. Fluoroscopy of a mouse with an implant placed in the femur.

We assessed the pain-stress and weight of each animal every 48 h on weekdays to ensure physical status. Evaluation of pain/stress was based on the presence or absence of six directly related behaviours in this species for the surgical procedure the animals underwent, i.e., limping, piloerection, lack of grooming, wound presence, passivity, and aggressiveness. In cases of sustained weight loss over time, the most appropriate refinement measures were taken to encourage the animal to eat. For this, they were offered an additional mixture of grains and vegetables (Vitakraft, Bremen, Germany). Five weeks (35 days) after surgery, all the animals were euthanised using hypercapnia. The right femur of each animal was then removed following sterile preparation of the knee, and the samples were sent for analysis. In case of the pre-euthanasia death of one of the mice in any group, the operated femur was alternatively used for microbiological or pathological studies.

4.3. Microbiological and Pathological Studies

After euthanasia and previous extraction of the femurs from Cal35-infected mice, joint fluid samples were taken using sterile swabs, and this fluid was used to make stamps on a slide for Gram staining. The 11 mice in the Cal-35-infected group were divided into two subgroups: 6 animals were used for microbiological studies and 5 for pathological studies. Three femurs from each noninfected group were used for microbiological studies.

Extracted bones were processed according to the methodology previously described by Aguilera-Correa et al. [30]. Briefly, using a hammer, each femur was divided into two samples in a sterile bag: (1) bone and adnexa and (2) implant. The bone was immersed in 2 mL of saline and sonicated using a sonicator at 22 °C for 5 min [48]. The resulting sonicate was diluted in a 10-fold dilution bank and seeded on chloramphenicol-gentamicin Sabouraud agar (bioMérieux, Marcy l'Etoile, France) using the plaque extension method, which consists of seeding 100 µL/plate of each dilution. The concentration of yeasts was estimated as CFU/g of bone and adnexa. The implant was sonicated in 2 mL of saline for 5 min to release the adhered yeast biofilm and to estimate biofilm concentration, measured as CFU/cm^2 of the implant. All plates were checked at 48 and 72 h.

The five femurs obtained from the Cal35-infected group were fixed in 4% paraformaldehyde for 48 h, decalcified in 10% ethylenediaminetetraacetic acid (EDTA) for 4 weeks, paraffin-infiltrated, and stained with haematoxylin-eosin. The presence of some necrotic trabecular bone and some repair areas, fibrosis, and adipose replacement of the bone marrow were identified and recorded. The presence of yeast was determined by using

Grocott's silver stain [49]. The presence/absence of round or ovoid structures, with or without signs of germination, was recorded.

Histopathological definitions were as follows:
- Acute osteomyelitis was defined as bone tissue evidencing moderate-to-high–intensity polymorphonuclear (PMN) inflammatory response with tissue necrosis phenomena and trapping of trabecular bone remains;
- Chronic osteomyelitis was defined as bone tissue that presents a variable inflammatory reaction, partially consisting of a PMN response, but mainly of plasma cells and lymphocytes;
- PJI was diagnosed when any type of osteomyelitis and the presence of yeast were evidenced.

4.4. Microcomputed Tomography

Eight bone samples from each noninfected group included in the aforementioned model were fixed in 10% formaldehyde for 48 h at 4 °C. After fixation, the samples were dehydrated in 96% ethanol for 48 h, changing the ethanol every 24 h, and in 100% ethanol for 48 h, changing the ethanol every 24 h. Hind legs were removed and fixed in 10% neutral buffered formalin. Before CT scanning, the paws were washed with running water for 15 min. Three-dimensional microcomputed tomographic imaging was performed with a CompaCT scanner (SEDECAL Madrid, Spain). Data were acquired with 720 projections by 360° scan, the integration time of 100 ms with three frames, a photon energy of 50 KeV, and current of 100 uA. The duration of imaging time was 20 min per scan. Three-dimensional renderings of images of hind paws were generated through original volumetric reconstructed images by MicroView software (GE Healthcare, Boston, MA, USA). Comparable regions of interest consisting of three metatarsal joints from each mouse were selected for analysis. Bone volume (BV), bone mass (BM), BMD (calculated as BM/BV mg/cm^3), and mean cortical thickness (mm) were quantified from micro-CT scans using GE MicroView software v2.2.

4.5. Immunohistochemistry

Five out of eight femurs used for microcomputed tomography from each group were decalcified in 10% EDTA for 4 weeks, paraffin-infiltrated, and stained with haematoxylin-eosin. In the noninfected groups, implants were removed and transversal sections in the knee condyles (5 μm) were made. Immunohistochemical analysis was carried out as previously described [50]. Briefly, sections were incubated with proteinase K Solution (20 μg/mL in Tris-EDTA Buffer, pH 8.0) for 15 min in a water bath at 37 °C for antigen retrieval after deparaffinisation and re-hydration. The blocking of nonspecific binding was performed with phosphate buffer saline (PBS), 3% bovine serum albumin (BSA) and 0.1% Triton X-100 for 1 h, and the primary antibodies anti-cathepsin K (1:25), cluster of differentiation 68 (CD68) (1:200), and alkaline phosphatase (ALP) 1:200 (all antibodies from Santa Cruz Biotechnology, Santa Cruz, CA, USA) were incubated overnight at 4 °C in a humidifying chamber. The secondary antibodies goat anti-rabbit-fluorescein isothiocyanate (FITC) (1:200) and goat anti-mouse FITC (1:200) (Invitrogen, Life Technologies, Carlsbad, CA, USA) were incubated for 1 h in the dark. Slides were mounted with Fluoroshield with 4′,6-diamidino-2-fenilindol (DAPI) mounting media (Sigma-Aldrich, St. Louis, MO, USA). Images were taken with the iScan Coreo Au scanner (Ventana Medical Systems, Roche Diagnostics, Basel, Switzerland) and visualised with Image Viewer v.3.1 software (Ventana Medical Systems, Roche Diagnostics, Basel, Switzerland). Images were taken at 4× or 10× magnification.

4.6. Statistical Analysis

The primary hypotheses were such that the anidulafungin-loaded sol-gel would prevent *C. albicans* PJI and that the anidulafungin-loaded sol-gel can be used without altering bone metabolism at any level. The secondary hypothesis was that the effect of anidulafungin-loaded sol-gel in preventing PJI could be evaluated by animal monitoring before euthanasia.

Statistical analyses were performed using Stata Statistical Software, Release 11 (StataCorp, College Station, TX, USA). Data were evaluated using a one-sided Wilcoxon non-parametric test to compare 2 groups or a one-sided proportion comparison Z-test. A log-rank test was used to perform a pairwise comparison of the Kaplan–Meier survival curves of two groups. Statistical significance was set at $p \leq 0.05$. Body weight was evaluated over time using a linear regression model. Microbiological results and weight values are represented as median and interquartile range. Other behavioural variables are represented as relative frequencies at each time point.

5. Conclusions

In conclusion, anidulafungin-loaded sol-gel can prevent PJI caused by *C. albicans* without compromising bone integrity.

6. Patents

The sol-gel used in this study is one of the products protected by the Spanish patent system with Publication Number 2686890, applied for 19 April 2017, and entitled Procedure for Obtaining a Sol-Gel Coating, Composition Coating and Use of the Same.

Author Contributions: Conceptualisation, J.J.A.-C. and J.E.; methodology, J.J.A.-C., H.G.-D. and A.M.; software, J.J.A.-C., A.M., R.A.C.-C. and F.M.; validation, J.J.A.-C., J.E., F.M. and R.A.C.-C.; formal analysis, J.J.A.-C., H.G.-D. and R.A.C.-C.; investigation, J.J.A.-C., H.G.-D., A.M., R.A.C.-C., B.T., F.M., V.F.-R., A.J.-M., E.C. and J.E.; resources, J.J.A.-C., H.G.-D., A.M., R.A.C.-C., B.T., F.M., V.F.-R., A.J.-M., E.C. and J.E.; data curation, J.J.A.-C., H.G.-D., A.M., R.A.C.-C., F.M. and J.E.; writing—original draft preparation, H.G.-D., J.J.A.-C., A.M., F.M. and R.A.C.-C.; writing—review and editing, J.J.A.-C., H.G.-D., A.M., R.A.C.-C., B.T., F.M., A.J.-M., E.C. and J.E.; visualisation, J.J.A.-C. and H.G.-D.; supervision, A.J.-M., E.C. and J.E.; project administration, J.J.A.-C., A.J.-M. and J.E.; funding acquisition, J.E., A.J.-M. and J.J.A.-C. All authors have read and agreed to the published version of the manuscript.

Funding: This research received financial support from the Mutua Madrileña Foundation (04078/001).

Institutional Review Board Statement: The use of yeast strains does not require approval by any research committee according to legislation in force. This study was approved by the Instituto de Investigación Sanitaria Fundación Jiménez Díaz (IIS-FJD) Animal Care and Use Committee (IRB number 04078-001), which includes ad hoc members for ethical issues. Animal care and maintenance complied with institutional guidelines as defined in national and international laws and policies (Spanish Royal Decree 53/2013, authorisation reference PROEX019/18 8 March 2018 granted by the Counsel for the Environment, Local Administration and Territorial Planning of the Community of Madrid and, Directive 2010/63/EU of the European Parliament and of the Council of 22 September 2010).

Informed Consent Statement: Not applicable.

Data Availability Statement: Data supporting reported results can be found by contacting with the corresponding authors.

Acknowledgments: We wish to acknowledge. Oliver Shaw for reviewing the manuscript for language-related aspects. The authors are also grateful to the Experimental Surgery and Animal Research Service, specifically Carlos Castilla-Reparaz and Carlos Carnero-Guerrero.

Conflicts of Interest: Jaime Esteban received travel grants from Pfizer and conference fees from bioMérieux and Heraeus. The funders had no role in the design of the study, the collection, analyses, or interpretation of data; the writing of the manuscript, or in the decision to publish the results. The remaining authors declare no conflict of interest.

References

1. Zhang, Y.; Jordan, J.M. Epidemiology of Osteoarthritis. *Clin. Geriatr. Med.* **2010**, *26*, 355–369. [CrossRef]
2. Tande, A.J.; Patel, R. Prosthetic Joint Infection. *Clin. Microbiol. Rev.* **2014**, *27*, 302–345. [CrossRef] [PubMed]

3. Chang, C.-H.; Lee, S.-H.; Lin, Y.-C.; Wang, Y.-C.; Chang, C.-J.; Hsieh, P.-H. Increased periprosthetic hip and knee infection projected from 2014 to 2035 in Taiwan. *J. Infect. Public Heal.* **2020**, *13*, 1768–1773. [CrossRef]
4. Kurtz, S.M.; Lau, E.; Watson, H.; Schmier, J.K.; Parvizi, J. Economic Burden of Periprosthetic Joint Infection in the United States. *J. Arthroplast.* **2012**, *27*, 61–65. [CrossRef] [PubMed]
5. Azzam, K.; Parvizi, J.; Jungkind, D.; Hanssen, A.; Fehring, T.; Springer, B.; Bozic, K.; Della Valle, C.; Pulido, L.; Barrack, R. Microbiological, Clinical, and Surgical Features of Fungal Prosthetic Joint Infections: A Multi-Institutional Experience. *J. Bone Jt. Surg. Am. Vol.* **2009**, *91*, 142–149. [CrossRef] [PubMed]
6. Kapadia, B.H.; Berg, R.A.; Daley, J.A.; Fritz, J.; Bhave, A.; Mont, M.A. Periprosthetic joint infection. *Lancet* **2016**, *387*, 386–394. [CrossRef]
7. Lerario, D.; Ferreira, S.; Miranda, W.; Chacra, A. Influence of dexamethasone and weight loss on the regulation of serum leptin levels in obese individuals. *Braz. J. Med Biol. Res.* **2001**, *34*, 479–487. [CrossRef] [PubMed]
8. Malkawi, A.K.; Alzoubi, K.H.; Jacob, M.; Matic, G.; Ali, A.; Al Faraj, A.; Almuhanna, F.; Dasouki, M.; Rahman, A.M.A. Metabolomics Based Profiling of Dexamethasone Side Effects in Rats. *Front. Pharmacol.* **2018**, *9*, 46. [CrossRef] [PubMed]
9. Marx, J.; Vudathala, D.; Murphy, L.; Rankin, S.; Hankenson, F.C. Antibiotic Administration in the Drinking Water of Mice. *J. Am. Assoc. Lab. Anim. Sci.* **2014**, *53*, 301–306. [PubMed]
10. Malani, P.N.; McNeil, S.A.; Bradley, S.F.; Kauffman, C.A. *Candida albicans* Sternal Wound Infections: A Chronic and Recurrent Complication of Median Sternotomy. *Clin. Infect. Dis.* **2002**, *35*, 1316–1320. [CrossRef]
11. Orlowski, H.L.P.; McWilliams, S.; Mellnick, V.M.; Bhalla, S.; Lubner, M.G.; Pickhardt, P.J.; Menias, C.O. Imaging Spectrum of Invasive Fungal and Fungal-like Infections. *Radiographics* **2017**, *37*, 1119–1134. [CrossRef]
12. Cheng, A.G.; McAdow, M.; Kim, H.K.; Bae, T.; Missiakas, D.M.; Schneewind, O. Contribution of Coagulases towards *Staphylococcus aureus* Disease and Protective Immunity. *PLoS Pathog.* **2010**, *6*, e1001036. [CrossRef]
13. Zawrotniak, M.; Wojtalik, K.; Rapala-Kozik, M. Farnesol, a Quorum-Sensing Molecule of Candida albicans Triggers the Release of Neutrophil Extracellular Traps. *Cells* **2019**, *8*, 1611. [CrossRef]
14. Mutua, V.; Gershwin, L.J. A Review of Neutrophil Extracellular Traps (NETs) in Disease: Potential Anti-NETs Therapeutics. *Clin. Rev. Allergy Immunol.* **2020**, 1–18. [CrossRef]
15. Schauer, C.; Janko, C.; Munoz, L.E.; Zhao, Y.; Kienhöfer, D.; Frey, B.; Lell, M.; Manger, B.; Rech, J.; Naschberger, E.; et al. Aggregated neutrophil extracellular traps limit inflammation by degrading cytokines and chemokines. *Nat. Med.* **2014**, *20*, 511–517. [CrossRef]
16. Karlowicz, M. Candidal renal and urinary tract infection in neonates. *Semin. Perinatol.* **2003**, *27*, 393–400. [CrossRef]
17. Pfaller, M.A.; Diekema, D.J. Epidemiology of Invasive Candidiasis: A Persistent Public Health Problem. *Clin. Microbiol. Rev.* **2007**, *20*, 133–163. [CrossRef]
18. Tsai, N.Y.; Laforce-Nesbitt, S.S.; Tucker, R.; Bliss, J.M. A Murine Model for Disseminated Candidiasis in Neonates. *Pediatr. Res.* **2011**, *69*, 189–193. [CrossRef]
19. Thorn, J.L.; Gilchrist, K.B.; Sobonya, R.E.; Gaur, N.K.; Lipke, P.N.; Klotz, S.A. Postmortem candidaemia: Marker of disseminated disease. *J. Clin. Pathol.* **2009**, *63*, 337–340. [CrossRef]
20. Gamaletsou, M.N.; Rammaert, B.; Bueno, M.A.; Sipsas, N.V.; Moriyama, B.; Kontoyiannis, D.P.; Roilides, E.; Zeller, V.; Tajaldeen, S.J.; Miller, A.O.; et al. Candida Arthritis: Analysis of 112 Pediatric and Adult Cases. *Open Forum Infect. Dis.* **2016**, *3*, ofv207. [CrossRef]
21. Komori, A.; Abe, T.; Kushimoto, S.; Ogura, H.; Shiraishi, A.; Ma, G.A.D.; Saitoh, D.; Fujishima, S.; Mayumi, T.; Gando, S.; et al. Clinical features of patients with candidemia in sepsis. *J. Gen. Fam. Med.* **2019**, *20*, 161–163. [CrossRef] [PubMed]
22. Kao, A.S.; Brandt, M.E.; Pruitt, W.R.; Conn, L.A.; Perkins, B.A.; Stephens, D.S.; Baughman, W.S.; Reingold, A.L.; Rothrock, G.A.; Pfaller, M.A.; et al. The Epidemiology of Candidemia in Two United States Cities: Results of a Population-Based Active Surveillance. *Clin. Infect. Dis.* **1999**, *29*, 1164–1170. [CrossRef] [PubMed]
23. Garcia-Casas, A.; Aguilera-Correa, J.; Mediero, A.; Esteban, J.; Jimenez-Morales, A. Functionalization of sol-gel coatings with organophosphorus compounds for prosthetic devices. *Colloids Surf. B Biointerfaces* **2019**, *181*, 973–980. [CrossRef] [PubMed]
24. Aguilera-Correa, J.J.; Vidal-Laso, R.; Carias-Cálix, R.A.; Toirac, B.; García-Casas, A.; Velasco-Rodríguez, D.; Llamas-Sillero, P.; Jiménez-Morales, A.; Esteban, J. A New Antibiotic-Loaded Sol-Gel can Prevent Bacterial Intravenous Catheter-Related Infections. *Materials* **2020**, *13*, 2946. [CrossRef]
25. Romera, D.; Toirac, B.; Aguilera-Correa, J.-J.; García-Casas, A.; Mediero, A.; Jiménez-Morales, A.; Esteban, J. A Biodegradable Antifungal-Loaded Sol–Gel Coating for the Prevention and Local Treatment of Yeast Prosthetic-Joint Infections. *Materials* **2020**, *13*, 3144. [CrossRef]
26. Poggioli, R.; Ueta, C.B.; Drigo, R.A.E.; Castillo, M.; Fonseca, T.L.; Bianco, A.C. Dexamethasone reduces energy expenditure and increases susceptibility to diet-induced obesity in mice. *Obesity* **2013**, *21*, E415–E420. [CrossRef]
27. Lazzarini, L.; Manfrin, V.; De Lalla, F. Candidal prosthetic hip infection in a patient with previous candidal septic arthritis. *J. Arthroplast.* **2004**, *19*, 248–252. [CrossRef]
28. Hwang, B.-H.; Yoon, J.-Y.; Nam, C.-H.; Jung, K.-A.; Lee, S.-C.; Han, C.-D.; Moon, S.-H. Fungal peri-prosthetic joint infection after primary total knee replacement. *J. Bone Jt. Surg. Br. Vol.* **2012**, *94*, 656–659. [CrossRef]

29. Dale, H.; Fenstad, A.M.; Hallan, G.; Havelin, L.I.; Furnes, O.; Overgaard, S.; Pedersen, A.B.; Kärrholm, J.; Garellick, G.; Pulkkinen, P.; et al. Increasing risk of prosthetic joint infection after total hip arthroplasty. *Acta Orthop.* **2012**, *83*, 449–458. [CrossRef]
30. Aguilera-Correa, J.J.; Garcia-Casas, A.; Mediero, A.; Romera, D.; Mulero, F.; Cuevas-López, I.; Jiménez-Morales, A.; Esteban, J. A New Antibiotic-Loaded Sol-Gel Can Prevent Bacterial Prosthetic Joint Infection: From in vitro Studies to an in vivo Model. *Front. Microbiol.* **2020**, *10*, 2335. [CrossRef]
31. Kim, S.-J.; Huh, J.; Odrobina, R.; Kim, J.H. Systemic Review of Published Literature on Candida Infection Following Total Hip Arthroplasty. *Mycopathology* **2014**, *179*, 173–185. [CrossRef]
32. Baker, D.G. Natural Pathogens of Laboratory Mice, Rats, and Rabbits and Their Effects on Research. *Clin. Microbiol. Rev.* **1998**, *11*, 231–266. [CrossRef]
33. Wright, A.M.; Mody, D.R.; Anton, R.C.; Schwartz, M.R. Aberrant staining with Grocott's methenamine silver: Utility beyond fungal organisms. *J. Am. Soc. Cytopathol.* **2017**, *6*, 223–227. [CrossRef]
34. Cobo, F.; Rodríguez-Granger, J.; López, E.M.; Jiménez, G.; Sampedro, A.; Aliaga-Martínez, L.; Navarro-Marí, J.M. Candida-induced prosthetic joint infection. A literature review including 72 cases and a case report. *Infect. Dis.* **2016**, *49*, 81–94. [CrossRef]
35. Riaz, T.; Tande, A.J.; Steed, L.L.; Demos, H.A.; Salgado, C.D.; Osmon, D.R.; Marculescu, C.E. Risk Factors for Fungal Prosthetic Joint Infection. *J. Bone Jt. Infect.* **2020**, *5*, 76–81. [CrossRef]
36. Grasso, R.J.; West, L.A.; Guay, R.C.; Klein, T.W. Inhibition of Yeast Phagocytosis by Dexamethasone in Macrophage Cultures: Reversibility of the Effect and Enhanced Suppression in Cultures of Stimulated Macrophages. *J. Immunopharmacol.* **1982**, *4*, 265–278. [CrossRef]
37. Swartjes, J.J.T.M.; Sharma, P.K.; Van Kooten, T.G.; Van Der Mei, H.C.; Mahmoudi, M.; Busscher, H.J.; Rochford, E.T.J. Current Developments in Antimicrobial Surface Coatings for Biomedical Applications. *Curr. Med. Chem.* **2015**, *22*, 2116–2129. [CrossRef]
38. Civantos, A.; Martínez-Campos, E.; Ramos, V.; Elvira, C.; Gallardo, A.; Abarrategi, A. Titanium Coatings and Surface Modifications: Toward Clinically Useful Bioactive Implants. *ACS Biomater. Sci. Eng.* **2017**, *3*, 1245–1261. [CrossRef]
39. Tsiapalis, D.; De Pieri, A.; Biggs, M.; Pandit, A.; Zeugolis, D.I. Biomimetic Bioactive Biomaterials: The Next Generation of Implantable Devices. *ACS Biomater. Sci. Eng.* **2016**, *3*, 1172–1174. [CrossRef]
40. Li, K.; Liu, S.; Hu, T.; Razanau, I.; Wu, X.; Ao, H.; Huang, L.; Xie, Y.; Zheng, X. Optimized Nanointerface Engineering of Micro/Nanostructured Titanium Implants to Enhance Cell–Nanotopography Interactions and Osseointegration. *ACS Biomater. Sci. Eng.* **2020**, *6*, 969–983. [CrossRef]
41. Siedenbiedel, F.; Tiller, J.C. Antimicrobial Polymers in Solution and on Surfaces: Overview and Functional Principles. *Polymer* **2012**, *4*, 46–71. [CrossRef]
42. Botequim, D.; Maia, J.; Lino, M.; Lopes, L.M.F.; Simões, P.N.; Ilharco, L.; Ferreira, L. Nanoparticles and Surfaces Presenting Antifungal, Antibacterial and Antiviral Properties. *Langmuir* **2012**, *28*, 7646–7656. [CrossRef]
43. Phelan, D.M.; Osmon, D.R.; Keating, M.R.; Hanssen, A.D. Delayed Reimplantation Arthroplasty for Candidal Prosthetic Joint Infection: A Report of 4 Cases and Review of the Literature. *Clin. Infect. Dis.* **2002**, *34*, 930–938. [CrossRef]
44. Arenas, M.A.; Pérez-Jorge, C.; Conde, A.; Matykina, E.; Hernández-López, J.M.; Perez-Tanoira, R.; de Damborenea, J.J.; Gómez-Barrena, E.; Esteban, J. Doped TiO2 anodic layers of enhanced antibacterial properties. *Colloids Surfaces B Biointerfaces* **2013**, *105*, 106–112. [CrossRef]
45. Walzer, P.D.; Runck, J.; Steele, P.; White, M.; Linke, M.J.; Sidman, C.L. Immunodeficient and immunosuppressed mice as models to test anti-Pneumocystis carinii drugs. *Antimicrob. Agents Chemother.* **1997**, *41*, 251–258. [CrossRef]
46. Slate, A.R.; Bandyopadhyay, S.; Francis, K.P.; Papich, M.G.; Karolewski, B.; Hod, E.A.; Prestia, K.A. Efficacy of Enrofloxacin in a Mouse Model of Sepsis. *J. Am. Assoc. Lab. Anim. Sci.* **2014**, *53*, 381–386. [PubMed]
47. Faul, F.; Erdfelder, E.; Lang, A.-G.; Buchner, A. G*Power 3: A flexible statistical power analysis program for the social, behavioral, and biomedical sciences. *Behav. Res. Methods* **2007**, *39*, 175–191. [CrossRef] [PubMed]
48. Esteban, J.; Gomez-Barrena, E.; Cordero, J.; Martín-De-Hijas, N.Z.; Kinnari, T.J.; Fernandez-Roblas, R. Evaluation of Quantitative Analysis of Cultures from Sonicated Retrieved Orthopedic Implants in Diagnosis of Orthopedic Infection. *J. Clin. Microbiol.* **2008**, *46*, 488–492. [CrossRef] [PubMed]
49. Grocott, B.R.G. A Stain for Fungi in Tissue Sections and Smears. *Am. J. Clin. Pathol.* **1955**, *25*, 975–979. [CrossRef] [PubMed]
50. Mediero, A.; Frenkel, S.R.; Wilder, T.; He, W.; Mazumder, A.; Cronstein, B.N. Adenosine A2A Receptor Activation Prevents Wear Particle-Induced Osteolysis. *Sci. Transl. Med.* **2012**, *4*, 135ra65. [CrossRef]

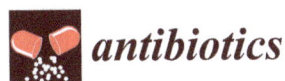

Article

Do Prosthetic Joint Infections Worsen the Functional Ambulatory Outcome of Patients with Joint Replacements? A Retrospective Matched Cohort Study

Isabel Mur [1,2,3], Marcos Jordán [4], Alba Rivera [5], Virginia Pomar [1,2], José Carlos González [4], Joaquín López-Contreras [1,2,3], Xavier Crusi [4], Ferran Navarro [5], Mercè Gurguí [1,2] and Natividad Benito [1,2,3,*]

[1] Infectious Disease Unit, Hospital de la Santa Creu i Sant Pau–Institut d'Investigació Biomèdica Sant Pau, 08025 Barcelona, Spain; imur@santpau.cat (I.M.); VPomar@santpau.cat (V.P.); jlcontreras@santpau.cat (J.L.-C.); MGurgui@santpau.cat (M.G.)
[2] Department of Medicine, Universitat Autònoma de Barcelona, 08193 Barcelona, Spain
[3] Bone and Joint Infection Study Group of the Spanish Society of Infectious Diseases and Clinical Microbiology (GEIO-SEIMC), 28003 Madrid, Spain
[4] Department of Orthopedic Surgery and Traumatology, Hospital de la Santa Creu i Sant Pau–Institut d'Investigació Biomèdica Sant Pau, 08025 Barcelona, Spain; MJordan@santpau.cat (M.J.); JGonzalezR@santpau.cat (J.C.G.); XCrusi@santpau.cat (X.C.)
[5] Department of Microbiology, Hospital Santa Creu i Sant Pau, Hospital de la Santa Creu i Sant Pau–Institut d'Investigació Biomèdica Sant Pau, Universitat Autònoma de Barcelona, 08025 Barcelona, Spain; mrivera@santpau.cat (A.R.); FNavarror@santpau.cat (F.N.)
* Correspondence: nbenito@santpau.cat; Tel.: +34-93-556-56-24; Fax: +34-93-553-71-40

Received: 10 November 2020; Accepted: 3 December 2020; Published: 5 December 2020

Abstract: Objectives: To assess the effect on the functional ambulatory outcome of postoperative joint infection (PJI) cured at the first treatment attempt versus not developing PJI in patients with hip and knee prostheses. Methods: In a single-hospital retrospectively matched cohort study, each patient with PJI between 2007 and 2016 was matched on age, sex, type of prosthesis and year of implantation with two other patients with uninfected arthroplasties. The definition of a PJI cure included infection eradication, no further surgical procedures, no PJI-related mortality and no suppressive antibiotics. Functional ambulatory status evaluated one year after the last surgery was classified into four simple categories: able to walk without assistance, able to walk with one crutch, able to walk with two crutches, and unable to walk. Patients with total hip arthroplasties (THAs), total knee arthroplasties (TKAs) and partial hip arthroplasties (PHAs) were analysed separately. Results: A total of 109 PJI patients (38 TKA, 41 THA, 30 PHA) and 218 non-PJI patients were included. In a model adjusted for clinically relevant variables, PJI was associated with a higher risk of needing an assistive device for ambulation (vs. walking without aid) among THA (adjusted odds ratio (OR) 3.10, 95% confidence interval (95% CI) 1.26–7.57; $p = 0.014$) and TKA patients (OR 5.40, 95% CI 2.12–13.67; $p < 0.001$), and with requiring two crutches to walk or being unable to walk (vs. walking unaided or with one crutch) among PHA patients (OR 3.05, 95% CI 1.01–9.20; $p = 0.047$). Conclusions: Ambulatory outcome in patients with hip and knee prostheses with postoperative PJI is worse than in patients who do not have PJI.

Keywords: prosthetic joint infection; arthroplasty infection; prosthetic joint infection functional outcome; prosthetic joint infection ambulatory outcome

1. Introduction

Hip and knee replacements are common and increasingly performed surgical procedures. The main indications for total hip arthroplasty (THA) and total knee arthroplasty (TKA) are to relieve pain and improve joint function in patients with advanced joint disease, while partial hip arthroplasties (PHAs) are mostly indicated for restoring function in elderly patients with displaced femoral neck fractures [1,2].

Prosthetic joint infection (PJI) is one of the most dreaded complications of these procedures. Eradication of infection requires surgery and antimicrobial therapy [3–5]. Surgical strategies include debridement with implant retention (DAIR) and prosthesis exchange. Cure at the first treatment attempt is critical because each treatment failure worsens tissue damage and functional integrity [6]. On rare occasions, resection of the prosthesis, arthrodesis or amputation is performed to eradicate infection but without restoring full function. Suppressive antibiotic therapy is an option that is not intended to eradicate infection but can minimise symptoms and sometimes preserve function when it is not possible to remove the prosthesis [7].

Unlike other infections, the goal of PJI treatment is not only to eradicate infection but also to relieve pain and maintain joint function; it is not always possible to achieve all these goals [3,4,8]. While PJI treatment success has been primarily defined as eradication of infection [9], few studies have analysed functional outcome, despite this being the main aim of prosthesis implantation. In terms of functional outcome, diverse results have been observed using different surgical procedures for PJI management as compared with uninfected primary arthroplasties [10–14]. The question of whether a PJI cured at the first therapeutic attempt, that is, in the best possible scenario, has a worse ambulatory outcome than an uninfected prosthetic joint, has not been specifically addressed and remains unresolved. Our objective is to assess the effect of postoperative PJI, as compared with not developing PJI, on functional ambulatory outcome in patients with hip and knee prostheses.

2. Methods

2.1. Setting and Study Design

This study was conducted at the Hospital de la Santa Creu i Sant Pau, a tertiary university hospital in Barcelona, Spain. Patients with PJI are treated by a multidisciplinary team, including medical and surgical specialists.

We used a retrospectively matched cohort study to compare the functional ambulatory outcome of hip and knee arthroplasty patients with (PJI cohort) or without (non-PJI cohort) postoperative PJI.

The Research Ethics Committee of our hospital approved the study.

2.2. Study Patients and Controls

Patients with the following criteria were included: (1) a diagnosis of postoperative PJI (excluding haematogenous infections) between January 2007 and December 2016, (2) PJI treatment was intended to eradicate the infection, and (3) the first planned treatment was successful. Since hematogenous PJIs can occur at any time after the index surgery, it would be very difficult to find suitable comparable patients with uninfected arthroplasties to match those with hematogenous PJIs occurring at very different times after prosthesis implantation in order to evaluate ambulatory outcome; for that reason, patients with hematogenous infections were excluded.

Each PJI patient was matched with two control patients with arthroplasties implanted at our institution, who had completed a minimum follow-up of 1 year after surgery without developing PJI. Exact matching was performed on patient sex and age (within a 5-year age range), type of prosthesis (THA, TKA or PHA), primary or revision arthroplasty and year of implantation. Controls for each case were sought by considering all the following patients who underwent the same type of arthroplasty implant; the first two patients who met all the remaining criteria were selected.

2.3. Definitions

The diagnosis of PJI was based on International Consensus Meeting for PJI criteria [15]. PJIs presenting within 1 month after surgery were classified as early postoperative infection [3]. When symptoms persisted for more than three weeks beyond one-month postintervention, the infection was defined as chronic [3]. Choice of the optimal surgical strategy for each patient was based on Zimmerli's algorithm, endorsed by the Infectious Diseases Society of America [3,5]. Despite the one-month postsurgery cut-off used to define chronic versus early PJI infection and the recommendation to remove the prosthesis in cases of chronic PJI, DAIR was allowed up to 3 months after prosthesis implantation, in accordance with Spanish guidelines and recent studies [4,16]. Mobile antibiotic-impregnated cement spacers were used in patients treated with two-stage exchange after removing the prosthesis. Infectious disease specialists selected and controlled antibiotic use. The duration of antimicrobial treatment, based on the Spanish guidelines for the management of PJI, typically ranged from 8 to 12 weeks following DAIR and 4–6 weeks after the first step of a two-stage prosthesis exchange [4]. Infectious disease specialists and orthopaedists followed PJI patients for a minimum of 2 years after ending antimicrobial therapy. Successful PJI treatment ("cure") was defined following a published consensus definition that included: (1) eradication of infection, characterised by no clinical failure (healed wound without fistula or drainage and painless joint), and no infection recurrence caused by the same organism strain, (2) no further surgical interventions due to infection (other than the one initially planned to treat PJI), and (3) no death caused by a condition directly related to PJI [9]. In addition, suppressive antibiotic therapy was considered a treatment failure. Only patients with PJI cured at the first treatment attempt were included in the current study; the first treatment attempt consisted of the first curative strategy utilised to treat the PJI and comprised a combination of both an appropriate surgical procedure (including DAIR, a one or two-stage prosthesis exchange) and antimicrobial therapy for a definite period of time; patients who required further surgery (such as spacer exchange) or a new course of antimicrobials after the first one ended were excluded. Treatment success was evaluated a minimum of 1 year after ending antimicrobial treatment (for PJIs treated with DAIR or a one-stage arthroplasty exchange) or after reimplantation surgery during a two-stage arthroplasty exchange (with negative intraoperative culture samples).

Under the supervision of a physiotherapist, all patients started full bodyweight bearing ambulation and physical therapy as soon as possible after surgery to facilitate recovery of function. Typically, the rehabilitation program begins from the first postoperative day after TKA and THA implantation (including new prostheses implanted in a one-step exchange or in the second stage of a two-step exchange). After DAIR, inpatient rehabilitation is commonly delayed for a few days (postoperative day 3–5), depending on wound evolution. Exercises to restore normal joint motion and strength are initiated in the hospital and continued upon discharge.

The Charlson comorbidity score and the American Society of Anesthesiologists (ASA) physical status classification system were used to evaluate baseline comorbidities and the patient's general health status, respectively [17,18].

2.4. Ambulatory Outcome

Functional ambulatory status was assessed 1 year after the last surgery. Due to the retrospective nature of the study and the fact that the evaluation of patients with arthroplasties was performed by different surgeons without a uniform scoring system, we classified the patient's ambulatory outcome in 4 simple categories: (1) able to ambulate without an assistive device, (2) able to walk with one crutch/stick, (3) able to walk with two crutches/sticks and (4) unable to walk. These categories were relative to the patient's normal outdoor ambulation capacity. Patients with TKA, THA, and PHA were analysed separately.

2.5. Statistical Analysis

Continuous variables were summarised as means and standard deviations and categorical variables as percentages relative to the total sample. We used the Wilcoxon and chi-square tests (or Fisher's exact tests when appropriate) to compare group differences for continuous and categorical variables, respectively. To evaluate whether PJI was an independent factor associated with a worse functional ambulatory outcome, any variable with a p-value less than 0.25 in univariate analysis, together with all clinically relevant variables, were included as covariates in an adjusted logistic regression model [19,20]. P-values of <0.05 were considered to be significant for all statistical tests. Data were analysed using IBM® SPSS®, version 26.0.

3. Results

3.1. Characteristics of Patients with Prosthetic Joint Infection

A total of 109 patients with postoperative PJI were included: 38 with TKA, 41 with THA, and 30 with PHA. As shown in Table 1, PHA patients were older and more frequently female than TKA and THA patients, who otherwise had similar demographic characteristics. Although most of the patients had early PJI, the percentage was higher in those with PHA. The commonest cause of infection was staphylococci (53.2%) followed by enterobacteria (25.7%). A total of 83 PJIs were treated with DAIR: 81 within the first month after joint replacement surgery (included as "early postoperative infections" in Table 1) and 2 in the second month after index surgery (included as "late chronic infections" in Table 1, in accordance with the above definitions of early and chronic PJIs). Prosthetic exchange was performed on 26 PJI patients (19 two-stage exchanges), 23 of them with chronic infections.

3.2. Patients with Infected versus Uninfected Hip and Knee Arthroplasties

Table 2 compares the characteristics and ambulatory outcomes of 109 patients with PJI (cases) and 218 patients without PJI (controls). Patients with PHA (both cases and controls) had more baseline comorbidities and a worse general medical status than those with TKA and THA. In addition, PHA was typically performed to treat hip fractures, whereas total knee and hip replacements were mostly performed for osteoarthritis. Because of these and other well-known differences between patients with PHA and those with THA [21–24], we analysed them in two separate groups. A detailed comparison of patients with infected versus uninfected TKA, THA and PHA is provided in Table 2. Within each group, patients with and without PJI showed no differences with respect to comorbidity burden and baseline health status, as measured by the Charlson and ASA scores. The indications for joint replacement in PJI and non-PJI patients were similar in the three groups, except for fractures and dislocations, which were more frequent in PJI patients in the THA group (all of these occurred in 7 patients with infected THAs).

Table 1. Characteristics of 109 patients with hip and knee prosthetic joint infection.

Variable	Patients with Prosthetic Total Knee Infection (n = 38)	Patients with Prosthetic Total Hip Infection (n = 41)	Patients with Prosthetic Partial Hip Infection (n = 30)
Age, years—mean (standard deviation)	74 (5.7)	72 (9)	83 (6.1)
Female gender—no. (%)	24 (63.3)	23 (56.1)	26 (86.7)
Primary arthroplasty—no. (%)	33 (86.8)	32 (78)	26 (86.7)
Early postoperative infection—no. (%)	27 (71.1)	29 (70.7)	28 (93.3)
Surgical treatment of early postoperative infections (EPI):			
• Debridement and implant retention—no. (% of EPI)	26 (96.3)	28 (96.6)	27 (96.4)
• Two-stage exchange no. (% of EPI)	1 (3.7)	1 (2.4)	1 (3.6)
• One-stage exchange no. (% of EPI)	-	-	-
Late chronic infection—no. (%)	11 (28.9)	12 (29.3)	2 (6.7)
Surgical treatment of late chronic infections (LCI):			
• Debridement and implant retention—no. (% of LCI)	1 (9.1)	1 (8.3)	-
• Two-stage exchange no. (% of LCI)	10 (90.9)	5 (41.7)	2 (100)
• One-stage exchange no. (% of LCI)	-	6 (50)	-
Culture-positive prosthetic joint infection—no. (%)	36 (94.7)	38 (92.7)	27 (90)
Microbial aetiology of prosthetic joint infection			
• *Staphylococcus aureus*—no. (%)	9 (25)	14 (36.8)	10 (37)
○ Methicillin-resistant *S. aureus*—no. (%)	5 (15.2)	2 (5.3)	5 (22.2)
• Coagulase negative staphylococci—no. (%)	10 (27.8)	10 (26.3)	5 (18.5)
• Enterobacteria—no. (%)	9 (25)	10 (26.3)	9 (33.3)
• Other microorganisms—no. (%)	14 (38.9)	10 (26.3)	6 (22.2)

Table 2. Characteristics of 327 patients with hip and knee arthroplasties, with and without prosthetic joint infection, matched 1:2 by gender, age ± 5 years, type of prosthesis, primary or revision arthroplasty and year of index surgery.

Variable	Total Knee Arthroplasty (n = 114)			Total Hip Arthroplasty (n = 123)			Partial Hip Arthroplasty (n = 90)		
	PJI (n = 38)	Non-PJI (n = 76)	p-Value*	PJI (n = 41)	Non-PJI (n = 82)	p-Value*	PJI (n = 30)	Non-PJI (n = 60)	p-Value*
Age, years—mean (standard deviation)	74 (5.7)	74 (5.8)	0.936	71 (9)	71 (8.3)	0.817	83 (6.1)	83 (6.0)	0.912
Charlson score ≥ 2—no. (%)	3 (7.9)	11 (15.8)	0.240	4 (9.8)	10 (12.2)	0.772	11 (36.7)	20 (33.3)	0.754
ASA > 2—no. (%)	11 (28.9)	24 (31.6)	0.774	13 (31.7)	28 (34.1)	0.787	17 (56.7)	39 (65)	0.442
Indications for arthroplasty									
• Osteoarthritis—no. (%)	32 (84.2)	66 (86.8)	0.703	28 (68.3)	64 (78)	0.240	-	-	-
• Aseptic loosening—no. (%)	4 (10.5)	9 (11.8)	1	4 (9.8)	14 (17.1)	0.279	2 (6.7)	3 (5)	1
• Periprosthetic fracture—no. (%)	1 (2.6)	1 (1.3)	1	2 (4.9)	2 (4.9)	1	2 (6.7)	4 (6.7)	1
• Fracture—no. (%)	0	0	-	4 (9.8)	0 (0)	**0.011**	26 (86.7)	52 (86.7)	1
• Dislocation—no. (%)	0	0	-	3 (7.3)	0 (0)	**0.035**	0 (0)	1 (1.7)	1
• Rheumatoid arthritis—no. (%)	1 (2.6)	0 (0)	0.333	-	-	-	-	-	-
Functional outcome									
• Able to walk without assistance—no. (%)	22 (57.9)	59 (77.6)	**0.028**	15 (36.6)	61 (74.4)	**<0.001**	2 (6.7)	7 (11.7)	0.712
• Walking with one crutch—no. (%)	10 (26.3)	16 (21.1)	0.528	21 (51.2)	16 (19.5)	**<0.001**	5 (16.7)	18 (30)	0.172
• Walking without assistance or with one crutch—no. (%)	32 (84.2)	75 (98.7)	**0.005**	36 (87.8)	77 (93.9)	0.299	7 (23.3)	25 (41.7)	0.087
• Walking with two crutches—no. (%)	6 (15.8)	1 (1.3)	**0.005**	5 (12.2)	5 (6.1)	0.299	16 (53.3)	25 (41.7)	0.295
• Unable to walk—no. (%)	0	0	-	0	0	-	7 (23.3)	10 (16.7)	0.446

Table 2. Cont.

Functional ambulatory outcome in matched pairs of patients in which those with PJI were treated with DAIR	PJI treated with DAIR (n = 27)	Non-PJI (matched with DAIR-treated PJI) (n = 54)		PJI treated with DAIR (n = 29)	Non-PJI (matched with DAIR-treated PJI) (n = 58)		PJI treated with DAIR (n = 27)	Non-PJI (matched with DAIR-treated PJI) (n = 54)	
• Able to walk without assistance—no. (%)	16 (59.3)	43 (79.6)	0.052	13 (44.8)	45 (77.6)	**0.002**	1 (3.7)	6 (11.1)	0.415
• Walking with one crutch—no. (%)	7 (25.9)	10 (18.5)	0.440	13 (44.8)	10 (17.2)	**0.006**	5 (18.5)	18 (33.3)	0.163
• Walking without assistance or with one crutch—no. (%)	23 (85.2)	53 (98.1)	**0.040**	26 (89.7)	55 (94.8)	0.396	6 (22.2)	24 (44.4)	0.051
• Walking with two crutches—no. (%)	4 (14.8)	1 (1.9)	**0.040**	3 (10.3)	3 (5.2)	0.396	14 (51.9)	20 (37.0)	0.203
• Unable to walk—no. (%)	0	0	-	0	0	-	7 (25.9)	10 (18.5)	0.440

Functional ambulatory outcome in matched pairs of patients in which those with PJI were treated with prosthesis exchange	PJI treated with prosthesis exchange (n = 11)	Non-PJI matched with exchange-treate PJI (n = 22)		PJI treated with prosthesis exchange (n = 12)	Non-PJI matched with exchange-treate PJI (n = 24)		PJI treated with prosthesis exchange (n = 3)	Non-PJI matched with exchange-treate PJI (n = 6)	
• Able to walk without assistance—no. (%)	6 (54.5)	16 (72.7)	0.437	2 (16.7)	16 (66.7)	**0.005**	1 (33.3)	1 (16.7)	1
• Walking with one crutch—no. (%)	3 (27.3)	6 (27.3)	1	8 (66.7)	8 (25)	**0.029**	0	0	-
• Walking without assistance or with one crutch—no. (%)	9 (81.8)	22 (100)	0.104	10 (83.3)	22 (91.7)	0.588	1 (33.3)	1 (16.7)	1
• Walking with two crutches—no. (%)	2 (18.2)	0	0.104	2 (16.7)	2 (8.3)	0.558	2 (66.7)	5 (83.3)	1
• Unable to walk—no. (%)	0	0	-	0	0	-	0	0	-

ASA = American Society of Anesthesiologists; DAIR = debridement, antibiotics and implant retention; PJI = prosthetic joint infection. * Results in bold refer to those that are statistically significant.

3.3. Functional Ambulatory Outcomes

Table 2 and Figure 1 show the functional ambulatory status of patients with and without PJI in univariate analysis.

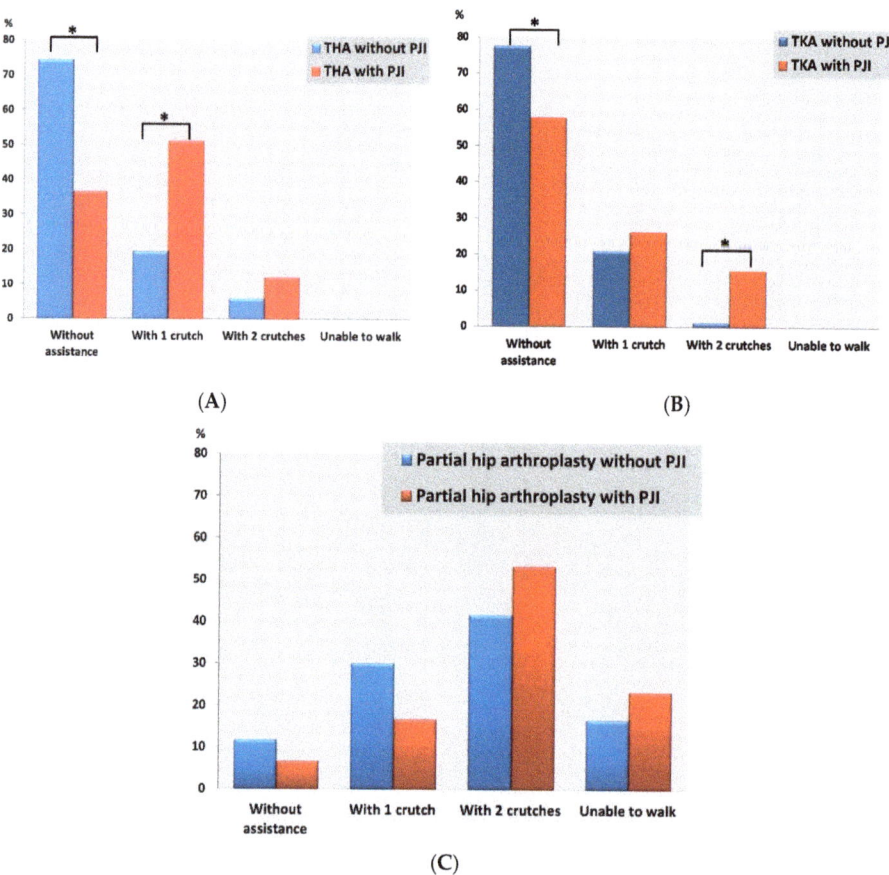

Figure 1. Functional ambulatory outcome in patients with total hip arthroplasty (**A**), patients with total knee arthroplasty (**B**), and patients with partial hip arthroplasty (**C**) with or without postoperative prosthetic joint infection. Total hip arthroplasty (THA), total knee arthroplasty (TKA) and PJI denote total hip arthroplasty, total knee arthroplasty and prosthetic joint infection, respectively. Statistically significant differences are marked with an asterisk (*).

Most TKA and THA patients (both with and without PJI) were able to walk unaided, but this was significantly more common in non-PJI patients in both the TKA and the THA group; otherwise, patients with TKA and PJI were almost twice as likely to require one or two crutches to walk (42.1% vs. 22.4%, $p = 0.028$), while patients with infected THAs were more than twice as likely to require an assistive device in order to walk than those with uninfected THAs (63.4% vs. 25.6%, $p < 0.001$). With respect to the matched pairs of TKA patients, in which those with PJI were treated with DAIR, differences in walking capacity between PJI and non-PJI patients remained, with non-PJI patients being more often able to walk unaided (79.6%% vs. 59.3, $p = 0.052$) or to walk without assistance or with one crutch (98.1% vs. 85.2%, $p = 0.040$). Regarding matched pairs of THA patients in which PJI patients were treated with DAIR, those with uninfected THAs were significantly more likely to ambulate unaided

(77.6% vs. 44.8%, $p = 0.002$). Patients with infected TKAs and THAs treated with prosthesis exchange were more likely to require crutches to walk than their matched pairs of patients with uninfected TKA and THA, although these differences were statistically significant only in the THA group.

Most PHA patients (both with and without PJI) needed two crutches to ambulate. No statistically significant differences were found between PJI and non-PJI patients in the four categories of ambulation capacity, although PHA patients without PJI were more commonly able to walk without assistance or with one crutch, while PJI patients more often required two crutches or were unable to walk ($p = 0.051$). In PHA patients, we further compared their ambulatory ability with that prior to PHA implantation, depending on whether or not they had postoperative PJI, and found no significant differences ($p = 0.965$): (1) 11 (39.3%) PJI vs. 22 (38.6%) non-PJI patients were observed to have the same walking ability as before; (2) walking ability decreased by one stage (e.g., from walking unaided to requiring the help of one crutch) in 9 (32.2%) PJI vs. 11 (36.8%) non-PJI patients; (3) walking ability decreased by two stages in 6 (21.4%) PJI vs. 10 (17.5%) non-PJI patients; (4) a three-stage deterioration was observed in 2 (7.1%) PJI vs. 4 (7%) non-PJI patients.

In patients with TKAs, the adjusted model for clinically relevant variables identified the following factors as being independently associated with a higher risk of needing an assistive device for ambulation (vs. walking without aid): Charlson score ≥2 and PJI (Table 3). Similarly, in analyses of THA patients, older age and PJI were independently associated with a worse ambulatory outcome, defined as requiring an assistive device to walk (Table 4). Considering patients with total hip and knee arthroplasties together, the adjusted model found that older age (odds ratio (OR) 1.07, confidence interval (95% CI) 1.03–1.12), Charlson score ≥2 (OR 3.52, 95% CI 1.45–8.55) and PJI (OR 3.91, 95% CI 2.10–7.37) were risk factors for needing crutches to walk (vs. walking unaided). In the PHA patient group, a worse functional status was defined as requiring two crutches to walk or being unable to walk; in this group of patients, PJI was also identified as an independent factor associated with a worse ambulatory outcome (Table 5). Since there was collinearity between the Charlson score and the ASA classification system used to evaluate the baseline health status of patients, only one of these variables was included in the final adjusted models (Tables 3–5).

Table 3. Factors associated with requiring an assistive device for ambulation versus walking without assistance in 114 patients undergoing total knee replacements one year after the last surgical procedure.

Variable	Univariate Analysis			Multivariate Analysis	
	Walking without Assistance (n = 81)	Walking with Crutches (n = 33)	p-Value	OR (95% CI) *	p-Value
Age, years—mean (standard deviation)	74 (5.8)	75 (5.5)	0.228	1.07 (0.98–1.16)	0.120
Female gender—no. (%)	48 (59.3)	24 (72.7)	0.176	1.90 (0.75–4.81)	0.175
Charlson score ≥ 2—no. (%)	8 (9.9)	7 (21.2)	0.129	**3.94 (1.15–13.53)**	0.029
ASA > 2—no. (%)	23 (28.4)	12 (36.4)	0.403	-	-
Revision arthroplasty (versus primary arthroplasty)—no. (%)	11 (13.6)	4 (12.1)	1	0.906 (0.25–3.28)	0.881
Urgent surgery (versus elective surgery)—no. (%)	2 (2.5)	0 (0)	1	-	-
Postoperative prosthetic joint infection—no. (%)	22 (27.2)	16 (48.5)	0.028	**3.10 (1.26–7.57)**	0.014

ASA = American Society of Anesthesiologists; CI = confidence interval; OR = odds ratio. * Results in bold refer to those that are statistically significant.

Table 4. Factors associated with requiring an assistive device for ambulation versus walking without assistance in 123 patients undergoing total hip replacements one year after the last surgical procedure.

Variable	Univariate Analysis			Multivariate Analysis	
	Walking without Assistance (n = 76)	Walking with Crutches (n = 47)	p-Value	OR (95% CI) *	p-Value
Age, years—mean (standard deviation)	69 (8.4)	74 (7.8)	0.001	**1.10 (1.03–1.16)**	0.003
Female gender—no. (%)	41 (53.9)	28 (59.6)	0.541	0.97 (0.39–2.45)	0.949
Charlson score ≥ 2—no. (%)	6 (7.9)	8 (17)	0.121	3.02 (0.76–12.01)	0.116
ASA > 2—no. (%)	22 (28.9)	19 (40.4)	0.189	-	-
Revision arthroplasty (versus primary arthroplasty)—no. (%)	13 (17.1)	14 (29.8)	0.099	1.04 (0.34–3.21)	0.942
Urgent surgery (versus elective surgery)—no. (%)	3 (3.9)	10 (21.3)	0.005	3.41 (0.66–17.70)	0.145
Postoperative prosthetic joint infection—no. (%)	15 (19.7)	26 (55.3)	<0.001	**5.40 (2.12–13.67)**	<0.001

ASA = American Society of Anesthesiologists; CI = confidence interval; OR = odds ratio. * Results in bold refer to those that are statistically significant.

Table 5. Factors associated with requiring two crutches to walk or not being able to walk versus walking without assistance or with one crutch in patients undergoing partial hip joint replacements one year after the last surgical procedure.

Variable	Univariate Analysis			Multivariate Analysis	
	Walking without Aid or with 1 Crutch (n = 32)	Walking with 2 Crutches or Not Able to Walk (n = 58)	p-Value	OR (95% CI) *	p-Value
Age, years—mean (standard deviation)	81 (6.0)	84 (5.7)	0.010	1.08–0.99 (1.18)	0.068
Female gender—no. (%)	27 (84.4)	51 (89.9)	0.748	1.02 (0.26–4.06)	0.973
Charlson score ≥ 2—no. (%)	7 (21.9)	24 (44.4)	0.062		
ASA > 2—no. (%)	31 (59.6)	41 (70.7)	0.026	2.59 (0.96–7.01)	0.062
Revision arthroplasty (versus primary arthroplasty)—no. (%)	5 (15.6)	7 (12.1)	0.748	2.75 (0.27–28.13)	0.393
Urgent surgery (versus elective surgery)—no. (%)	28 (87.5)	57 (98.3)	0.052	22.29 (0.77–641.97)	0.070
Postoperative prosthetic joint infection (versus uninfected arthroplasty)—no. (%)	7 (21.9)	23 (39.7)	0.087	**3.054 (1.01–9.20)**	**0.047**

ASA = American Society of Anesthesiologists; CI = confidence interval; OR = odds ratio. * Results in bold refer to those that are statistically significant.

4. Discussion

In patients with hip and knee replacements, we found that having postoperative PJI —even if successfully treated at the first attempt— was associated with a worse functional ambulatory outcome when compared with not having PJI. Patients with total hip and knee prostheses with PJI more often needed an assistive device to walk than patients without PJI. Patients with PHA and PJI were more likely to need two crutches to walk or to be unable to walk than those without PJI.

Although restoring or improving joint function is one of the main goals of joint replacement surgical procedures, few studies have evaluated the effect of PJI on the functional status of patients with hip and knee prosthesis. The studies are heterogeneous, and most of them have important methodological drawbacks that make it difficult to interpret the results. Furthermore, since there are no specific measures to determine functional outcome after PJI [25], different studies have employed a variety of measures, generally extrapolated from those used in total hip and knee arthroplasties. There is also no gold standard outcome measure for arthroplasties [25], which makes it even more difficult to interpret and compare the results of different reports.

Some studies without control groups have evaluated functional outcomes in patients with PJI treated with specific surgical strategies. According to some of them, both DAIR [26] and one-stage arthroplasty exchange [27] showed satisfactory functional results in patients with THA and PJI. A comparison of one- and two-stage arthroplasty exchanges in infected THA patients found better results with the single-stage exchange [28]. Other studies have assessed the functional outcomes of arthroplasty exchanges performed for PJI (septic revision) compared with joint revision surgery performed for noninfectious reasons (aseptic revision) in TKA and THA, with conflicting results. Thus, the results of septic revision were reported to be mostly inferior [29–32] but also similar [33–36] and even superior [37] to those of aseptic revision. The variety of indications for aseptic revision in different studies could explain, at least in part, these contradictory results [32].

In recent years, a few studies have evaluated functional outcomes after using different surgical procedures to treat PJI compared with uninfected primary THA and TKA. While some studies showed similar results after PJIs successfully treated with DAIR, as compared with non-PJI patients [10–12,14], another one found inferior outcomes in the former group [13]. Overall, the results were worse in PJI patients treated with a two-stage arthroplasty exchange than in uninfected patients [11–13,38]. The main limitations of these studies were small sample sizes, functional outcomes evaluated at different follow-up times in PJI and non-PJI patients, and failure to adjust for other variables.

We did not set out to compare the functional results of PJIs according to surgical treatment, since surgical indication is based on algorithms, mainly determined by nonmodifiable circumstances such as time after index arthroplasty [5,16]. Our aim was to assess the influence of PJIs on functional ambulatory outcome in patients with hip and knee arthroplasties, even in the best possible scenario of infections successfully treated at the first therapeutic attempt. This question has never specifically been addressed or resolved. Our study demonstrated a worse ambulatory outcome in PJI than in non-PJI patients one year after the last surgery and after adjusting for other relevant factors influencing the outcome. Due to the well-known differences between patients with PHA and those with THA, we evaluated TKA, THA and PHA groups separately. Although this reduced the statistical power of the total sample size, we found that, in each group, PJI negatively affected the ambulatory outcome of these patients. Furthermore, older age and worse baseline comorbidities were also found to be associated with poorer ambulatory capacity in patients with infected total hip and knee arthroplasties, as previously observed [10]. These factors did not reach the level of statistical significance in the group of patients with PHA, although its smaller sample size limits the value of these results.

Our study has limitations. Firstly, it has the limitations intrinsic to the retrospective design of the study, although it would be difficult and take a long time to find such a large number of patients with PJI and apply the rigorous criteria required in the current investigation using a prospective design. Due to the retrospective study design, we used a very simple scale for functional outcomes focused on walking capacity. More sophisticated outcome measures using quantitative scoring systems have been used in previous studies, some of them specifically for total knee or hip arthroplasties [25]. Although they are a priori more appropriate and precise measures, they also have some disadvantages. First, the heterogeneity of the measures used prevents comparison between studies; furthermore, the clinical interpretation of quantitative measures is not always clear, and statistically significant differences between quantitative measures may not have clinical relevance. Our simple scale of four categories is clinically relevant and easily interpretable. Nevertheless, beyond ambulation capacity, there are other dimensions that are also important when evaluating the results of elective total joint arthroplasties, such as the patient's quality of life, level of satisfaction and other organ-specific measures [25], but these fall outside the scope of the present study. Furthermore, PJI is an important psychosocial stressor for many patients, which could have influenced their ambulatory outcome, although we could not assess this possibility [39]. Finally, preoperative walking capacity was often not available in the records of patients undergoing total hip and knee arthroplasties, and we cannot, therefore, completely exclude potential baseline differences between infected and noninfected patients. Our study has several strengths. This study evaluating the effect of PJIs on the functional ambulatory result of knee and hip arthroplasties has the largest number of patients. We also evaluated populations that have not been included in previous studies, such as patients with PHA. Finally, our study has overcome some of the methodological limitations of previous studies, making its conclusions more robust.

The results of the present study demonstrate conclusively that having a PJI diminishes the functional ambulatory result that implantation of a hip or knee prosthesis sets out to achieve. It is important to keep this in mind when planning treatment for PJIs and to advise and inform the patient accordingly. These results underscore the need to continue investing effort in the prevention of PJI.

Author Contributions: I.M. and N.B. conceived and designed the study and conducted the literature search. N.B. analysed the data. I.M., N.B., M.J., J.C.G., and X.C. interpreted the results. I.M. drafted the report. I.M., A.R., and V.P. collected the data and critically revised the report. M.J., J.C.G., J.L.-C., X.C., F.N., and M.G. critically revised the report for important intellectual content. N.B. supervised the study and critically revised the report. All authors have read and agreed to the published version of the manuscript.

Funding: This research was funded by the Instituto de Salud Carlos III, Spanish Ministry of Economy and Competitiveness (grant number PI15/1026) and cofunded by European Regional Development Fund/European Social Fund "Investing in your future".

Conflicts of Interest: All authors report no conflicts of interest relevant to this article.

References

1. Pivec, R.; Johnson, A.J.; Mears, S.C.; Mont, M.A. Hip arthroplasty. *Lancet* **2012**, *380*, 1768–1777. [CrossRef]
2. Carr, A.J.; Robertsson, O.; Graves, S.; Price, A.J.; Arden, N.K.; Judge, A.; Beard, D.J. Knee replacement. *Lancet* **2012**, *379*, 1331–1340. [CrossRef]
3. Zimmerli, W.; Sendi, P. Orthopaedic biofilm infections. *APMIS* **2017**, *125*, 353–364. [CrossRef] [PubMed]
4. Ariza, J.; Cobo, J.; Baraia-Etxaburu, J.; Benito, N.; Bori, G.; Cabo, J.; Corona, P.; Esteban, J.; Horcajada, J.P.; Lora-Tamayo, J.; et al. Executive summary of management of prosthetic joint infections. Clinical practice guidelines by the Spanish Society of Infectious Diseases and Clinical Microbiology (SEIMC). *Enferm. Infecc. Microbiol. Clin.* **2017**, *35*, 189–195. [CrossRef] [PubMed]
5. Osmon, D.R.; Berbari, E.F.; Berendt, A.R.; Lew, D.; Zimmerli, W.; Steckelberg, J.M.; Rao, N.; Hanssen, A.; Wilson, W.R. Infectious Diseases Society of America Diagnosis and management of prosthetic joint infection: Clinical practice guidelines by the Infectious Diseases Society of America. *Clin. Infect. Dis.* **2013**, *56*, e1–e25. [CrossRef] [PubMed]
6. Zimmerli, W.; Sendi, P. Orthopedic Implant–Associated Infections. In *Mandell, Douglas, and Bennett's Principles and Practice of Infectious Diseases*; Elsevier Inc.: Oxford, UK, 2020; pp. 1430–1442.
7. Escudero-Sanchez, R.; Senneville, E.; Digumber, M.; Soriano, A.; del Toro, M.D.; Bahamonde, A.; del Pozo, J.L.; Guio, L.; Murillo, O.; Rico, A.; et al. Suppressive antibiotic therapy in prosthetic joint infections: A multicentre cohort study. *Clin. Microbiol. Infect.* **2020**, *26*, 499–505. [CrossRef]
8. Tande, A.J.; Patel, R. Prosthetic Joint Infection. *Clin. Microbiol. Rev.* **2014**, *27*, 302–345. [CrossRef]

9. Diaz-Ledezma, C.; Higuera, C.A.; Parvizi, J. Success after treatment of periprosthetic joint infection: A Delphi-based international multidisciplinary consensus. *Clin. Orthop. Relat. Res.* **2013**, *471*, 2374–2382. [CrossRef]
10. Aboltins, C.; Dowsey, M.M.; Peel, T.; Lim, W.K.; Parikh, S.; Stanley, P.; Choong, P.F. Early prosthetic hip joint infection treated with debridement, prosthesis retention and biofilm-active antibiotics: Functional outcomes, quality of life and complications. *Intern. Med. J.* **2013**, *43*, 810–815. [CrossRef]
11. Dzaja, I.; Howard, J.; Somerville, L.; Lanting, B. Functional outcomes of acutely infected knee arthroplasty: A comparison of different surgical treatment options. *Can. J. Surg.* **2015**, *58*, 402–407. [CrossRef]
12. Herman, B.V.; Nyland, M.; Somerville, L.; MacDonald, S.J.; Lanting, B.A.; Howard, J.L. Functional outcomes of infected hip arthroplasty: A comparison of different surgical treatment options. *Hip Int.* **2017**, *27*, 245–250. [CrossRef] [PubMed]
13. Grammatopoulos, G.; Bolduc, M.E.; Atkins, B.L.; Kendrick, B.J.L.; McLardy-Smith, P.; Murray, D.W.; Gundle, R.; Taylor, A.H. Functional outcome of debridement, antibiotics and implant retention in periprosthetic joint infection involving the hip. *Bone Jt. J.* **2017**, *99B*, 614–622. [CrossRef] [PubMed]
14. Barros, L.H.; Barbosa, T.A.; Esteves, J.; Abreu, M.; Soares, D.; Sousa, R. Early Debridement, antibiotics and implant retention (DAIR) in patients with suspected acute infection after hip or knee arthroplasty—Safe, effective and without negative functional impact. *J. Bone Jt. Infect.* **2019**, *4*, 300–305. [CrossRef]
15. Parvizi, J.; Tan, T.L.; Goswami, K.; Higuera, C.; Della Valle, C.; Chen, A.F.; Shohat, N. The 2018 Definition of Periprosthetic Hip and Knee Infection: An Evidence-Based and Validated Criteria. *J. Arthroplasty* **2018**, *33*, 1309–1314. [CrossRef] [PubMed]
16. Löwik, C.A.M.; Parvizi, J.; Jutte, P.C.; Zijlstra, W.P.; Knobben, B.A.S.; Xu, C.; Goswami, K.; Belden, K.A.; Sousa, R.; Carvalho, A.; et al. Debridement, Antibiotics, and Implant Retention Is a Viable Treatment Option for Early Periprosthetic Joint Infection Presenting More Than 4 Weeks After Index Arthroplasty. *Clin. Infect. Dis.* **2020**, *71*, 630–636. [CrossRef]
17. Charlson, M.E.; Pompei, P.; Ales, K.L.; MacKenzie, C.R. A new method of classifying prognostic comorbidity in longitudinal studies: Development and validation. *J. Chronic Dis.* **1987**, *40*, 373–383. [CrossRef]
18. Hooper, G.J.; Rothwell, A.G.; Hooper, N.M.; Frampton, C. The Relationship Between the American Society of Anesthesiologists Physical Rating and Outcome Following Total Hip and Knee Arthroplasty. *J. Bone Jt. Surg. Am. Vol.* **2012**, *94*, 1065–1070. [CrossRef]
19. Hosmer, D.W.; Lemeshow, S.; Sturdivant, R. Model-building strategies and methods for logistic regression. In *Applied Logistic Regression*; Hosmer, D.W., Lemeshow, S., Sturdivant, R., Eds.; John Wiley & Sons, Inc.: Hoboken, NJ, USA, 2013; pp. 89–152. ISBN 9780761922087.
20. Sjölander, A.; Greenland, S. Ignoring the matching variables in cohort studies—When is it valid and why? *Stat. Med.* **2013**, *32*, 4696–4708. [CrossRef]
21. Lora-Tamayo, J.; Euba, G.; Ribera, A.; Murillo, O.; Pedrero, S.; García-Somoza, D.; Pujol, M.; Cabo, X.; Ariza, J. Infected hip hemiarthroplasties and total hip arthroplasties: Differential findings and prognosis. *J. Infect.* **2013**, *67*, 536–544. [CrossRef]
22. del Toro, M.D.; Nieto, I.; Guerrero, F.; Corzo, J.; del Arco, A.; Palomino, J.; Nuño, E.; Lomas, J.M.; Natera, C.; Fajardo, J.M.; et al. Are hip hemiarthroplasty and total hip arthroplasty infections different entities? The importance of hip fractures. *Eur. J. Clin. Microbiol. Infect. Dis.* **2014**, *33*, 1439–1448. [CrossRef]
23. Le Manach, Y.; Collins, G.; Bhandari, M.; Bessissow, A.; Boddaert, J.; Khiami, F.; Chaudhry, H.; De Beer, J.; Riou, B.; Landais, P.; et al. Outcomes after hip fracture surgery compared with elective total hip replacement. *JAMA J. Am. Med. Assoc.* **2015**, *314*, 1159–1166. [CrossRef] [PubMed]
24. Grammatico-Guillon, L.; Perreau, C.; Miliani, K.; L'Heriteau, F.; Rosset, P.; Bernard, L.; Lepelletier, D.; Rusch, E.; Astagneau, P. Association of Partial Hip Replacement with Higher Risk of Infection and Mortality in France. *Infect. Control Hosp. Epidemiol.* **2017**, *38*, 123–125. [CrossRef] [PubMed]
25. Puhto, A.-P.; Parra Aguilera, S.; Diaz-Ledezma, C. What quality of life measures should be used when determining the functional outcomes of periprosthetic joint infection treatment? In *Proceedings of the Second International Consensus Meeting on Musculoeskeletal Infection*; Parvizi, J., Gehrke, T., Eds.; Data Trace Publishing Company: Brooklandville, MD, USA, 2018; pp. 249–251. ISBN 878-1-57400-157-0.
26. Westberg, M.; Grøgaard, B.; Snorrason, F. Early prosthetic joint infections treated with debridement and implant retention. *Acta Orthop.* **2012**, *83*, 227–232. [CrossRef] [PubMed]

27. Kuiper, J.W.P.; Rustenburg, C.M.E.; Willems, J.H.; Verberne, S.J.; Peters, E.J.G.; Saouti, R. Results and Patient Reported Outcome Measures (PROMs) after One-Stage Revision for Periprosthetic Joint Infection of the Hip: A Single-centre Retrospective Study. *J. Bone Jt. Infect.* **2018**, *3*, 143–149. [CrossRef] [PubMed]
28. Oussedik, S.I.S.; Dodd, M.B.; Haddad, F.S. Outcomes of revision total hip replacement for infection after grading according to a standard protocol. *J. Bone Joint Surg. Br.* **2010**, *92*, 1222–1226. [CrossRef]
29. Barrack, R.L.; Engh, G.; Rorabeck, C.; Sawhney, J.; Woolfrey, M. Patient satisfaction and outcome after septic versus aseptic revision total knee arthroplasty. *J. Arthroplasty* **2000**, *15*, 990–993. [CrossRef]
30. Boettner, F.; Cross, M.B.; Nam, D.; Kluthe, T.; Schulte, M.; Goetze, C. Functional and Emotional Results Differ After Aseptic vs. Septic Revision Hip Arthroplasty. *HSS J.* **2011**, *7*, 235–238. [CrossRef]
31. Wang, C.J.; Hsieh, M.C.; Huang, T.W.; Wang, J.W.; Chen, H.S.; Liu, C.Y. Clinical outcome and patient satisfaction in aseptic and septic revision total knee arthroplasty. *Knee* **2004**, *11*, 45–49. [CrossRef]
32. Van Kempen, R.W.T.M.; Schimmel, J.J.P.; Van Hellemondt, G.G.; Vandenneucker, H.; Wymenga, A.B. Reason for revision TKA predicts clinical outcome: Prospective evaluation of 150 consecutive patients with 2-years followup knee. *Clin. Orthop. Relat. Res.* **2013**, *471*, 2296–2302. [CrossRef]
33. Ghanem, E.; Restrepo, C.; Joshi, A.; Hozack, W.; Sharkey, P.; Parvizi, J. Periprosthetic infection does not preclude good outcome for revision arthroplasty. *Clin. Orthop. Relat. Res.* **2007**, *461*, 54–59. [CrossRef]
34. Romanò, C.L.; Romanò, D.; Logoluso, N.; Meani, E. Septic versus aseptic hip revision: How different? *J. Orthop. Traumatol.* **2010**, *11*, 167–174. [CrossRef] [PubMed]
35. Rajgopal, A.; Vasdev, A.; Gupta, H.; Dahiya, V. Revision Total Knee Arthroplasty for Septic versus Aseptic Failure. *J. Orthop. Surg.* **2013**, *21*, 285–289. [CrossRef] [PubMed]
36. Konrads, C.; Franz, A.; Hoberg, M.; Rudert, M. Similar Outcomes of Two-Stage Revisions for Infection and One-Stage Revisions for Aseptic Revisions of Knee Endoprostheses. *J. Knee Surg.* **2019**, *32*, 897–899. [CrossRef] [PubMed]
37. Patil, N.; Lee, K.; Huddleston, J.I.; Harris, A.H.S.; Goodman, S.B. Aseptic versus septic revision total knee arthroplasty: Patient satisfaction, outcome and quality of life improvement. *Knee* **2010**, *17*, 200–203. [CrossRef] [PubMed]
38. De Man, F.H.R.; Sendi, P.; Zimmerli, W.; Maurer, T.B.; Ochsner, P.E.; Ilchmann, T. Infectiological, functional, and radiographic outcome after revision for prosthetic hip infection according to a strict algorithm. *Acta Orthop.* **2011**, *82*, 27–34. [CrossRef] [PubMed]
39. Knebel, C.; Menzemer, J.; Pohlig, F.; Herschbach, P.; Burgkart, R.; Obermeier, A.; von Eisenhart-Rothe, R.; Mühlhofer, H.M.L. Peri-Prosthetic Joint Infection of the Knee Causes High Levels of Psychosocial Distress: A Prospective Cohort Study. *Surg. Infect. (Larchmt)* **2020**. [CrossRef]

Publisher's Note: MDPI stays neutral with regard to jurisdictional claims in published maps and institutional affiliations.

© 2020 by the authors. Licensee MDPI, Basel, Switzerland. This article is an open access article distributed under the terms and conditions of the Creative Commons Attribution (CC BY) license (http://creativecommons.org/licenses/by/4.0/).

MDPI
St. Alban-Anlage 66
4052 Basel
Switzerland
Tel. +41 61 683 77 34
Fax +41 61 302 89 18
www.mdpi.com

Antibiotics Editorial Office
E-mail: antibiotics@mdpi.com
www.mdpi.com/journal/antibiotics

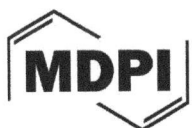

www.ingramcontent.com/pod-product-compliance
Lightning Source LLC
LaVergne TN
LVHW070656100526
838202LV00013B/979